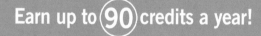
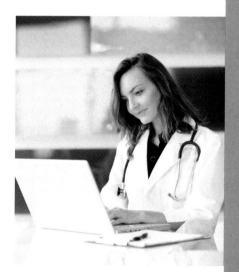

MR Imaging of the Prostate

Editor

AYTEKIN OTO

RADIOLOGIC CLINICS
OF NORTH AMERICA

www.radiologic.theclinics.com

Consulting Editor
FRANK H. MILLER

March 2018 • Volume 56 • Number 2

ELSEVIER

1600 John F. Kennedy Boulevard • Suite 1800 • Philadelphia, Pennsylvania, 19103-2899

http://www.theclinics.com

RADIOLOGIC CLINICS OF NORTH AMERICA Volume 56, Number 2
March 2018 ISSN 0033-8389, ISBN 13: 978-0-323-58172-1

Editor: John Vassallo (j.vassallo@elsevier.com)
Developmental Editor: Donald Mumford

Radiologic Clinics of North America (ISSN 0033-8389) is published bimonthly by Elsevier Inc., 360 Park Avenue South, New York, NY 10010-1710. Months of issue are January, March, May, July, September, and November. Periodicals postage paid at New York, NY and additional mailing offices. Subscription prices are USD 493 per year for US individuals, USD 889 per year for US institutions, USD 100 per year for US students and residents, USD 573 per year for Canadian individuals, USD 1136 per year for Canadian institutions, USD 680 per year for international individuals, USD 1136 per year for international institutions, and USD 315 per year for Canadian and international students/residents. To receive student and resident rate, orders must be accompanied by name of affiliated institution, date of term and the signature of program/residency coordinatior on institution letterhead. Orders will be billed at individual rate until proof of status is received. Foreign air speed delivery is included in all *Clinics* subscription prices. All prices are subject to change without notice. **POSTMASTER:** Send address changes to *Radiologic Clinics of North America*, Elsevier Health Sciences Division, Subscription Customer Service, 3251 Riverport Lane, Maryland Heights, MO63043. **Customer Service: Telephone: 1-800-654-2452** (U.S. and Canada); **1-314-447-8871** (outside U.S. and Canada). **Fax: 1-314-447-8029. E-mail: journalscustomerservice-usa@elsevier.com (for print support); journalsonlinesupport-usa@elsevier.com (for online support).**

Reprints. For copies of 100 or more of articles in this publication, please contact the Commercial Reprints Department, Elsevier Inc., 360 Park Avenue South, New York, New York 10010-1710. Tel.: +1-212-633-3874; Fax: +1-212-633-3820; E-mail: reprints@elsevier.com.

Radiologic Clinics of North America also published in Greek Paschalidis Medical Publications, Athens, Greece.

Radiologic Clinics of North America is covered in *MEDLINE/PubMed (Index Medicus), EMBASE/Excerpta Medica, Current Contents/Life Sciences, Current Contents/Clinical Medicine, RSNA Index to Imaging Literature, BIOSIS, Science Citation Index,* and *ISI/BIOMED.*

Printed in the United States of America.

Contributors

CONSULTING EDITOR

FRANK H. MILLER, MD
Chief, Body Imaging Section and
Fellowship Program, Medical Director
of MRI, Professor, Department of
Radiology, Northwestern University
Feinberg School of Medicine, Chicago,
Illinois, USA

EDITOR

AYTEKIN OTO, MD, MBA
Professor of Radiology and Surgery,
Vice Chair for Business Development,
Section Chief of Abdominal Imaging
and Chief of Body MR, Department of
Radiology, The University of Chicago, Chicago,
Illinois, USA

AUTHORS

AMIR A. BORHANI, MD
Department of Radiology, University
of Pittsburgh, Pittsburgh, Pennsylvania,
USA

PETER L. CHOYKE, MD
Molecular Imaging Program, National Cancer
Institute, National Institutes of Health,
Bethesda, Maryland, USA

PIET DIRIX, MD
Department of Radiation Oncology, Iridium
Cancer Network, Department of Molecular
Imaging, Pathology, Radiotherapy and
Oncology (MIPRO), University of Antwerp,
Antwerp, Belgium

SASHA C. DRUSKIN, MD
James Buchanan Brady Urological Institute,
The Johns Hopkins University School of
Medicine, Baltimore, Maryland, USA

PETAR DUVNJAK, MD
Assistant Professor, Department of Radiology,
Medical College of Wisconsin, Milwaukee,
Wisconsin, USA (formerly Fellow in Abdominal
Imaging, Department of Radiology, Duke
University Medical Center, Durham, North
Carolina, USA)

SCOTT E. EGGENER, MD
Professor of Surgery and Radiology, Section
of Urology, The University of Chicago, The
University of Chicago Medicine, Chicago,
Illinois, USA

ALESSANDRO FURLAN, MD
Department of Radiology, University
of Pittsburgh, Pittsburgh, Pennsylvania,
USA

SONIA GAUR, BS
Molecular Imaging Program, National Cancer
Institute, National Institutes of Health,
Bethesda, Maryland, USA

RAJAN T. GUPTA, MD
Associate Professor, Department of Radiology,
Duke University Medical Center, Assistant
Professor, Department of Surgery, Division
of Urologic Surgery, Duke Prostate Center,
Duke University Medical Center, Duke Cancer
Institute, Durham, North Carolina, USA

JAMIE N. HOLTZ, MD
Department of Radiology, Duke
University Medical Center, Durham, North
Carolina, USA

JIAOTI HUANG, MD, PhD
Professor and Chair, Department of
Pathology, Duke University Medical Center,
Duke Cancer Institute, Durham, North Carolina,
USA

GARY LINEY, PhD
Medical Physics, Ingham Institute for Applied
Medical Research and Liverpool Cancer
Therapy Centre, New South Wales, Australia

CYNTHIA MÉNARD, MD
Centre Hospitalier de l'Université de
Montréal (CHUM), Montréal, Canada;
TECHNA Institute, University of Toronto,
Toronto, Canada

KATARZYNA J. MACURA, MD, PhD
Professor of Radiology, Urology, and
Oncology, Department of Radiology and
Radiological Science, The James Buchanan
Brady Urological Institute, Johns Hopkins
School of Medicine, Baltimore, Maryland, USA

PATRICK MCLAUGHLIN, MD
Department of Radiation Oncology,
University of Michigan, Ann Arbor, Michigan,
USA

SHERIF G. NOUR, MD, FRCR
Divisions of Abdominal Imaging, Interventional
Radiology and Image-Guided Medicine,
Director, Interventional MRI Program,
Associate Professor, Department of Radiology
and Imaging Sciences, Emory University
Hospital, Emory University School of Medicine,
Atlanta, Georgia, USA

TUFVE NYHOLM, PhD
Department of Radiation Sciences, Umeå
University, Umeå, Sweden

AYTEKIN OTO, MD, MBA
Professor of Radiology and Surgery,
Vice Chair for Business Development,
Section Chief of Abdominal Imaging and
Chief of Body MR, Department of Radiology,
The University of Chicago, Chicago, Illinois,
USA

ERIC PAULSON, PhD
Radiation Oncology, Radiology, and
Biophysics, Medical College of Wisconsin,
Milwaukee, Wisconsin, USA

THOMAS J. POLASCIK, MD, FACS
Professor, Department of Surgery,
Division of Urologic Surgery, Duke Prostate
Center, Duke University Medical Center,
Duke Cancer Institute, Durham, North Carolina,
USA

ANDREI S. PURYSKO, MD
Section of Abdominal Imaging, Imaging
Institute, Cleveland Clinic, Cleveland, Ohio,
USA

JOSEPH F. RODRIGUEZ, MD
Resident Physician, Section of
Urology, The University of Chicago, The
University of Chicago Medicine, Chicago,
Illinois, USA

ANDREW B. ROSENKRANTZ, MD
Department of Radiology, NYU Langone
Medical Center, New York, New York, USA

SARADWATA SARKAR, PhD
Principal Scientist, Research and
Development, Eigen, Grass Valley, California,
USA

ARIEL A. SCHULMAN, MD
Fellow in Urologic Oncology, Department of
Surgery, Division of Urologic Surgery, Duke
Prostate Center, Duke University Medical
Center, Durham, North Carolina, USA

STEPHEN THOMAS, MD
Department of Radiology, The University of
Chicago, Chicago, Illinois, USA

BARIS TURKBEY, MD
Molecular Imaging Program, National Cancer
Institute, National Institutes of Health,
Bethesda, Maryland, USA

UULKE A. VAN DER HEIDE, PhD
Department of Radiation Oncology, The Netherlands Cancer Institute, Amsterdam, The Netherlands

SADHNA VERMA, MD, FSAR
Professor, Department of Radiology, Adjunct Professor of Urology and Radiation Oncology, The University of Cincinnati College of Medicine, Cincinnati, Ohio, USA

ANTONIO C. WESTPHALEN, MD, PhD
Departments of Radiology and Biomedical Imaging and Urology, University of California San Francisco, San Francisco, California, USA

JOSEPH H. YACOUB, MD
Assistant Professor, Department of Radiology, Loyola University Chicago, Stritch School of Medicine, Maywood, Illinois, USA

Contents

> The diagnosis and management of prostate cancer have substantially changed over the last 3 decades. Serum prostate-specific antigen (PSA) was adopted for screening in the 1990s after it was found to be a sensitive indicator of disease. Because of a lack of specificity for significant disease, indiscriminate PSA testing led to overdiagnosis and overtreatment. Several biomarkers have been developed that are superior to PSA in stratifying a man's risk for harboring potentially lethal prostate cancer.

> McNeal first described the zonal anatomy of the prostate about 40 years ago, outlining 4 zones of the prostate and defining their relation to the urethra and the ejaculatory ducts. The zonal anatomy remains the accepted model for describing the prostate, and the zones are well depicted on MR imaging, including the central zone, which until recently was grouped with the transition zone in the radiology literature. An accurate understanding of the zonal anatomy and periprostatic anatomy is key for accurate interpretation of the prostate MR imaging.

 Video content accompanies this article at http://www.radiologic.theclinics.com.

> Multiparametric MR imaging provides detailed anatomic assessment of the prostate as well as information that allows the detection and characterization of prostate cancer. To obtain high-quality MR imaging of the prostate, radiologists must understand sequence optimization to overcome commonly encountered technical challenges. This article discusses the techniques that are used in state-of-the-art MR imaging of the prostate, including imaging protocols, hardware considerations, and important aspects of patient preparation, with an emphasis on the recommendations provided in the prostate imaging-reporting and data system version 2 guidelines.

> Multiparametric MR imaging of the prostate is a complex study that combines anatomic and functional imaging. The complexity of this technique, along with an increasing demand, has brought new challenges to imaging interpretation. The Prostate Imaging Reporting and Data System provides radiologists with guidelines

to standardize interpretation. This article discusses the interpretation of the pulse sequences recommended in the Prostate Imaging Reporting and Data System version 2 guidelines, reviews advanced quantitative imaging tools, and discusses future directions.

Petar Duvnjak, Ariel A. Schulman, Jamie N. Holtz, Jiaoti Huang, Thomas J. Polascik, and Rajan T. Gupta

Meaningful changes to the approach of prostate cancer staging and management have been made over the past decade with increasing demand for high-quality multiparametric MR imaging (mpMRI) of the prostate. This article focuses on the evolving paradigm of prostate cancer staging, with emphasis on the role of mpMRI on staging and its integration into clinical decision making. Current prostate cancer staging systems are defined and mpMRI's role in the detection of non–organ-confined disease and how it has an impact on the selection of appropriate next steps are discussed. Several imaging pitfalls, limitations, and future directions of mpMRI also are discussed.

Sasha C. Druskin and Katarzyna J. Macura

The current prostate cancer management paradigm has been criticized in recent years for contributing to the overdiagnosis and overtreatment of the disease. Active surveillance is an avenue by which to reduce overtreatment, but patient selection and monitoring remain a challenge. The use of prostate MR imaging has been growing in recent years and has been incorporated into prostate cancer screening and patient selection and monitoring for active surveillance. This article discusses the current evidence for the use of MR imaging in each of those settings.

Sonia Gaur and Baris Turkbey

Prostate multiparametric MR imaging (mpMRI) plays an important role in local evaluation after treatment of prostate cancer. After radical prostatectomy, radiation therapy, and focal therapy, mpMRI can be used to visualize normal posttreatment changes and to diagnose locally recurrent disease. An understanding of the various treatments and expected changes is essential for complete and accurate posttreatment mpMRI interpretation.

Stephen Thomas and Aytekin Oto

Multiparametric MR imaging is widely embraced for the diagnosis, staging, and surveillance of prostate cancer. However, normal anatomic structures and many benign entities have overlapping imaging features with prostate cancer. Although some of these entities require biopsy and histopathologic diagnosis, some have characteristic imaging features that are suggestive of their diagnosis. Knowledge of these pitfalls is important in establishing a correct diagnosis and avoiding unnecessary biopsies, as these entities are encountered routinely in clinical practice.

Conventional ultrasound-guided prostate biopsies have multiple limitations leading to underdetection of clinically significant prostate cancer (PCa) and overdetection of clinically insignificant PCa. Multiparametric MR imaging of the prostate offers better localization of prostatic tumors in comparison with ultrasound imaging and can help address these limitations. MR imaging–identified lesions can be targeted for biopsy directly in-gantry or indirectly using a fusion of MR imaging and ultrasound imaging. The fusion may be performed by the operator visually or using a software fusion device. In this article, the authors review the various techniques for MR imaging–targeted prostate biopsies and their clinical impact for PCa diagnosis.

Focal treatment of prostate cancer has evolved from a concept to a practice in the recent few years and is projected to fill an existing need, bridging the gap between conservative and radical traditional treatment options. With its low morbidity and rapid recovery time compared with whole-gland treatment alternatives, focal therapy is poised to gain more acceptance among patients and health care providers. As the experience with focal treatment matures and evidence continues to accrue, the landscape of this practice might look quite different in the future.

The use of prostate MR imaging in radiotherapy continues to evolve. This article describes its current application in the selection of treatment regimens, integration in treatment planning or simulation, and assessment of response. An expert consensus statement from the annual MR in RT symposium is presented, as a list of 21 key quality indicators for the practice of MR imaging simulation in prostate cancer. Although imaging requirements generally follow PIRADSv2 guidelines, additional requirements specific to radiotherapy planning are described. MR imaging–only workflows and MR imaging–guided treatment systems are expected to replace conventional computed tomography–based practice, further adding specific requirements for MR imaging in radiotherapy.

MR imaging is an important part of prostate cancer diagnosis. Variations in quality and skill in general practice mean results are not as impressive as they were in academic centers. This observation provides an impetus to improve the method. Improved quality assurance will likely result in better outcomes. Improved characterization of clinically significant prostate cancer may assist in making MR imaging more useful. Improved methods of registering MR imaging with transrectal ultrasound imaging and robotic arms controlling the biopsy can reduce the impact of inexperienced operators and make the entire system of MR imaging–guided biopsies more robust.

PROGRAM OBJECTIVE

The objective of the *Radiologic Clinics of North America* is to keep practicing radiologists and radiology residents up to date with current clinical practice in radiology by providing timely articles reviewing the state of the art in patient care.

TARGET AUDIENCE

Practicing radiologists, radiology residents, and other healthcare professionals who provide patient care utilizing radiologic findings.

LEARNING OBJECTIVES

Upon completion of this activity, participants will be able to:
1. Review prostate cancer and the role of biomarkers in screening and diagnosis.
2. Discuss the multi-parametric MRI of the prostate, screening and surveillance, and prostate zonal anatomy.
3. Recognize MRI targeted prostate biopsies and pitfalls in interpretation.

ACCREDITATION

The Elsevier Office of Continuing Medical Education (EOCME) is accredited by the Accreditation Council for Continuing Medical Education (ACCME) to provide continuing medical education for physicians.

The EOCME designates this enduring material for a maximum of 15 *AMA PRA Category 1 Credit*(s)™. Physicians should claim only the credit commensurate with the extent of their participation in the activity.

All other healthcare professionals requesting continuing education credit for this enduring material will be issued a certificate of participation.

DISCLOSURE OF CONFLICTS OF INTEREST

The EOCME assesses conflict of interest with its instructors, faculty, planners, and other individuals who are in a position to control the content of CME activities. All relevant conflicts of interest that are identified are thoroughly vetted by EOCME for fair balance, scientific objectivity, and patient care recommendations. EOCME is committed to providing its learners with CME activities that promote improvements or quality in healthcare and not a specific proprietary business or a commercial interest.

The planning committee, staff, authors and editors listed below have identified no financial relationships or relationships to products or devices they or their spouse/life partner have with commercial interest related to the content of this CME activity:
Peter L. Choyke, MD; Piet Dirix, MD; Sasha C. Druskin, MD; Petar Duvnjak, MD; Sonia Gaur, BS; Jamie N. Holtz, MD; Jiaoti Huang, MD, PhD; Gary Liney, PhD; Leah Logan; Patrick McLaughlin, MD; Cynthia Ménard, MD; Frank H. Miller, MD; Sherif G. Nour, MD, FRCR; Tufve Nyholm, PhD; Eric Paulson, PhD; Thomas J. Polascik, MD, FACS; Andrei S. Purysko, MD; Joseph F. Rodriguez, MD; Saradwata Sarkar, PhD; Ariel A. Schulman, MD; Karthik Subramaniam; Stephen Thomas, MD; Baris Turkbey, MD; Uulke A. van der Heide, PhD; Sadhna Verma, MD, FSAR; John Vassallo; Joseph H. Yacoub, MD.

The planning committee, staff, authors and editors listed below have identified financial relationships or relationships to products or devices they or their spouse/life partner have with commercial interest related to the content of this CME activity:
Amir A. Borhani, MD, is a consultant/advisor for Guerbet, LLC and receives royalties from Elsevier.
Scott E. Eggener, MD, is on the speakers' bureau for MDx Health and OPKO Health.
Alessandro Furlan, MD, is a consultant/advisor for General Electric and Elsevier/Amirsys, with research support from General Electric and receives royalties from Elsevier/Amirsys.
Rajan T. Gupta, MD, is on the speakers' bureau, is a consultant/advisor for Bayer Pharma AG and is a consultant/advisor for Invivo Corporation, Halyard Health, Siemens AG.
Katarzyna J. Macura, MD, PhD, has research support from Profound Medical Corp.
Aytekin Oto, MD, MBA, is a consultant/advisor for and receives research support from Profound Medical Corp., receives research support from Philips Healthcare and Guerbet, LLC.
Andrew B. Rosenkrantz, MD, receives royalties from Thieme Medical Publishers.
Antonio C. Westphalen, MD, PhD, is a consultant/advisor for 3D Biopsy LLC, Scientific Advisory Board.

UNAPPROVED/OFF-LABEL USE DISCLOSURE

The EOCME requires CME faculty to disclose to the participants:
1. When products or procedures being discussed are off-label, unlabelled, experimental, and/or investigational (not US Food and Drug Administration [FDA] approved); and
2. Any limitations on the information presented, such as data that are preliminary or that represent ongoing research, interim analyses, and/or unsupported opinions. Faculty may discuss information about pharmaceutical agents that is outside of FDA-approved labelling. This information is intended solely for CME and is not intended to promote off-label use of these medications. If you have any questions, contact the medical affairs department of the manufacturer for the most recent prescribing information.

TO ENROLL

To enroll in the *Radiologic Clinics of North America* Continuing Medical Education program, call customer service at 1-800-654-2452 or sign up online at http://www.theclinics.com/home/cme. The CME program is available to subscribers for an additional annual fee of USD 327.60.

METHOD OF PARTICIPATION

In order to claim credit, participants must complete the following:
1. Complete enrolment as indicated above.
2. Read the activity.
3. Complete the CME Test and Evaluation. Participants must achieve a score of 70% on the test. All CME Tests and Evaluations must be completed online.

CME INQUIRIES/SPECIAL NEEDS

For all CME inquiries or special needs, please contact elsevierCME@elsevier.com.

RADIOLOGIC CLINICS OF NORTH AMERICA

ISSUE OF RELATED INTEREST

PET Clinics, April 2017 (Vol. 12, Issue 2)
Prostate Cancer Imaging and Therapy
Richard P. Baum and Cristina Nanni, *Editors*
Available at: www.pet.theclinics.com

Preface
Prostate MR Imaging

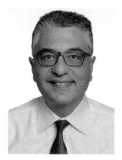

Aytekin Oto, MD, MBA
Editor

Prostate cancer is the third leading cause of cancer death in men and an important public health problem in the United States. MR imaging is currently the best modality for imaging of the prostate. Prostate MR has been performed for close to 40 years, but only after development of a multi-parametric prostate MR protocol (including T2, Diffusion weighted and Dynamic contrast enhanced MRI) has it been widely embraced world-wide in the last decade. The publication of PI-RADS Version-2 guidelines by the ACR has been another important milestone toward standardization of this test. During the last decade, improved performance of prostate MR imaging and its combination with MR-ultrasound (US) fusion biopsy has led to a paradigm shift in the diagnosis of prostate cancer. MR-targeted biopsies have started to replace random transrectal US-guided biopsies. Prostate MR has also been used for the triage and follow-up of patients with active surveillance. All of these new indications have increased the prostate MR volumes in radiology departments and hence the need for radiologists who are competent and experienced in interpretation of these studies. Rapid advancement of the field has also resulted in substantial publications and an accelerated pace in creation of new knowledge in the field. This issue of *Radiologic Clinics of North America* focusing on prostate MR imaging is therefore very timely and aims to fill the gap in the education of radiologists in this relatively new field as well as to serve as an updated reference resource summarizing the current knowledge and status of prostate MR imaging.

I am deeply indebted to the distinguished contributors to this issue for sharing their outstanding expertise and insights along with their terrific illustrations. Our goal was to provide a 360° view of prostate MR imaging with this issue. We covered basic concepts of prostate MR imaging, including anatomy, technique, interpretation tips/strategies, and pitfalls. Articles addressing the role and performance of prostate MRI for conventional (staging and recurrence) and emerging indications (targeted biopsy and focal therapy) are included in this issue. Perspectives from urologists and radiation oncologists are important highlights of the issue, completing the 360° view. A brief glimpse at the future of prostate MR imaging in this issue will help radiologists to better prepare themselves to the upcoming challenges. Overall, I am confident that this issue of *Radiologic Clinics of North America* will be a comprehensive and valuable resource for radiologists for years to come.

I would like to thank Dr Frank Miller and Elsevier for the opportunity to compile this issue on prostate MR imaging. I also would like to acknowledge my section at the University of Chicago for their invaluable support and friendship. Last, I would like to thank my family for their love, encouragement, and continuous support.

Aytekin Oto, MD, MBA
Department of Radiology
University of Chicago
5841 South Maryland Avenue, MC 2026
Chicago, IL 60637, USA

E-mail address:
aoto@radiology.bsd.uchicago.edu

Radiol Clin N Am 56 (2018) xiii
https://doi.org/10.1016/j.rcl.2017.12.001
0033-8389/18/© 2017 Elsevier Inc. All rights reserved.

radiologic.theclinics.com

Prostate Cancer and the Evolving Role of Biomarkers in Screening and Diagnosis

Joseph F. Rodriguez, MD*, Scott E. Eggener, MD

KEYWORDS

- Prostate • Cancer • Biomarkers • Screening • PSA

KEY POINTS

- Prostate-specific antigen (PSA) testing has contributed to a decline in prostate cancer–specific mortality observed over the last 30 years.
- PSA lacks specificity and leads to overdiagnosis and overtreatment when used indiscriminately.
- Harms from screening can be reduced by advocating active surveillance for low-risk cancers.
- There are several serologic and pathologic biomarkers with higher specificity than PSA that can limit unnecessary biopsies and inform treatment decisions.

INTRODUCTION

Prostate cancer will account for ~26,000 deaths in the United States in 2017.[1] The current, age-adjusted mortality of 19 per 100,000 men is a 50% improvement compared with the early 1990s.[2] Modifications in screening, diagnosis, and management have dramatically impacted incident rates and survival. Recent efforts have focused on limiting the diagnosis and treatment of indolent disease, while treating those with more aggressive features within a window of curative potential. Consequently, several biomarkers have been developed to more selectively identify men likely to benefit from timely diagnosis and effective treatment. The authors review the evolution of prostate cancer risk assessment in the United States with an emphasis on biomarkers.

BACKGROUND

Autopsy studies have identified prostate cancer in ~5% of specimens from men younger than 30 to ~60% from those aged greater than 79 years.[3] Pathologic examination after biopsy or surgery identifies patterns used to grade disease. Gleason score is based on the 2 most prevalent of these patterns and often informs prognosis more than tumor stage.[4] Gleason 6 (3 + 3) represents the most indolent pattern, whereas Gleason 10 (5 + 5) represents the most aggressive. In 2014, grade groups 1 to 5 were established to simplify pathologic interpretation for patients and physicians and have been validated to predict risk of recurrence (Table 1).[5,6]

The natural history of prostate cancer varies widely by stage and grade.[7] Men with metastatic disease have a median survival of 30 months. In contrast, men with low-grade organ-confined

Disclosures: None (J.F. Rodriguez). S.E. Eggener has served as a research investigator and speaker for MDx Health and OPKO health.
Section of Urology, University of Chicago, The University of Chicago Medicine, 5841 South Maryland Avenue, MC 6038, Chicago, IL 60637, USA
* Corresponding author.
E-mail address: tony.rodriguez17@gmail.com

Radiol Clin N Am 56 (2018) 187–196
https://doi.org/10.1016/j.rcl.2017.10.002
0033-8389/18/© 2017 Elsevier Inc. All rights reserved.

Table 1
Gleason grade groupings and risk of biochemical recurrence following radical prostatectomy

Grade Group	Gleason Score	Hazard Ratio for Recurrence
1	≤6	(Reference)
2	3 + 4	1.9
3	4 + 3	5.1
4	8	8.0
5	9–10	11.7

Data from Epstein JI, Zelefsky MJ, Sjoberg DD, et al. A contemporary prostate cancer grading system: a validated alternative to the Gleason score. Eur Urol 2016;69(3):428–35.

disease can often live decades without any treatment. Popiolek and colleagues[8] closely followed a population-based cohort of 223 Swedish men diagnosed with localized disease for 30 years until 99% had died. There was no screening, and these men were untreated except with hormonal therapy if they developed symptomatic local progression or metastases. All patients with poorly differentiated tumors died within 10 years of cancer or other causes, but 64% of men never required hormonal therapy. Although overall survival declined steadily over the observation period, cancer-specific mortality increased rapidly from 15 to 20 years after diagnosis, illustrating the oft-prolonged natural history expected from low-grade, localized disease.

PROSTATE CANCER IN THE "PRE–PROSTATE-SPECIFIC ANTIGEN ERA"

Through the 1980s, prostate cancer diagnosis was often not made until a patient was symptomatic from advanced disease, and 5-year relative survival was 70%.[2] For nonmetastatic disease, up to 50% of men did not undergo any primary treatment.[9] Prostatectomy was associated with 3% mortality, high rates of total incontinence, and universal impotence.[10] The introduction of serum prostate-specific antigen (PSA) in the latter part of the decade spurred a dramatic shift.[11]

The addition of PSA to the digital rectal examination (DRE) significantly improved the sensitivity of screening, and as early as 1992, organizations recommended PSA testing for men over the age of 50.[12–14] Urologists began adopting surgical techniques pioneered by Patrick Walsh to decrease the morbidity of radical prostatectomy, including the use of nerve sparing for potency preservation.[15,16] With an increasing pool of patients diagnosed with localized disease and an improved surgical treatment option, rates of radical prostatectomy increased by a factor of 6.[17]

The latter half of the 1990s showed declining rates of prostate cancer mortality and advanced disease, but there was a disproportionately larger increase in cancer incidence and use of radical treatment.[18] Refinements to therapy, such as minimally invasive approaches to surgery and less toxic radiation delivery methods, decreased morbidity, but treatments were still associated with a risk of incontinence, erectile dysfunction, cystitis, proctitis, and urethral strictures.

In the "PSA era," many questioned whether benefits of screening outweighed the harms of overtreatment.[19,20] Two prospective randomized trials were therefore conducted to answer this question: the Prostate, Lung, Colorectal and Ovarian Cancer Screening Trial in the United States (PLCO) and the European Randomized Study of Screening for Prostate Cancer (ERSPC) in multiple European countries.

PROSTATE-SPECIFIC ANTIGEN SCREENING TRIALS

In the PLCO trial, more than 75,000 men aged 55 to 74 years were randomly assigned to annual screening with PSA and DRE or usual care.[21] Men with suspicious DRE or PSA greater than 4 ng/mL were advised to undergo diagnostic evaluation. In 2009, the first results were reported after a median follow-up of 11.5 years. Through year 10 of the study, there were 92 prostate cancer deaths in the screening arm and 82 in the control arm (rate ratio 1.11; 95% confidence interval [CI], 0.83–1.50) with no apparent benefit to screening.

In the ERSPC trial, greater than 160,000 men aged 55 to 69 years were randomized to PSA screening (typically every 2–4 years) or usual care.[22] Most centers involved used PSA greater than 3.0 ng/mL as a cutoff to recommend diagnostic evaluation, although there was some variation between sites. With a median follow-up of 9 years, there was a 20% decreased mortality in the screened group (95% CI 0.65–0.98; adjusted $P = .04$). Given low prostate cancer–specific mortalities overall, this translated into the requirement of 1410 men screened and 48 men diagnosed to prevent 1 death from prostate cancer. An updated report in 2014 with 13 years median follow-up suggests a number needed to screen of 781 and a number needed to diagnose of 27 to prevent one death from prostate cancer.[23]

The contradictory results of PLCO and ERSPC can be explained by high rates of PSA testing in the United States around the study period contaminating the control arm. Contamination in PLCO has been estimated to be as high as 90%.[24] In addition, participant survey data reveal that when considering the 3 years before PLCO randomization, the control patients had more cumulative PSA testing than those assigned to screening.[24] In contrast, contamination in ERSPC is estimated to be 23% to 40%.[23]

The Göteborg trial, designed and conducted independently from ERSPC but from which a subset of patients is included in ERSPC data, bears mentioning given its low rate of contamination in control patients (estimated 3%).[25] A population-based registry was used to randomly select 20,000 of the Göteborg, Sweden's 32,298 men aged 50 to 64 years. Half were invited for PSA screening every 2 years until age 69. About three-quarters of invited men participated, and after 14 years of follow-up (with 78% of men meeting this endpoint), the relative risk reduction for prostate cancer–specific mortality was 42%. These results suggest a number needed to invite to screening of 293, and a number needed to diagnose of 12 to prevent 1 prostate cancer death.

Based on concerns for overdiagnosis and overtreatment, in 2008, the US Preventive Services Task Force (USPSTF) recommended against PSA screening for patients 75 years and older.[26] This was followed in 2012 by a "grade D" recommendation discouraging PSA screening for all men.[27] At the time of writing this review, a draft statement by the USPSTF softened this position and recommended shared patient-physician decision making weighing benefits and harms of screening for patients aged 55 to 69 years (grade C),[28] consistent with current recommendations from both the American Cancer Society and the American Urological Association.[29,30]

REDUCING OVERTREATMENT THROUGH ACTIVE SURVEILLANCE

One way to reduce prostate cancer overtreatment as a result of screening is to discourage immediate therapy for patients with suspected indolent disease. Active surveillance (AS) is a serial monitoring program with treatment initiated if prompted by new information suggesting a higher volume or higher grade cancer. Various eligibility recommendations exist for AS but generally consist of men with Gleason 6 disease, which has been shown to be nearly incapable of metastasizing when appropriately classified.[31,32] For men with shorter life expectancies and Gleason 3 + 4 disease, AS may also be considered.[33]

Several AS cohorts have demonstrated its safety.[33–39] The most mature data come from Klotz and colleagues,[33] who report the survival of 993 men on AS after a median follow-up from first biopsy of 6.4 years and a maximum follow-up of 20 years. All men with Gleason ≤6 disease and PSA less than 10 ng/mL were eligible in addition to men with Gleason 3 + 4 disease and/or PSA 10 to 20 ng/mL if life expectancy was less than 10 years. They were followed with PSA testing every 3 to 6 months and biopsies every 3 to 4 years with the decision to treat based on PSA kinetics or histologic upgrading. This group is notable in that it had the least restrictive inclusion criteria as well as less intensive follow-up compared with other cohorts. Nevertheless, cancer-specific survival at 10 and 15 years was 98.1% and 94.3%, respectively, with more than half of patients remaining untreated.

In contrast, the Johns Hopkins AS cohort was restricted to men with low-volume Gleason 6 disease and PSA density less than 0.15 ng/mL.[34] Follow-up included yearly biopsies. The latest report from this group followed 1298 men for a median of 5 years and maximum of 18 years. Cancer-specific survival at 15 years was 99.9% with 50% of men remaining untreated at 10 years and 43% remaining untreated at 15 years.

PROSTATE-SPECIFIC ANTIGEN LACKS SPECIFICITY

Another way to limit prostate cancer overtreatment is to improve upon the specificity of PSA. This serves the additional benefit of avoiding biopsies, which are associated with increasing complications in the era of antibiotic resistance.[40]

In addition to malignancy, benign prostate enlargement, prostatitis, and increasing age can all increase PSA.[41,42] To improve the test characteristics of PSA, age-specific and race-specific cutoffs have been explored with minimal gains in accuracy.[43,44] PSA kinetics including PSA velocity have been associated with subsequent death from prostate cancer, but specificity remained poor within the "gray zone" of PSA values (4–10 ng/mL).[45] The comparison of free PSA, PSA unbound to proteins, to total PSA (%fPSA) has also been studied. A meta-analysis reports the area under the curve (AUC) for the receiver operator characteristic curve of free PSA to be 0.70.[46] Given low specificity within the PSA gray zone however, %fPSA only significantly impacts the decision to pursue prostate biopsy at extreme values.

Over the last decade, research has moved away from total PSA derivatives in search of novel biomarkers to improve specificity of prostate cancer testing. There are multiple urine, blood, and tissue-based assays now available to more accurately stratify risk of significant prostate cancer.

PROSTATE CANCER ANTIGEN 3 TEST

Prostate cancer antigen 3 test (PCA3) was the first urine-based, commercially available test specific for prostate cancer (Progensa PCA3; Hologic Inc, Bedford, MA, USA).[47] Following DRE with prostatic massage, this assay measures RNA from the PCA3 gene as well as PSA in a patient's urine. The PCA3 gene is specifically overexpressed in prostate cancer and unaffected by prostate volume or inflammation.[48,49] In the United States, it was US Food and Drug Administration approved in 2012 for use in patients older than age 50 years with a prior negative biopsy but persistent clinical suspicion of prostate cancer.

PCA3 was first reported as a marker for prostate cancer in men with prior negative biopsies in 2007.[50] The largest study of PCA3 comprised greater than 1000 men with prior negative biopsy and a cancer prevalence of 18% on repeat biopsy. A direct correlation was observed between PCA3 and cancer detection. Sensitivity was 48%, whereas specificity was 79% at a previously established cutoff score. Negative predictive value (NPV), a useful metric for a test primarily used to "rule-out" disease, was 88%, which has been validated in other studies.[51,52] Studies of PCA3 correlation with Gleason score have shown mixed results,[50,53–55] and one study showed a strong correlation between PCA3 and extracapsular extension.[56]

TMPRSS2:ERG

PCA3 testing has been recently studied in combination with measurement of TMPRSS2:ERG, an androgen-regulated gene fused to an oncogene that is present in about 50% of prostate cancers.[57] It can be measured in post-DRE urine in the same way as PCA3 and is more specific than PSA for the detection of prostate cancer.[51] Although studies have shown mixed results in its ability to selectively identify aggressive disease,[58–61] others show in combination with PCA3 it can have clinical utility.[62,63]

Researchers at the University of Michigan (MLabs, Ann Arbor, MI) have developed a risk assessment tool marketed as "Mi-Prostate Score" or "MiPS," which combines measurement of urinary PSA, PCA3, and TMPRSS2:ERG.[62] Models were constructed for the prediction of prostate cancer as well as the prediction of Gleason ≥ 7 cancer from 711 patients. These models were then tested in a validation cohort of 1225 patients and compared with algorithms incorporating information from a nomogram based on clinical data with or without each component of MiPS. The highest AUC for predicting any cancer as well as Gleason ≥ 7 cancer was the MiPS + nomogram model with AUCs of 0.76 and 0.78, respectively. Using the MiPs + nomogram model and a risk tolerance of up to 15% for Gleason greater than 6 tumor on subsequent biopsy, 36% of biopsies could be avoided while delaying the diagnosis of high-grade disease in 1.6% of patients. Extrapolating from these data, which are based upon an 18% prevalence of high-grade disease, the NPV is 96%.

DLX1 AND HOXC6 (SelectMDx)

Another novel post-DRE urinary biomarker has recently come to market (SelectMDx; MDxHealth, Inc, Irvine, CA, USA). The test measures messenger RNA levels of 2 genes upregulated in Gleason ≥ 7 (DLX1 and HOXC6) relative to a reference gene.[64] An algorithm incorporates measured gene expression with clinical factors, including family history, history of prior biopsies, PSA density, and DRE findings, to predict likelihood of both low- and high-grade prostate cancer. Notable is the inclusion of PSA density in this test, which was reported by transrectal ultrasound.

The test was developed and validated in separate multicenter, prospective cohorts of consecutive men undergoing biopsy for PSA ≥ 3 ng/mL, abnormal DRE, or positive family history.[65] In a validation cohort of 386 patients, the developed algorithm performed with an AUC of 0.86 (95% CI, 0.80–0.92) for the detection of Gleason ≥ 7 cancer. Another model was created excluding DRE findings, and although it did not perform as well in the model cohort (n = 519), it was superior in the validation cohort to the original model (AUC 0.90, $P = .03$). This model performed with an AUC of 0.87 when it did not include urinary biomarkers in the validation cohort, and there was no statistically significant improvement when PCA3 measurement was incorporated. Although the investigators make the point that this demonstrates the utility of DLX1 and HOXC6 assessment over PCA3, it is notable the model without biomarkers performed with a very high AUC in this cohort. Given the AUC was much lower for risk assessment based on the prostate cancer prevention trial risk calculator 2.0 (AUC = 0.77), which does not consider PSA density, it is possible the subsequently shown superiority of the urinary-biomarker test was largely the result of incorporation of PSA density data as opposed to DLX1 and HOXC6 expression. Regardless of the primary driver of this effect, the investigators estimate that with a cutoff NPV of 98%, for Gleason score ≥ 7 cancer, total biopsies could be reduced by 42%.

PSA ISOFORMS AND PROSTATE HEALTH INDEX

The measurement of blood-based biomarkers offers an alternative to transcription-mediated assays performed on post-DRE urine. PSA isoforms have been incorporated into testing panels to improve specificity for prostate cancer. The Prostate Health Index (PHI; Beckman Coulter, Inc, Brea, CA) incorporates the measurement of PSA, %fPSA, and [−2]pro-PSA ("pro-two-PSA") to predict prostate cancer risk.

The trial leading to its approval was a multicenter validation study of nearly 900 men aged greater than 50 years with normal DRE, no history of prostate cancer, and PSA 2 to 10 ng/mL who had blood drawn before prostate biopsy.[66] Nearly 80% of these were initial biopsies, and analysis was conducted with bootstrapping to set the prevalence of cancer at 25%. The AUC was greater for PHI than for %fPSA (×3) (0.70 vs 0.65, $P = .004$). With sensitivity set to 90%, PHI would avoid 26% of biopsies compared with 18% for free PSA ($P = .04$). Higher PHI scores were also associated with Gleason ≥7 cancers. A subsequent study reported on patients in the same cohort with PSA 4 to 10 ng/mL and found an AUC of 0.70 for detecting Gleason ≥7 cancer compared with 0.67 for %free PSA.[67] Using a cutoff with a sensitivity of 90% for Gleason ≥7 disease, 30% of biopsies could be avoided versus 22% for % free PSA. A meta-analysis including 8 studies supports these findings.[68]

4-KALLIKREIN PANEL

A 4-kallikrein panel has been developed as an alternative to the PHI. Similar to PHI, this panel measures prostate-specific kallikrein levels in the blood. These 4 kallikreins are total PSA, free PSA, intact PSA, and human kallikrein 2. The test incorporates patient age, history of prostate biopsy, and presence of palpable abnormality to estimate an individual's risk of having Gleason ≥7 disease on prostate biopsy.

The 4-kallikrein panel was first validated to improve accuracy over serum PSA for the prediction of biopsy results in several cohorts from the previously mentioned ERSPC screening trial.[69–74] Subsequently, it was tested in men undergoing biopsy as part of the UK-based ProtecT study, in which men aged 50 to 69 years were invited for prostate biopsy if serum PSA was greater than 3 ng/mL.[75] In the 6129 men with blood available for analysis, approximately one-third had prostate cancer and approximately one-third of those men had Gleason ≥7. The AUC for the detection of

Gleason ≥7 cancer was improved to 0.82 (from 0.74, $P<.001$) over the base model, which included age and total PSA.

A US-based, prospective study of 1012 men scheduled for prostate biopsy regardless of PSA or clinical findings recently validated 4- kallikrein.[76] It showed superiority of the kallikrein panel model to predict significant cancer risk over the Prostate Cancer Prevention Trial Risk Calculator 2.0 (includes age, race, family history, PSA, prior biopsy, palpable nodule).[76] If the decision to biopsy was based on ≥9% risk of Gleason ≥7 prostate cancer in this study, then 43% of biopsies could have been avoided at the expense of delaying the diagnosis of 2.4% of patients with Gleason ≥7 disease. Similar test characteristics have been demonstrated in a community cohort from Sweden.[77]

EPIGENETICS & CONFIRMMDX

A tissue-based, epigenetic assay has been developed to risk-stratify patients who may harbor prostate cancer in the setting of a prior negative biopsy.[78] A "field effect" has been observed in normal prostate epithelium up to 3 mm away from cancerous tissue whereby genes associated with the cell cycle and DNA repair have been silenced by methylation.[79] By measuring these changes in negative biopsy tissue, this test seeks to determine risk of unbiopsied prostate cancer. If risk is sufficiently low, a patient could be more safely spared from repeat biopsy.

A validation study of the assay included 350 patients from multiple US centers with serial biopsies. Two controls (negative biopsy followed by negative biopsy) were enrolled per case, and subsequently cancer prevalence was set to 18%, which is consistent with clinical experience.[80,81] The NPV was 88% with a sensitivity of 62%. With the assay calibration used in this study, there was no ability to distinguish risk for high- versus low-grade disease. However, a separate study with altered calibration did show an association between methylation levels and high-grade cancer.[82]

TISSUE-BASED GENOMIC TESTS

The previously discussed biomarkers have thus far been discussed for their utility in men considering prostate biopsy. These assays have also been explored for prognostic value in patients with known cancer.[83–85] The information provided on tumor aggressiveness could be used to refine AS selection criteria or to identify patients who may benefit from early treatment, including with possible adjuvant therapies. In addition to the blood and urine based previously discussed, there are several tissue-based genomic assays available to inform decisions.

A cell-cycle progression score (Prolaris, Myriad Genetics) has been developed based upon the expression levels of 31 genes found upregulated in aggressive prostate cancer.[86] Tissues from either biopsy or prostatectomy are analyzed to estimate the 10-year risk of prostate cancer–specific mortality. This assay has been found to subclassify low-risk men better than currently available clinical paradigms and may help determine those patients best managed with AS.[87,88]

The Genomic Prostate Score (OncotypeDx GPS; Genomic Health, Inc) measures the expression of 17 genes involved in multiple neoplastic pathways. Results are reported on a scale of 0 to 100, with 100 representing an aggressive tumor. For each 20-point increase, the risk for Gleason ≥ 7 and/or pathologic T3 (extracapsular extension) approximately doubles.[89] Notably, in multiple validation cohorts, relatively few clinically low-risk patients reached a score greater than 40.[89,90] Decision-curve analysis found a net benefit, however, to the genomic score over clinical factors alone for all outcomes measured.

Another genomic classifier (Decipher GenomeDx Biosciences, San Diego, CA, USA) based on 22 genes has been found to predict both metastasis at 5 years and prostate cancer–specific mortality at 10 years.[91,92] These genes were selected by measuring differential expression levels in samples enriched with aggressive disease, and many actually produce noncoding RNA.[93] Scores are reported from 0 to 1, with 1 representing the highest risk. An increase in score by 0.1 reflects a 30% increased hazard of metastasis.[94] One application of the genomic classifier is to risk-stratify patients with adverse pathologic features following prostatectomy to determine those most likely to benefit from adjuvant or salvage radiation therapy.[95,96] Although the most robust data supporting the use of this genomic classifier come from the analysis of prostatectomy specimens, it has also been shown to predict risk of metastasis from biopsy samples.[94,97]

SUMMARY

Over the last 30 years, the diagnosis and management of prostate cancer have evolved substantially, and there has been a decrease in prostate cancer mortality. PSA screening has likely been a major contributor to this decrease, but has also led to the overtreatment of many men due to a lack of specificity for aggressive disease and the protracted course of most prostate cancers. By improving patient risk-stratification through the selective use of biomarkers, and encouraging AS when appropriate, overdiagnosis and overtreatment can be limited while preserving reductions in morbidity and mortality realized over the last 3 decades.

REFERENCES

1. Siegel RL, Miller KD, Jemal A. Cancer statistics, 2017. CA Cancer J Clin 2017;67(1):7–30.
2. Cancer Statistics Review, 1975-2013-SEER Statistics. Available at: https://seer.cancer.gov/csr/1975_2013/. Accessed March 7, 2017.
3. Bell KJ, Mar CD, Wright G, et al. Prevalence of incidental prostate cancer: a systematic review of autopsy studies. Int J Cancer 2015;137(7):1749.
4. Gleason DF. Histologic grading of prostate cancer: a perspective. Hum Pathol 1992;23(3):273–9.
5. Epstein JI, Egevad L, Amin MB, et al. The 2014 International Society of Urological Pathology (ISUP) consensus conference on Gleason grading of prostatic carcinoma: definition of grading patterns and proposal for a new grading system. Am J Surg Pathol 2016;40(2):244–52.
6. Epstein JI, Zelefsky MJ, Sjoberg DD, et al. A contemporary prostate cancer grading system: a validated alternative to the Gleason score. Eur Urol 2016;69(3):428–35.
7. Kessler B, Albertsen P. The natural history of prostate cancer. Urol Clin North Am 2003;30(2):219–26.
8. Popiolek M, Rider JR, Andrén O, et al. Natural history of early, localized prostate cancer: a final report from three decades of follow-up. Eur Urol 2013; 63(3):428–35.
9. Prostate Cancer Trends, 1973-1995-SEER Publications. Available at: https://seer.cancer.gov/archive/publications/prostate/. Accessed April 13, 2017.
10. Denmeade SR, Isaacs JT. A history of prostate cancer treatment. Nat Rev Cancer 2002;2(5):389–96.
11. Stamey TA, Yang N, Hay AR, et al. Prostate-specific antigen as a serum marker for adenocarcinoma of the prostate. N Engl J Med 1987;317(15):909–16.
12. History of ACS recommendations for the early detection of cancer in people without symptoms. Available at: https://www.cancer.org/healthy/find-cancer-early/cancer-screening-guidelines/chronological-history-of-acs-recommendations.html. Accessed April 17, 2017.
13. Hankey BF, Feuer EJ, Clegg LX, et al. Cancer surveillance series: interpreting trends in prostate cancer—part I: evidence of the effects of screening in recent prostate cancer incidence, mortality, and survival rates. J Natl Cancer Inst 1999;91(12):1017–24.
14. Catalona WJ, Richie JP, Ahmann FR, et al. Comparison of digital rectal examination and serum prostate

specific antigen in the early detection of prostate cancer: results of a multicenter clinical trial of 6,630 men. J Urol 1994;151(5):1283–90.

15. Walsh PC, Lepor H, Eggleston JC. Radical prostatectomy with preservation of sexual function: anatomical and pathological considerations. Prostate 1983;4(5):473–85.

16. Reiner WG, Walsh PC. An anatomical approach to the surgical management of the dorsal vein and Santorini's plexus during radical retropubic surgery. J Urol 1979;121(2):198–200.

17. Lu-Yao GL, McLerran D, Wasson J, et al. An assessment of radical prostatectomy: time trends, geographic variation, and outcomes. JAMA 1993; 269(20):2633–6.

18. Newcomer LM, Stanford JL, Blumenstein BA, et al. Temporal trends in rates of prostate cancer: declining incidence of advanced stage disease, 1974 to 1994. J Urol 1997;158(4):1427–30.

19. Whitmore WF. Management of clinically localized prostatic cancer: an unresolved problem. JAMA 1993;269(20):2676–7.

20. Woolf SH. Screening for prostate cancer with prostate-specific antigen—an examination of the evidence. N Engl J Med 1995;333(21):1401–5.

21. Andriole GL, Crawford ED, Grubb RLI, et al. Mortality results from a randomized prostate-cancer screening trial. N Engl J Med 2009;360(13):1310–9.

22. Schröder FH, Hugosson J, Roobol MJ, et al. Screening and prostate-cancer mortality in a randomized European study. N Engl J Med 2009; 360(13):1320–8.

23. Schröder FH, Hugosson J, Roobol MJ, et al. Screening and prostate cancer mortality: results of the European Randomised Study of Screening for Prostate Cancer (ERSPC) at 13 years of follow-up. Lancet 2014;384(9959):2027–35.

24. Shoag JE, Mittal S, Hu JC. Reevaluating PSA testing rates in the PLCO trial. N Engl J Med 2016;374(18): 1795–6.

25. Hugosson J, Carlsson S, Aus G, et al. Mortality results from the Göteborg randomised population-based prostate-cancer screening trial. Lancet Oncol 2010;11(8):725–32.

26. U.S. Preventive Services Task Force. Screening for prostate cancer: U.S. Preventive Services Task Force recommendation statement. Ann Intern Med 2008;149(3):185–91.

27. Moyer VA, U.S. Preventive Services Task Force. Screening for prostate cancer: U.S. Preventive Services Task Force recommendation statement. Ann Intern Med 2012;157(2):120–34.

28. Draft Recommendation Statement: Prostate Cancer: Screening - US Preventive Services Task Force. Available at: https://www.uspreventiveservicestaskforce. org/Page/Document/RecommendationStatementDraft /prostate-cancer-screening1. Accessed May 2, 2017.

29. Carter HB. American Urological Association (AUA) guideline on prostate cancer detection: process and rationale. BJU Int 2013;112(5):543–7.

30. Wolf AMD, Wender RC, Etzioni RB, et al. American Cancer Society guideline for the early detection of prostate cancer: update 2010. CA Cancer J Clin 2010;60(2):70–98.

31. Eggener SE, Scardino PT, Walsh PC, et al. Predicting 15-year prostate cancer specific mortality after radical prostatectomy. J Urol 2011;185(3):869–75.

32. Ross HM, Kryvenko ON, Cowan JE, et al. Do adenocarcinomas of the prostate with Gleason score (GS) ≤6 have the potential to metastasize to lymph nodes? Am J Surg Pathol 2012;36(9):1346–52.

33. Klotz L, Vesprini D, Sethukavalan P, et al. Long-term follow-up of a large active surveillance cohort of patients with prostate cancer. J Clin Oncol 2015;33(3): 272–7.

34. Tosoian JJ, Mamawala M, Epstein JI, et al. Intermediate and longer-term outcomes from a prospective active-surveillance program for favorable-risk prostate cancer. J Clin Oncol 2015;33(30):3379–85.

35. Dall'Era MA, Konety BR, Cowan JE, et al. Active surveillance for the management of prostate cancer in a contemporary cohort. Cancer 2008;112(12): 2664–70.

36. Bokhorst LP, Valdagni R, Rannikko A, et al. A decade of active surveillance in the PRIAS study: an update and evaluation of the criteria used to recommend a switch to active treatment. Eur Urol 2016;70(6):954–60.

37. Soloway MS, Soloway CT, Eldefrawy A, et al. Careful selection and close monitoring of low-risk prostate cancer patients on active surveillance minimizes the need for treatment. Eur Urol 2010;58(6):831–5.

38. Selvadurai ED, Singhera M, Thomas K, et al. Medium-term outcomes of active surveillance for localised prostate cancer. Eur Urol 2013;64(6):981–7.

39. Godtman RA, Holmberg E, Khatami A, et al. Outcome following active surveillance of men with screen-detected prostate cancer. Results from the Göteborg randomised population-based prostate cancer screening trial. Eur Urol 2013;63(1):101–7.

40. Nam RK, Saskin R, Lee Y, et al. Increasing hospital admission rates for urological complications after transrectal ultrasound guided prostate biopsy. J Urol 2013;189(1 Suppl):S12–8.

41. Bozeman CB, Carver BS, Eastham JA, et al. Treatment of chronic prostatitis lowers serum prostate specific antigen. J Urol 2002;167(4):1723–6.

42. Punglia RS, D'Amico AV, Catalona WJ, et al. Impact of age, benign prostatic hyperplasia, and cancer on prostate-specific antigen level. Cancer 2006;106(7): 1507–13.

43. Oesterling JE, Jacobsen SJ, Chute CG, et al. Serum prostate-specific antigen in a community-based population of healthy men: establishment

of age-specific reference ranges. JAMA 1993; 270(7):860–4.

44. Moul JW. Targeted screening for prostate cancer in African-American men. Prostate Cancer Prostatic Dis 2000;3(4):248–55.

45. Carter HB, Ferrucci L, Kettermann A, et al. Detection of life-threatening prostate cancer with prostate-specific antigen velocity during a window of curability. J Natl Cancer Inst 2006;98(21):1521–7.

46. Lee R, Localio AR, Armstrong K, et al, Free PSA Study Group. A meta-analysis of the performance characteristics of the free prostate-specific antigen test. Urology 2006;67(4):762–8.

47. Hessels D, Klein Gunnewiek JMT, van Oort I, et al. DD3PCA3-based molecular urine analysis for the diagnosis of prostate cancer. Eur Urol 2003;44(1):8–16.

48. Bussemakers MJ, van Bokhoven A, Verhaegh GW, et al. DD3: a new prostate-specific gene, highly overexpressed in prostate cancer. Cancer Res 1999;59(23):5975–9.

49. de Kok JB, Verhaegh GW, Roelofs RW, et al. DD3PCA3, a very sensitive and specific marker to detect prostate tumors. Cancer Res 2002;62(9):2695–8.

50. Marks LS, Fradet Y, Lim Deras I, et al. PCA3 molecular urine assay for prostate cancer in men undergoing repeat biopsy. Urology 2007;69(3):532–5.

51. Salagierski M, Schalken JA. Molecular diagnosis of prostate cancer: PCA3 and TMPRSS2:ERG gene fusion. J Urol 2012;187(3):795–801.

52. Wei JT, Feng Z, Partin AW, et al. Can urinary PCA3 supplement PSA in the early detection of prostate cancer? J Clin Oncol 2014;32(36):4066–72.

53. Haese A, de la Taille A, van Poppel H, et al. Clinical utility of the PCA3 urine assay in European men scheduled for repeat biopsy. Eur Urol 2008;54(5):1081–8.

54. Deras IL, Aubin SMJ, Blase A, et al. PCA3: a molecular urine assay for predicting prostate biopsy outcome. J Urol 2008;179(4):1587–92.

55. Aubin SMJ, Reid J, Sarno MJ, et al. PCA3 molecular urine test for predicting repeat prostate biopsy outcome in populations at risk: validation in the placebo arm of the dutasteride REDUCE trial. J Urol 2010;184(5):1947–52.

56. Whitman EJ, Groskopf J, Ali A, et al. PCA3 score before radical prostatectomy predicts extracapsular extension and tumor volume. J Urol 2008;180(5):1975–9.

57. Tomlins SA, Rhodes DR, Perner S, et al. Recurrent fusion of TMPRSS2 and ETS transcription factor genes in prostate cancer. Science 2005;310(5748):644–8.

58. Pettersson A, Graff RE, Bauer SR, et al. The TMPRSS2:ERG rearrangement, ERG expression, and prostate cancer outcomes: a cohort study and meta-analysis. Cancer Epidemiol Biomarkers Prev 2012;21(9):1497–509.

59. Rubio-Briones J, Fernández-Serra A, Calatrava A, et al. Clinical implications of TMPRSS2-ERG gene fusion expression in patients with prostate cancer treated with radical prostatectomy. J Urol 2010;183(5):2054–61.

60. Attard G, Clark J, Ambroisine L, et al. Duplication of the fusion of TMPRSS2 to ERG sequences identifies fatal human prostate cancer. Oncogene 2008;27(3):253–63.

61. Demichelis F, Fall K, Perner S, et al. TMPRSS2:ERG gene fusion associated with lethal prostate cancer in a watchful waiting cohort. Oncogene 2007;26(31):4596–9.

62. Tomlins SA, Day JR, Lonigro RJ, et al. Urine TMPRSS2:ERG plus PCA3 for individualized prostate cancer risk assessment. Eur Urol 2016;70(1):45–53.

63. Leyten GHJM, Hessels D, Jannink SA, et al. Prospective multicentre evaluation of PCA3 and TMPRSS2-ERG gene fusions as diagnostic and prognostic urinary biomarkers for prostate cancer. Eur Urol 2014;65(3):534–42.

64. Leyten GHJM, Hessels D, Smit FP, et al. Identification of a candidate gene panel for the early diagnosis of prostate cancer. Clin Cancer Res 2015;21(13):3061–70.

65. Van Neste L, Hendriks RJ, Dijkstra S, et al. Detection of high-grade prostate cancer using a urinary molecular biomarker–based risk score. Eur Urol 2016;70(5):740–8.

66. Catalona WJ, Partin AW, Sanda MG, et al. A multicenter study of [−2]pro-prostate-specific antigen (PSA) in combination with PSA and free PSA for prostate cancer detection in the 2.0 to 10.0 ng/mL PSA range. J Urol 2011;185(5):1650–5.

67. Loeb S, Sanda MG, Broyles DL, et al. The Prostate Health Index selectively identifies clinically significant prostate cancer. J Urol 2015;193(4):1163–9.

68. Filella X, Giménez N. Evaluation of [−2] proPSA and Prostate Health Index (PHI) for the detection of prostate cancer: a systematic review and meta-analysis. Clin Chem Lab Med 2012;51(4):729–39.

69. Vickers AJ, Cronin AM, Aus G, et al. A panel of kallikrein markers can reduce unnecessary biopsy for prostate cancer: data from the European Randomized Study of Prostate Cancer Screening in Göteborg, Sweden. BMC Med 2008;6:19.

70. Vickers AJ, Cronin AM, Roobol MJ, et al. A four-kallikrein panel predicts prostate cancer in men with recent screening: data from the European Randomized Study of Prostate Cancer Screening, Rotterdam. Clin Cancer Res 2010;16(12):3232–9.

71. Vickers AJ, Cronin AM, Aus G, et al. Impact of recent screening on predicting the outcome of prostate cancer biopsy in men with elevated PSA: data

from the European Randomized Study of Prostate Cancer Screening in Gothenburg, Sweden. Cancer 2010;116(11):2612–20.

72. Benchikh A, Savage C, Cronin A, et al. A panel of kallikrein markers can predict outcome of prostate biopsy following clinical work-up: an independent validation study from the European Randomized Study of Prostate Cancer screening, France. BMC Cancer 2010;10:635.

73. Gupta A, Roobol MJ, Savage CJ, et al. A four-kallikrein panel for the prediction of repeat prostate biopsy: data from the European Randomized Study of Prostate Cancer Screening in Rotterdam, Netherlands. Br J Cancer 2010;103(5):708–14.

74. Vedder MM, de Bekker-Grob EW, Lilja HG, et al. The added value of percentage of free to total prostate-specific antigen, PCA3, and a kallikrein panel to the ERSPC risk calculator for prostate cancer in prescreened men. Eur Urol 2014;66(6): 1109–15.

75. Bryant RJ, Sjoberg DD, Vickers AJ, et al. Predicting high-grade cancer at ten-core prostate biopsy using four kallikrein markers measured in blood in the ProtecT study. J Natl Cancer Inst 2015;107(7).

76. Parekh DJ, Punnen S, Sjoberg DD, et al. A multi-institutional prospective trial in the USA confirms that the 4Kscore accurately identifies men with high-grade prostate cancer. Eur Urol 2015;68(3): 464–70.

77. Braun K, Sjoberg DD, Vickers AJ, et al. A four-kallikrein panel predicts high-grade cancer on biopsy: independent validation in a community cohort. Eur Urol 2016;69(3):505–11.

78. Stewart GD, Van Neste L, Delvenne P, et al. Clinical utility of an epigenetic assay to detect occult prostate cancer in histopathologically negative biopsies: results of the MATLOC study. J Urol 2013;189(3): 1110–6.

79. Mehrotra J, Varde S, Wang H, et al. Quantitative, spatial resolution of the epigenetic field effect in prostate cancer. Prostate 2008;68(2):152–60.

80. Djavan B, Zlotta A, Remzi M, et al. Optimal predictors of prostate cancer on repeat prostate biopsy: a prospective study of 1,051 men. J Urol 2000; 163(4):1144–8 [discussion: 1148–9].

81. Roehl KA, Antenor JAV, Catalona WJ. Serial biopsy results in prostate cancer screening study. J Urol 2002;167(6):2435–9.

82. Van Neste L, Partin AW, Stewart GD, et al. Risk score predicts high-grade prostate cancer in DNA-methylation positive, histopathologically negative biopsies. Prostate 2016;76(12):1078–87.

83. Stattin P, Vickers AJ, Sjoberg DD, et al. Improving the specificity of screening for lethal prostate cancer using prostate-specific antigen and a panel of kallikrein markers: a nested case–control study. Eur Urol 2015;68(2):207–13.

84. Ploussard G, Durand X, Xylinas E, et al. Prostate cancer antigen 3 score accurately predicts tumour volume and might help in selecting prostate cancer patients for active surveillance. Eur Urol 2011;59(3): 422–9.

85. Tosoian JJ, Loeb S, Feng Z, et al. Association of [-2] proPSA with biopsy reclassification during active surveillance for prostate cancer. J Urol 2012; 188(4):1131–6.

86. Warf MB, Reid JE, Brown KL, et al. Analytical validation of a cell cycle progression signature used as a prognostic marker in prostate cancer. J Mol Biomark Diagn 2015;6(4).

87. Cooperberg MR, Simko JP, Cowan JE, et al. Validation of a cell-cycle progression gene panel to improve risk stratification in a contemporary prostatectomy cohort. J Clin Oncol 2013;31(11): 1428–34.

88. Cuzick J, Stone S, Fisher G, et al. Validation of an RNA cell cycle progression score for predicting death from prostate cancer in a conservatively managed needle biopsy cohort. Br J Cancer 2015; 113(3):382–9.

89. Klein EA, Cooperberg MR, Magi-Galluzzi C, et al. A 17-gene assay to predict prostate cancer aggressiveness in the context of Gleason grade heterogeneity, tumor multifocality, and biopsy undersampling. Eur Urol 2014;66(3):550–60.

90. Cullen J, Rosner IL, Brand TC, et al. A biopsy-based 17-gene genomic prostate score predicts recurrence after radical prostatectomy and adverse surgical pathology in a racially diverse population of men with clinically low- and intermediate-risk prostate cancer. Eur Urol 2015; 68(1):123–31.

91. Karnes RJ, Choeurng V, Ross AE, et al. Validation of a genomic risk classifier to predict prostate cancer-specific mortality in men with adverse pathologic features. Eur Urol 2017. [Epub ahead of print].

92. Karnes RJ, Bergstralh EJ, Davicioni E, et al. Validation of a genomic classifier that predicts metastasis following radical prostatectomy in an at risk patient population. J Urol 2013;190(6):2047–53.

93. Erho N, Crisan A, Vergara IA, et al. Discovery and validation of a prostate cancer genomic classifier that predicts early metastasis following radical prostatectomy. PLoS One 2013;8(6):e66855.

94. Spratt DE, Yousefi K, Deheshi S, et al. Individual patient-level meta-analysis of the performance of the decipher genomic classifier in high-risk men after prostatectomy to predict development of metastatic disease. J Clin Oncol 2017;35(18):1991–8.

95. Freedland SJ, Choeurng V, Howard L, et al. Utilization of a genomic classifier for prediction of metastasis following salvage radiation therapy after radical prostatectomy. Eur Urol 2016;70(4): 588–96.

96. Dalela D, Santiago-Jiménez M, Yousefi K, et al. Genomic classifier augments the role of pathological features in identifying optimal candidates for adjuvant radiation therapy in patients with prostate cancer: development and internal validation of a multivariable prognostic model. J Clin Oncol 2017; 35(18):1982–90.

97. Klein EA, Haddad Z, Yousefi K, et al. Decipher genomic classifier measured on prostate biopsy predicts metastasis risk. Urology 2016;90:148–52.

MR Imaging of Prostate Zonal Anatomy

Joseph H. Yacoub, MD[a],*, Aytekin Oto, MD, MBA[b]

KEYWORDS

- Prostate anatomy • Prostate zones • Prostate MR Imaging • Multiparametric MR Imaging

KEY POINTS

- The prostate is divided into 4 zones peripheral zone, central zone, transition zone and the anterior fibromuscular stroma, which are well-depicted on MR imaging.
- The urethra, verumontanum, and ejaculatory ducts are the key anatomic reference points.
- Multiple layers of fascia, collectively called the periprostatic fascia, surround the prostate and contain the neurovascular bundles.
- Prostate pathology correlates with anatomy. Benign prostatic hyperplasia occurs almost exclusively in the transition zone.
- Roughly two-thirds of prostate cancer occurs in the peripheral zone, one-third in the transition zone, and less than 5% in the central zone.

INTRODUCTION

The prostate gland is a cone-shaped organ in the subperitoneal space located posterior to the pubic symphysis and anterior to the rectum. The base of the cone is attached to the neck of the bladder with the prostatic urethra entering near the anterior surface of the base. The apex rests on the superior surface of the urogenital diaphragm and contacts the medial surface of the levator ani muscles[1] (Fig. 1). The normal prostate measures approximately 4 × 3 × 3 cm, weighing roughly 15 to 20 g.[2] The median volume measured by MR imaging in a group of 420 healthy volunteers age 21 to 25 was 11.5 mL (range, 1.6–20.6).[3] In contrast, in 503 patients referred to MR imaging with mean and median age of 60 years (range, 38–83) the median prostate volume was 39.6 mL (range, 13.0–169.8).[4]

For more than one-half of the twentieth century, the idea of prostatic lobes dominated the understanding of the prostatic anatomy.[5] In a series of articles starting the late 1960s and spanning the 1970s and 1980s, John McNeal pioneered a new understanding of the prostate based on zones instead of lobes,[5,6] which became known as the zonal anatomy of the prostate[7] and remains the main model of understanding the prostate anatomy until now. McNeal described 4 distinct zones of the prostate namely, the peripheral zone (PZ), the central zone (CZ), the transition zone, and the anterior fibromuscular stroma (AFMS).

McNeal's analysis of the anatomy and histology of the prostate was timely for radiology, because the early studies on MR imaging that emerged in the 1980s benefiting from the newly recognized zonal anatomy of the prostate. Before MR imaging, computed tomography scans and ultrasound imaging were limited in their ability to depict the zonal anatomy of the prostate.[8,9]

Disclosures: None.
[a] Department of Radiology, Loyola University Chicago, Stritch School of Medicine, 2160 South 1st Avenue, Maywood, IL 60153, USA; [b] Department of Radiology, University of Chicago, 5841 South Maryland Avenue, MC 2026, Chicago, IL 60637, USA
* Corresponding author.
E-mail address: joeyacoub@gmail.com

Radiol Clin N Am 56 (2018) 197–209
https://doi.org/10.1016/j.rcl.2017.10.003

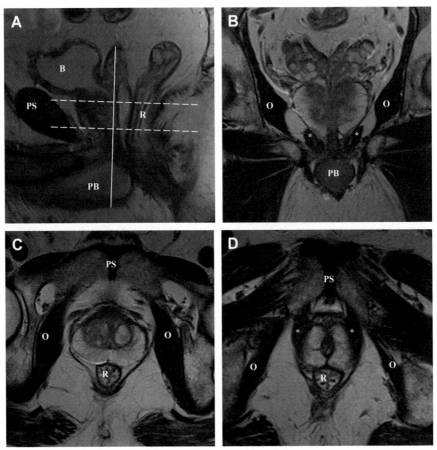

Fig. 1. Prostate location and MR imaging planes. B, bladder; O, obturator internus; PB, penile bulb; PS, pubic symphysis; R, rectum. Sagittal T2-weighted turbo spin echo (TSE) image (*A*) shows the relationship of the prostate to the bladder (B) and rectum (R). Anteriorly, the prostate is separated from the pubic symphysis (PS) by an area of fat. The coronal plane is acquired parallel to the rectal surface of the prostate (*solid line*) and the axial plane is acquired perpendicular to it (*dashed line*). Coronal T2-weighted TSE image (*B*) demonstrates the relationship of the prostate to the levator ani muscle (*asterisks*). Axial T2-weighted TSE images obtained at the mid gland (*C*) and apex (*D*) show the relationship of the prostate to the pubic symphysis (PS) and rectum (R) as well as the levator ani muscles (*asterisks*).

In this article, we review the anatomy of the prostate and focus on correlating the anatomic descriptions with the appearance of the prostate on MR imaging. Some general conventions are used when referring to the prostate on pathologic sections or imaging. The prostate is divided into 3 roughly equal parts along its craniocaudal extent, namely the base, mid, and apex. There are no anatomic delimiters between those parts. On MR imaging, the coronal plane is angled parallel to the rectal surface of the prostate and the axial plane is acquired perpendicular to that (see **Fig. 1**). This coronal plane roughly parallels the plane of the distal urethra, which is the anatomic plane that McNeal used to describe the relationships of the prostate zones.[7]

THE ANATOMIC REFERENCE POINTS
The Urethra and Verumontanum

The prostatic urethra is the primary anatomic reference point in the prostate. When assessed in the sagittal plane, the urethra makes a 35° angulation at the midpoint of its course from the bladder neck (proximal) to the apex (distal) near the location of the verumontanum,[7,10–12] dividing the urethra into 2 nearly equal segments that are commonly referred to as the proximal and distal urethra.[2,7] The angulation can be variable between individuals and is affected by the development of benign prostatic hyperplasia (BPH).[10,13] The preprostatic (internal) sphincter is a well-developed smooth muscle sphincter that completely envelops the proximal urethra from the base of the gland to the base of the verumontanum.[7] The periurethral gland region consists of scattered tiny ducts and abortive acinar systems confined by the periurethral smooth muscle of the preprostatic sphincter.[10] This complete cylindrical barrier can explain the limited development of the periurethral ducts.[7] Anteriorly the fibers of preprostatic sphincter do not form complete rings, but terminate within the tissue of the AFMS.[10] On dynamic imaging of the prostate during ejaculation, the preprostatic sphincter can be seen contracting for the duration of ejaculation at around the same time the ejaculate reaches the distal urethra,[14] thus preventing retrograde ejaculation.[10]

The verumontanum is an exaggerated area of glandular–stromal tissue protruding from the posterior urethral wall into its lumen.[10,12] The verumontanum lies entirely in the distal urethral segment with its base at the level of the angulation of the urethra.[11] Distal to the verumontanum, the distal urethra is partially encircled by a similar sphincter of striated muscles that forms a semicircular band discontinuous posteriorly. The striated muscles around the distal urethra blend distally with the external sphincter beyond the apex of the prostate.[11] The external (distal) urethral sphincter is also semicircular, incomplete posteriorly, where its bundles anchor into the anterior surface of the PZ.[1] It is located just distal to the prostate apex in a close anatomic relation to the pelvic floor, but is independent of the pelvic floor muscles.[15,16] The external sphincter surrounds the membranous urethra extending from the prostate apex to the entry of the urethra into the penile bulb. The length of membranous urethra is variable. In 1 study, it ranged from 6 to 24 mm.[17] A longer membranous urethra was associated with significantly more rapid return of urinary continence after surgery.[17] Damage to this sphincter during transurethral resection of the prostate, or more commonly during radical prostatectomy, may lead to urinary incontinence.[1,16]

On MR imaging, the urethra can usually be delineated. The distal urethra is more readily visible with high signal intensity center surrounded by the lower signal intensity urethral muscle wall and periurethral tissue.[2,11] The verumontanum demonstrates high T2 signal[11] and, in the study by Vargas and colleagues,[18] it was identified on MR imaging in 93% of patients (Fig. 2).

Ejaculatory Ducts and Seminal Vesicles

The paired ejaculatory ducts are also important landmarks in identifying the zonal anatomy of the prostate.[19] As the vas deferens enters the posterior prostate base, it merges with the duct of the ipsilateral seminal vesicle to form the ejaculatory duct.[19] The ejaculatory duct courses caudally from the base of the prostate to the verumontanum along the same plane of the distal urethra, although usually offset a few millimeters posteriorly.[10] The orifices of the ejaculatory ducts open in the mid convexity of the verumontanum.[7]

On MR imaging, the ejaculatory duct can demonstrate either low or high T2 signal

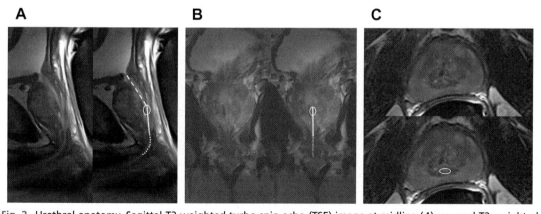

A   **B**   **C**

Fig. 2. Urethral anatomy. Sagittal T2-weighted turbo spin echo (TSE) image at midline (A), coronal T2-weighted TSE image in the plane of the distal urethra (B) and axial T2-weighted TSE image at the mid gland at the level of verumontanum (C) demonstrate the urethral anatomy. The urethra is demarcated on the image replicas. The proximal urethra is demarcated by a dashed line extending from the base of the bladder to the verumontanum. A white ellipse demarcates the verumontanum, which is located at the superior most aspect of the distal urethra. The distal urethra is demarcated by a solid white line. The external urethral sphincter is demarcated by a doted line. It surrounds the membranous urethra extending from the prostate apex to the base of the penis and it varies in length between individuals. The proximal and distal urethra make angle of approximately 35°, which also varies between individual and is affected by the presence of benign prostatic hyperplasia.

intensity.[11] The seminal vesicles demonstrate high T2 signal owing to their fluid content (**Fig. 3**). MR imaging of the seminal vesicle before and after ejaculation demonstrates a decrease in the size of the seminal vesicle after ejaculation in the majority of patients.[14] Some centers instruct patients to abstain from ejaculation for about 2 days before getting a prostate MR imaging to maximize the distention of the seminal vesicle and improve assessment for seminal vesicle invasion.

THE PROSTATE ZONES

Based on McNeal's description of the prostate, the ducts radiating from different parts of the urethra form the different zones of the prostate. Two sets of ducts arise from the proximal urethral segment. As mentioned, very tiny ducts arising from the proximal urethral segment are confined by the preprostatic sphincter and, therefore, the periurethral gland region remains very small in size, only a fraction of the size of the surrounding transition zone. More distally within the proximal urethral segment, a second set of ducts leave the posterolateral recesses of the urethral wall at a single point at the lower border of the preprostatic sphincter, just proximal to the point of urethral angulation.[7] These ducts extend laterally and then curve sharply anteromedially, forming the transition zone.[7,12] The directions of growth of these ducts is toward the bladder intimately related to the preprostatic sphincter.[7]

Two sets of ducts arise from the distal urethral segment. Ducts arising from the convexity of the verumontanum, clustered in a small circle around the ejaculatory duct orifices, branch directly toward the base of the prostate along the course of the ejaculatory ducts in the coronal plane and form the CZ of the gland.[7] Finally, 2 rows of duct buds in the lateral recess of the posterior urethral wall of the verumontanum and distal urethra radiate laterally forming the PZ.[7] The more proximal ducts that have their orifices at the base of the verumontanum become larger than the more apical ducts and fan out more proximally and laterally above the level of the verumontanum, explaining the superior extension of the PZ to near the base the gland posterior to the CZ.[7]

Fig. 4 is a schematic of the zonal anatomy of the prostate demonstrating the relative locations and relationships of the PZ, CZ, transitional zone (TZ), and the AFMS.

Peripheral Zone

The PZ is the major glandular component of the prostate gland,[12] making up about 70% of the glandular tissue.[7] Using the standard sector map described in the Prostate Imaging, Reporting and Data System Version 2 (PI-RADS v2),[20] the PZ can be subdivided into 3 sections—the posterior medial, posterior lateral, and anterior section—in the apex, mid, and base of the gland on each side of the midline (**Fig. 5**). The anterior sections on both sides appear as 2 horns and hence the commonly used term of anterior horns. In the apex, the 2 anterior horns curve anterior medially to nearly abut each other anterior to the urethra, forming a near complete ring of PZ that surrounds the urethra and abuts the AFMS.[12] In the mid gland, the PZ encompass the posterior, the lateral, and the majority of the anterolateral tissue.[12] The

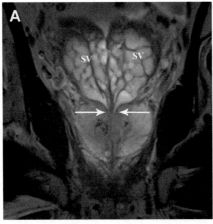
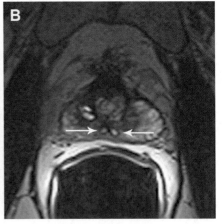

Fig. 3. Seminal vesicles (SV) and ejaculatory ducts. Coronal T2-weighted turbo spin echo image (*A*) and axial 3-dimensional T2-weighted near the mid of the gland (*B*) demonstrate the ejaculatory ducts (*arrows*) coursing from the point of insertion of the SV to the verumontanum (not shown). The course of the ejaculatory ducts is in the same plane as the distal urethra, possibly offset by few millimeters posteriorly.

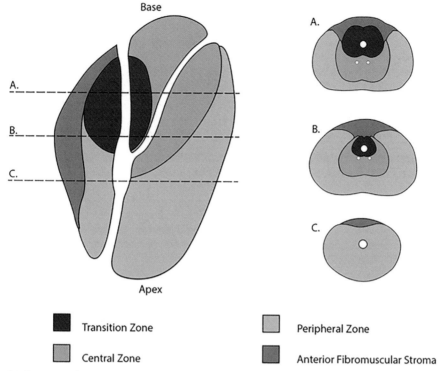

Base

A.

B.

C.

Apex

A.

B.

C.

| | Transition Zone | | Peripheral Zone |
| | Central Zone | | Anterior Fibromuscular Stroma |

Fig. 4. (A–C) Schematic of the zonal anatomy of the prostate. The schematic demonstrates the relationships of the peripheral zone, central zone, transitional zone, and anterior fibromuscular stroma.

anterior horns may curve anteromedially, but not to the point of touching each other. Toward the base, the PZ surrounds the CZ and TZ.[21] The anterior horns are less reaching anteriorly and the CZ largely replaces the posteromedial segments. As the TZ enlarges owing to BPH, the anterior horns of the PZ become compressed toward the most lateral portions of the gland.[12] On MR imaging, the normal PZ has a high T2 signal, which can be delineated easily from other zones or surrounding structures (see **Fig. 5**; **Fig. 6**).

Central Zone

The CZ is a flattened, cone-shaped glandular tissue surrounding the ejaculatory ducts most prominent at the base of the prostate, with its apex at the verumontanum.[10,21,22] It accounts for 25% of the glandular prostate in young adults[7] and its

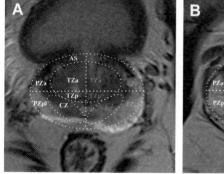
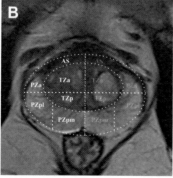
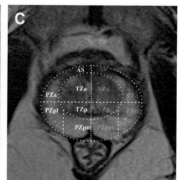

Fig. 5. Sector map superimposed on T2-weighted turbo spin echo images of the prostate base (*A*), mid gland (*B*), and apex (*C*). AS, anterior fibromuscular stroma; PZa, peripheral zone anterior horn; PZpl, peripheral zone posterior lateral; PZpm, peripheral zone posterior medial; TZa, transition zone anterior; TZp, transition zone posterior.

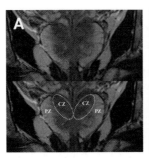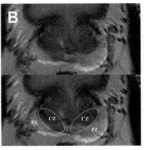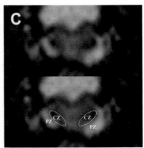

Fig. 6. The central zone (CZ) and the peripheral zone (PZ). Coronal T2-weighted turbo spin echo (TSE) image in the plane of the distal urethra (*A*), axial T2-weighted TSE image at the base (*B*), and axial apparent diffusion coefficient (ADC) map at the base (*C*) demonstrate the appearance of the CZ, which is demarcated by the dashed oval on image replicas. Relative to the PZ, the CZ seems to be darker on T2-weighted images and the ADC map.

volume decreases gradually after age 35.[22] According to McNeal, there are "dramatic" histologic difference between the CZ and PZ.[7] Compared with the PZ, the acini of the CZ are larger and more irregular.[7,21] Numerous epithelial covered ridges or septa project from the walls of the acini into the lumen, forming a characteristic Roman bridge architecture and intraglandular lacuna.[7,23] The basal cell layer of the CZ is prominent.[7,23] The epithelial cells seem to be more crowded, containing more opaque granular eosinophilic cytoplasm.[7] The stroma of the CZ is compact in distinction to the stroma of the PZ, which is made of loosely arranged and randomly interwoven muscle bundles.[21] These histologic differences between the CZ and the PZ, in particular the more compact stroma and decreased luminal fluid content, may account for the differing MR imaging characteristics.[11,24,25] The histologic differences between the CZ and the rest of the glandular tissue of the prostate can be explained by the embryologic origin of these zones. Whereas the PZ and the TZ are derivatives of the urogenital sinus, the CZ is a derivative of the Wolffian duct and, therefore, has some histologic characteristics that resemble the seminal vesicles and the ejaculatory ducts.[22,26]

On MR imaging, the distinction between the CZ and PZ has long been recognized—since the earliest papers on MR imaging of the prostate. Hricak and colleagues[11] reported that, on T2-weighted sequences obtained on 0.3-Telsa magnets, the CZ was identified in 31 of 32 men aged 25 to 35 years, but only in 8 of 23 men aged 40 years or older. A decrease in the size of the CZ with age, as well as compression and effacement of the CZ by an enlarging adjacent TZ, accounts for the decreasing visibility of the CZ with age.[2] In contrast, the distinction of the CZ and the TZ on MR imaging has only become widely accepted recently. Early studies of prostate MR

imaging suggested that the CZ could not be delineated from the TZ, except by anatomic location.[11] Subsequently, the term central gland was coined to refer to the combined CZ and TZ, and became widely used,[2,18,27] spreading with it the notion the central gland is a single imaging entity. More recently, Vargas and colleagues[18] have shown that in a population undergoing MR imaging for the assessment of prostate cancer with a mean age of 60 years, the CZ was visible, at least partially, in 81% to 84% of patients. Similarly, in a comparable population, Hansford and colleagues[25] were able to identify the CZ in 92% to 93% of patients on T2-weighted images and 78% to 88% of patients on apparent diffusion coefficient (ADC) maps. They suggested that readers with varying prostate MR imaging experiences could fairly reliably identify the CZ. The PI-RADS v2 has since discouraged the use of the term central gland, because it is not reflective of the zonal anatomy as visualized or reported on pathologic specimens.[20]

On MR imaging, the CZ is identified surrounding the ejaculatory ducts from the base of the prostate to the verumontanum on either sides of midline, demonstrating homogenous low signal intensity on T2-weighted images and a low ADC[18,25] (see Fig. 6). Gupta and colleagues[28] have shown that the ADC of benign CZ is lower than the ADC of other zones of the prostate and overlaps with the ADC of prostate cancer tissue. The T2 signal and ADC appearance of benign CZ can, therefore, masquerade as prostate cancer. Knowledge of the zonal anatomy of the prostate and the ability to identify the CZ is, therefore, very important. If the CZ is not recognized, it may be overcalled as prostate cancer owing to its imaging characteristics. The CZ can be best depicted and distinguished from the PZ on coronal images along the same plane of the distal urethra[11,18] (see **Fig. 6**). The symmetric appearance on either side of midline is particularly useful in differentiating the CZ from other causes of T2 and ADC signal changes. Occasionally, the normal CZ may seem to be asymmetric, either owing to slight angulation of the axis of the prostate relative to the imaging planes or owing to asymmetric compression of the CZ by the enlarging TZ, posing an imaging challenge.[29] On dynamic contrast-enhanced imaging, the CZ demonstrated either type 1 or type 2, but not type 3, curves.[25] This feature may be useful when trying to differentiate the CZ from a suspected tumor at the base.

Transition Zone

Two small lobes located anteromedially in the mid and base of the gland surrounding the proximal urethral form the TZ. The acini and ducts of the TZ are similar to the those of the PZ; however, they are less numerous and are surrounded by more dense stroma.[30] In young adults, the TZ constitutes only 5% of the glandular tissue of the prostate[7] and is of a homogenous, low T2 signal.[11] In our experience, a majority of patients presenting for prostate MR imaging have some degree of BPH and, therefore, the appearance of the TZ varies significantly from this classic description. The TZ can grow significantly in size owing to BPH, resulting in significant deformity of the prostate. For example, whereas the normal TZ is confined to the mid and base of the gland above the level of verumontanum, in a majority of patients the enlarged TZ deforms the gland and extends below the level of the verumontanum, reaching the level of the apex in some cases.[31]

The TZ is well-demarcated from the PZ by a concentric band of fibromuscular tissue and compressed glandular tissue, which becomes more pronounced in the setting of BPH.[2,11,22] This band has been historically called the "surgical capsule"[22] (Fig. 7). It has low signal intensity on both T2-weighted images and ADC maps owing to the dense compacted fibromuscular tissue.[22] Owing to a combination of its curving contour and volume averaging artifact, it may seem to be focally thickened laterally on axial images near the base, mimicking a focal tumor. Recognizing the location, looking for symmetry, and recognizing its linear morphology on the coronal plane can avoid this pitfall.

Anterior Fibromuscular Stroma

The AFMS is the main nonglandular tissue of the prostate. It is made of smooth muscles blending with muscle fibers surrounding the urethra to form a band of fibromuscular tissue. Superiorly, it blends with the smooth muscles and skeletal muscles of the bladder, bladder neck, and preprostatic sphincter. It descends as an apron of muscular tissue, forming the entire anterior surface of the prostate and contacting the urethra again at its distal end in the prostate apex.[7,10,12,22] Its bulk and consistency vary considerably from the base to the apex.[12] Its lateral margins blend with the prostate capsule and it is inseparably fused to the glandular prostate.[7,10]

On MR imaging, it demonstrated markedly low T2 signal, low ADC, and low diffusion-weighting imaging signal,[11,22,32] and is often hypovascular[22] demonstrating type 1 enhancement pattern on

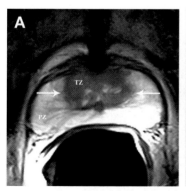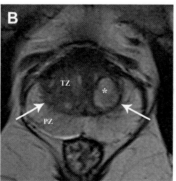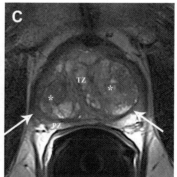

Fig. 7. Transition zone (TZ) and surgical capsule. T2-weighted turbo spin echo axial images from 3 different patients demonstrate varying sizes of the TZ. The first patient (*A*) has a normal size TZ, the second patient has moderately enlarged TZ containing few benign prostatic hyperplasia (BPH) nodules (*B*), and the third patient has a markedly enlarged TZ with numerous BPH nodules (*C*). BPH nodules of various sizes in the second and third patients (*asterisks*) have heterogeneous T2 signal and well-defined capsules. This appearance of the TZ in setting of BPH with multiple, well-defined BPH nodules has been described as organized chaos. The surgical capsule is the dark line demarcating the TZ from the PZ (*arrows*). It becomes more evident in the setting of BPH (*B, C*). PZ, peripheral zone.

dynamic contrast-enhanced MR imaging.[32] It decreases in thickness in men with advancing age and prostate size likely owing to the compressive effects of BPH.[22,27]

Prostate Capsule

Although not considered a zone of the prostate, we describe the capsule in this section because of its inseparable relation to the prostate glandular tissue and the AFMS. The "capsule" is made up of a band of concentrically placed fibromuscular tissue that is an inseparable component of the prostatic stroma about 0.5 mm in thickness.[8,30,33] It is, therefore, not a true capsule in the anatomic or histologic sense, for which reason some authors prefer to call it a pseudocapsule.[1] However, others have used the term pseudocapsule to refer to the "surgical capsule" discussed elsewhere in this article.[20] To avoid potential confusion, we avoid the use of the term pseudocapsule in this article. The capsule surrounds the entire prostate, blending with the AFMS anteriorly with 2 notable defects. At the prostate apex, there is a defect in the capsule anteriorly and laterally,[10,33] where the prostate stroma blends with the muscle fibers of the urinary sphincter.[15] It is, therefore, difficult to define the exact boundaries of the prostate in this area,[2,10] creating a challenge for the pathologist in assessing the pathologic stage of prostate cancer at this region.[1,34] At the base of the gland, there is a second defect at the bladder neck and where the ejaculatory ducts enter the prostate, creating similar difficulties.[10] Multiple vessels and nerves penetrate the prostate capsule at the lateral portion of the prostate,[15] which can form routes for spread of prostate cancer outside the capsule.

On MR imaging, the capsule appears as a thin rim of dark T2 signal surrounding the prostate that servers as a landmark to assess to extracapsular extension of tumor[20] (Fig. 8). In the early literature on MR imaging of the prostate, the capsule was reportedly inconsistently visualized,[11,24] seen only 31% of the patients in 1 study using a mix of 0.35-T and 1.5-T magnets.[11] More modern literature focuses on the accuracy of MR imaging for the detection of extracapsular extension, with no specific reports on the rate of complete visualization of the prostate capsule. The capsule demonstrates delayed but persistent contrast enhancement.

PERIPROSTATIC ANATOMY
Periprostatic Fascia

There is a variation in the terminology used in the surgical literature to describe the fascia surrounding the prostate and, despite extensive research, the exact details remain controversial.[15] Walz and colleagues[15] categorize the layers of the fascia as parietal fascia that they collectively call the parietal endopelvic fascia or "endopelvic fascia" for short, and the visceral prostatic fascia (PF). The parietal endopelvic fascia is primarily composed of the levator ani fascia. The PF covers the prostate capsule with the neurovascular structures found merged into or sandwiched between the levator ani fascia and the PF. Both the parietal endopelvic fascia and the PF together can be referred to as the periprostatic fascia. Walz and colleagues[15] use the term periprostatic fascia to signify all fasciae around the prostate that are external to the prostate capsule and further divide the periprostatic fascia into 3 components based

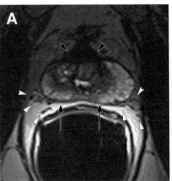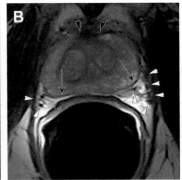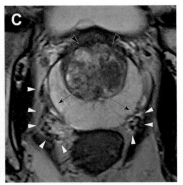

Fig. 8. Capsule and neurovascular bundles. Axial T2-weighted images from 3 different patients (*A–C*) demonstrate the appearance of the prostate capsule, which appears as a thin black line surrounding the prostate (*black arrows*). In the anterior most aspect of the prostate, the capsule blends with the anterior fibromuscular stroma (*black arrow heads*). The neurovascular bundle is located posterolateral to the prostate and appears as a cluster of dark T2 foci (*white arrow heads*), which likely represent nerve bundles and their associated vascular structures. There is significant variability in the appearance of the neurovascular bundle between patients, as is evident from these images.

on their locations, namely, anterior, lateral, and posterior. It is important to recognize that each of those components could be multilayered. These fasciae are generally not well-delineated on MR imaging. Perhaps the most relevant of the fasciae from an imaging standpoint is the posterior PF and seminal vesicle fascia, which cover the posterior prostate surface and seminal vesicle, separating them from the rectum. Together, they are referred to as Dennonvillier's fascia, which was described in the prostate MR imaging literature as having a lower signal intensity than either the rectal wall or PZ of the prostate gland[11,35] (Fig. 9). The Dennonvillier's fascia is often fused with the prostate capsule posteriorly at midline.[15] Toward the posterolateral aspect of the prostate, the Dennonvillier's fascia is separated from the prostate by areolar connective tissue containing the neurovascular bundle (NVB).[15]

Neurovascular Bundles

The nerve fibers that ultimately supply the corpora cavernosa distal to the prostate apex arise from the pelvic plexus, which is located lateral to the rectum at the level of the seminal vesicles.[15] These nerve fibers are accompanied by vascular structure as they course inferiorly forming the NVB. The NVB course posterolateral to the prostate at the 5 o'clock and 7 o'clock positions in triangular areas formed between the layers of the

periprostatic fascia. The medial wall of the triangle is formed by the PF, which is intimately attached to the prostatic capsule. The lateral wall is formed by the lateral fascia, and the posterior wall by Dennonvillier's fascia. The triangular area is wide toward the base and becomes narrow toward the apex.[36] As the NVB descend, they course slightly medially approaching the midline and each other toward the apex of the gland. In the apical region, the NVB is located very close to the urethral sphincter and the prostate apex.[15] Small branches arise from the NVB along their course and arborize over the prostate surface, and giving rise to smaller branches that penetrate the capsule in no consistent way, tethering the bundles to the posterolateral surface of the prostate.[10,15,36] Some small branches may also supply the urethral sphincter.[15]

The neural anatomy may, however, vary substantially. Kiyoshima and colleagues[37] reported that 52% of prostates lacked a definite NVB formation, and vessels and nerves were spread throughout the lateral aspect. The nerve fibers have been shown to disperse along the lateral surface of the prostate from the 7 o'clock to 10 o'clock positions and from the 5 o'clock to 2 o'clock positions.[15] Similar findings were reported by Lee and colleagues,[38] who also observed that a significant portion of the nerves (approximately 20%) were on the anterior surface of the prostate. Nerve sparing surgical approaches that aim at preserving the erectile function after prostatectomy will at a minimum try to preserve the NVB at the 5 o'clock and 7 o'clock positions with the surrounding Dennonvillier's fascia and lateral fascia. Modifications of surgical techniques that aim at preserving more nerve fibers closer to the prostate surface and along the lateral surface of the prostate have been described.[15,39] The 6 o'clock position anterior to the rectum has been consistently describe as sparse in nerve fibers.[10,15]

Axial MR images can delineate triangular regions posterolateral to the prostate at the 5 o'clock and 7 o'clock positions that house the NVB. These regions demonstrate fat signal containing small punctate dark structures that likely represent components of the NVB coursing perpendicular to the plane of the image. In our experience, a well-defined singular bundle is rarely, if ever, seen and more often it appears as a cluster of punctate structures with intervening fat signal. Of note, the nerve fibers are microscopic and are not seen during routine surgery; therefore, the dark punctate structures seen on MR imaging likely represent a combination of vessels and bundles of nerves (see Fig. 8).

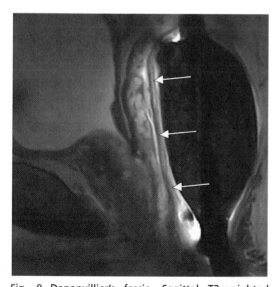

Fig. 9. Denonvillier's fascia. Sagittal T2-weighted turbo spin echo image at midline demonstrate a dark vertical line (arrows) interposed between the rectum and the prostate/seminal vesicle, which represents the posterior prostatic fascia and seminal vesicle fascia (pPF/SVF), also referred to as Denonvillier's fascia.

Periprostatic Lymphatic and Vasculature

The lymphatic of the prostate accompanies the veins draining primarily to the obturator, internal iliac, external iliac, common iliac, and presacral lymph nodes.[2] Periprostatic lymph nodes are uncommon, only found in 4.4% of prostatectomy specimen in 1 study[40] and more typically near the base. When present on the surgical specimens, they can be malignantly involved in up to 15% of patients in 1 study.[41] The periprostatic lymph nodes are occasionally seen on MR imaging,[22] but distinguishing malignant from benign is not reliably possible.

The arterial supply of the prostate is highly variable, with multiple common patterns described and multiple additional uncommon patterns.[42] Recognizing the specific pattern of arterial supply has become important with the advent of prostate arterial embolization as a potential treatment for BPH. These arteries, however, are not readily recognizable on a standard prostate MR imaging protocol. The prostate is surrounded by periperostatic vessels that supply and drain the penis. These vessels are becoming of increasing relevance in prostate radiotherapy. According to Lee and colleagues,[43] vasculogenic causes seem to be predominant in radiation-induced erectile dysfunction and, therefore, vessel-sparing radiotherapy techniques have been devised to reduce the rate of erectile dysfunction. The internal pudendal artery supplies the cavernosal erectile tissue often originating from the anterior division of the internal iliac artery and coursing through the greater and lesser sciatic foramina and then coursing inferior to the prostate before entering the corpus cavernosum. The internal pudendal artery does not come in close contact with the prostate; however, anatomic variations of the pudendal artery, such as the accessory pudendal artery, can course closer to the prostate apex potentially making vessel-sparing radiation unfeasible.[43] Few papers have described the use of MR angiography to identify the penile arterial anatomy before surgery[44] and before vessel-sparing radiotherapy.[43] The dorsal venous complex is located just anterior to the prostate[11,43] and provides venous drainage for the penis.

THE ANATOMY–PATHOLOGY CONNECTION
Prostate Anatomy and Prostate Cancer

Around two-thirds of all prostate cancers occur in the PZ, compared with roughly one-quarter or one-third in the TZ.[1,34,45] Cohen and colleagues[45] further showed that, when tumor is present in the

TZ, it represents the index lesion only 41% of the time. This distribution has implication on detection and diagnosis of prostate cancer. Systematic transrectal ultrasound–guided biopsy, which has been the main stay of diagnosis, preferentially sampled the posterior prostate. Anterior TZ tumors were largely undersampled in the era of systematic transrectal ultrasound–guided biopsy.[46,47] MR imaging is now playing an increasing role in the detection of prostate cancer[48,49] and the guidance of targeted biopsy of suspicious lesions.[50] Accurate localization of suspicious lesions on MR imaging to the appropriate zone is essential for assessing the likelihood of cancer[20] and subsequent decisions of target biopsy. In contrast, prostate cancer rarely occurs in the CZ, with CZ cancer accounting for 2.5% to 8.0% of prostate cancers.[34,45,51] Cohen and colleagues[45] further note that, when CZ cancer is present, it represented the index tumor 93.6% of the time. CZ cancer has been shown to be more aggressive with a higher clinical stage at diagnosis and higher rates of capsular penetration, positive margin, and seminal vesicle invasion.[18,45,51] The clinical outcomes for these cancers were significantly worse.[45] Although the normal CZ and PZ are histologically different, tumors arising in the CZ are indistinguishable from PZ tumors of similar grade.[23,45] In addition, because of the lack of a clearly delineated boundary between the PZ and the CZ, a pathologist may not routinely recognize or report the zonal origin of CZ tumors on prostatectomy specimens. Recognizing the tumor's zone of origin depends on the identification of morphologic features in the normal prostate tissue adjacent to the tumor. Preoperative MR imaging could play a role in suggesting the CZ origin of the tumor, which could guide the surgical approach and affect the prognosis of the patient. As mentioned, the CZ poses challenges on imaging owing to the overlap between T2-weighted and ADC characteristics of normal CZ and prostate cancer. Furthermore, available guidelines are very brief on the assessment of the CZ.[20] The inherent difficulties of assessing this region of the prostate call for a consistent understanding and reporting of the anatomy by radiologist and pathologists.

Prostate Anatomy and Benign Prostatic Hyperplasia

Benign prostatic hyperplasia (BPH) refers to the stromal and glandular epithelial hyperplasia that exclusively occurs in the TZ.[7,10,21] The glands themselves remain normal; thus, it is the overall architecture and organization that defines BPH.[21] BPH is common in men older than 40 years of age, and increases in prevalence with advancing age. Therefore, it is present to various degrees in a majority of patients presenting for MR imaging. Different patterns of BPH have been described on ultrasound examinations and adapted to MR imaging.[52,53] As the TZ grows, it deforms the prostate and the adjacent zones. The PZ can become more compressed with increasing splaying of the anterior horns, which becomes even more compressed laterally and absent anteriorly. The CZ also gradually atrophies with age and becomes increasingly more difficult to delineate. The AFMS becomes thinner as it is compressed anteriorly. The TZ itself extends closer to the apex below the level of the verumontanum. Superiorly, the enlarged TZ can protrude into the bladder, a finding that is called the "median lobe" in the surgical literature, possibly a carry-over term from the old lobar anatomy of the prostate, and has more recently been called pedunculated enlargement in the radiology literature[13,52] (Fig. 10). Intravesical prostate protrusion (IPP) may correlate with lower urinary tract symptoms (LUTS)[13] and may have implications on the technical difficulty and length of robotic assisted prostatectomies.[54–56]

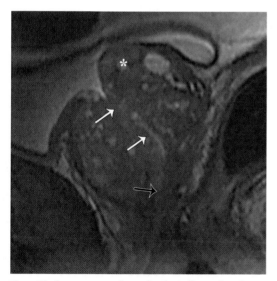

Fig. 10. Reconstructed sagittal 3-dimensional T2-weighted image demonstrates a markedly enlarge transitional zone secondary to benign prostatic hyperplasia with intravascular prostate protrusion (*asterisk*), which has been described as pedunculated enlargement and is also referred to as median lobe in the surgical literature. The proximal (*white arrows*) and distal urethra (*black arrow*) can be somewhat delineated on the image.

Prostate Anatomy and Atrophy

There are variety of causes that lead to atrophy in the prostate, including inflammation, radiation, antiandrogens, chronic ischemia, and age-related androgen withdrawal.[10,22] Atrophy is characterized by crowded glands with scant cytoplasm and crowding of the nuclei. McNeal[10] specifically noted that atrophy of the CZ has the most dramatic alteration of the architecture. Although diffuse atrophy is often attributed to age-related factors,[10] according to McNeal focal atrophy suggests previous inflammation.[10] On MR imaging, atrophy is nonspecific in appearance and usually appears as loss of normal T2 signal of the PZ with an associated loss of volume. There can be a moderate degree of associated restricted diffusion and, therefore, focal atrophy can mimic prostate cancer on MR imaging.[22]

SUMMARY

The zonal anatomy of the prostate is of much relevance in assessing prostate pathology. Radiologists should be aware of zonal prostate anatomy because each zone has distinct, multiparametric characteristics on MR imaging. The notion that the TZ and CZ are indistinguishable on MR imaging has largely been replaced by the recognition that the CZ can be identified in the majority of cases. Despite the complexity of the periprostatic fascia and nerves, MR imaging can provide a simplified view of the periprostatic anatomy that allows for preoperative staging.

REFERENCES

1. Lee CH, Akin-Olugbade O, Kirschenbaum A. Overview of prostate anatomy, histology, and pathology. Endocrinol Metab Clin North Am 2011;40(3):565–75.
2. Coakley FV, Hricak H. Radiologic anatomy of the prostate gland: a clinical approach. Radiol Clin North Am 2000;38(1):15–30.
3. Ren J, Liu H, Wang H, et al. MRI to predict prostate growth and development in children, adolescents and young adults. Eur Radiol 2014;25(2):516–22.
4. Turkbey B, Huang R, Vourganti S, et al. Age-related changes in prostate zonal volumes as measured by high-resolution magnetic resonance imaging (MRI): a cross-sectional study in over 500 patients. BJU Int 2012;110(11):1642–7.
5. Cunha GR, Ricke WA. A historical perspective on the role of stroma in the pathogenesis of benign prostatic hyperplasia. Differentiation 2011;82(4–5):168–72.
6. Selman SH. The McNeal prostate: a review. Urology 2011;78(6):1224–8.

7. McNeal JE. The zonal anatomy of the prostate. Prostate 1981;2(1):35–49.

8. Villers A, Terris MK, McNeal JE, et al. Ultrasound anatomy of the prostate: the normal gland and anatomical variations. J Urol 1990;143(4):732–8.

9. Mirowitz SA, Hammerman AM. CT depiction of prostatic zonal anatomy. J Comput Assist Tomogr 1992; 16(3):439–41.

10. McNeal JE. Normal histology of the prostate. Am J Surg Pathol 1988;12:619–33.

11. Hricak H, Dooms GC, McNeal JE, et al. MR imaging of the prostate gland: normal anatomy. Am J Roentgenol 1987;148(1):51–8.

12. Fine SW, Reuter VE. Anatomy of the prostate revisited: Implications for prostate biopsy and zonal origins of prostate cancer. Histopathology 2012;60(1): 142–52.

13. Guneyli S, Ward E, Peng Y, et al. MRI evaluation of benign prostatic hyperplasia: correlation with international prostate symptom score. J Magn Reson Imaging 2017;45(3):917–25.

14. Medved M, Sammet S, Yousuf A, et al. MR imaging of the prostate and adjacent anatomic structures before, during, and after ejaculation: qualitative and quantitative evaluation. Radiology 2014;271(2): 452–60.

15. Walz J, Burnett AL, Costello AJ, et al. A critical analysis of the current knowledge of surgical anatomy related to optimization of cancer control and preservation of continence and erection in candidates for radical prostatectomy. Eur Urol 2010;57(2):179–92.

16. Stolzenburg JU, Schwalenberg T, Horn LC, et al. Anatomical landmarks of radical prostatectomy. Eur Urol 2007;51(3):629–39.

17. Coakley FV, Eberhardt S, Kattan MW, et al. Urinary continence after radical retropubic prostatectomy: relationship with membranous urethral length on preoperative endorectal magnetic resonance imaging. J Urol 2002;168(3):1032–5.

18. Vargas HA, Akin O, Franiel T, et al. Normal central zone of the prostate and central zone involvement by prostate cancer: clinical and MR imaging implications. Radiology 2012;262(3):894–902.

19. Nunes LW, Schiebler MS, Rauschning W, et al. The normal prostate and periprostatic structures: correlation between MR images made with an endorectal coil and cadaveric microtome sections. Am J Roentgenol 1995;164(4):923–7.

20. Weinreb JC, Barentsz JO, Choyke PL, et al. PI-RADS prostate imaging - reporting and data system: 2015, version 2. Eur Urol 2016;69(1):16–40.

21. Aaron LT, Franco OE, Hayward SW. Review of prostate anatomy and embryology and the etiology of benign prostatic hyperplasia. Urol Clin North Am 2016;43(3):279–88.

22. Kitzing YX, Prando A, Varol C, et al. Benign conditions that mimic prostate carcinoma: MR imaging features with histopathologic correlation. Radiographics 2016;36(1):162–75.

23. Srodon M, Epstein JI. Central zone histology of the prostate: a mimicker of high-grade prostatic intraepithelial neoplasia. Hum Pathol 2002;33(5):518–23.

24. Sommer FG, McNeal JE, Carrol CL. MR depiction of zonal anatomy of the prostate at 1.5 T. J Comput Assist Tomogr 1986;10(6):983–9.

25. Hansford BG, Karademir I, Peng Y, et al. Dynamic contrast-enhanced MR imaging features of the normal central zone of the prostate. Acad Radiol 2014;21(5):569–77.

26. Quick CM, Gokden N, Sangoi AR, et al. The distribution of PAX-2 immunoreactivity in the prostate gland, seminal vesicle, and ejaculatory duct: comparison with prostatic adenocarcinoma and discussion of prostatic zonal embryogenesis. Hum Pathol 2010; 41(8):1145–9.

27. Allen KS, Kressel HY, Arger PH, et al. Age-related changes of the prostate: evaluation by MR imaging. Am J Roentgenol 1989;152(1):77–81.

28. Gupta RT, Kauffman CR, Garcia-Reyes K, et al. Apparent diffusion coefficient values of the benign central zone of the prostate: comparison with low- and high-grade prostate cancer. Am J Roentgenol 2015;205(2):331–6.

29. Yu J, Fulcher AS, Turner MA, et al. Prostate cancer and its mimics at multiparametric prostate MRI. Br J Radiol 2014;87(1037). 20130659.

30. Villers A, Steg A, Boccon-Gibod L. Anatomy of the prostate: review of the different models. Eur Urol 1991;20(4):261–8.

31. Hansford BG, Peng Y, Jiang Y, et al. Revisiting the central gland anatomy via MRI: does the central gland extend below the level of verumontanum? J Magn Reson Imaging 2014;39(1):167–71.

32. Ward E, Baad M, Peng Y, et al. Multi-parametric MR imaging of the anterior fibromuscular stroma and its differentiation from prostate cancer. Abdom Radiol (NY) 2017;42(3):926–34.

33. Ayala AG, Ro JY, Babaian R, et al. The prostatic capsule: does it exist? Its importance in the staging and treatment of prostatic carcinoma. Am J Surg Pathol 1989;13(1):21–7.

34. McNeal JE, Redwine EA, Freiha FS, et al. Zonal distribution of prostatic adenocarcinoma. Am J Surg Pathol 1988;12:897–906.

35. Dooms GC, Hricak H. Magnetic resonance imaging of the pelvis: prostate and urinary bladder. Urol Radiol 1986;8(1):156–65.

36. Tewari A, Peabody JO, Fischer M, et al. An operative and anatomic study to help in nerve sparing during laparoscopic and robotic radical prostatectomy. Eur Urol 2003;43(5):444–54.

37. Kiyoshima K, Yokomizo A, Yoshida T, et al. Anatomical features of periprostatic tissue and its surroundings: a histological analysis of 79 radical retropubic

prostatectomy specimens. Jpn J Clin Oncol 2004;
34(8):463–8.

38. Lee SB, Hong SK, Choe G, et al. Periprostatic distribution of nerves in specimens from non–nerve-
sparing radical retropubic prostatectomy. Urology
2008;72(4):878–81.

39. Savera AT, Kaul S, Badani K, et al. Robotic radical
prostatectomy with the "veil of Aphrodite" technique:
histologic evidence of enhanced nerve sparing. Eur
Urol 2006;49(6):1065–74.

40. Kothari PS, Scardino PT, Ohori M, et al. Incidence,
location, and significance of periprostatic and peri-
seminal vesicle lymph nodes in prostate cancer.
Am J Surg Pathol 2001;25(11):1429–32.

41. Yuh B, Wu H, Ruel N, et al. Analysis of regional
lymph nodes in periprostatic fat following robot-
assisted radical prostatectomy. BJU Int 2012;
109(4):603–7.

42. Carnevale FC, Soares GR, de Assis AM, et al.
Anatomical variants in prostate artery embolization:
a pictorial essay. Cardiovasc Intervent Radiol 2017;
40(9):1321–37.

43. Lee JY, Spratt DE, Liss AL, et al. Vessel-sparing radiation and functional anatomy-based preservation
for erectile function after prostate radiotherapy. Lancet Oncol 2017;17(5):e198–208.

44. Thai CT, Karam IM, Nguyen-Thi PL, et al. Pelvic
magnetic resonance imaging angioanatomy of the
arterial blood supply to the penis in suspected
prostate cancer patients. Eur J Radiol 2015;84(5):
823–7.

45. Cohen RJ, Shannon BA, Phillips M, et al. Central
zone carcinoma of the prostate gland: a distinct tumor type with poor prognostic features. J Urol
2008;179(5):1762–7.

46. Lawrentschuk N, Haider MA, Daljeet N, et al. "Prostatic evasive anterior tumours": the role of magnetic
resonance imaging. BJU Int 2010;105(9):1231–6.

47. Bott SR, Young MP, Kellett MJ, et al. Anterior prostate cancer: is it more difficult to diagnose? BJU
Int 2002;89(9):886–9.

48. Heidenreich A, Bellmunt J, Bolla M, et al. EAU
guidelines on prostate cancer. part 1: screening,
diagnosis, and treatment of clinically localised disease. Eur Urol 2011;59(1):61–71.

49. Eberhardt SC, Carter S, Casalino DD, et al. ACR
appropriateness criteria prostate cancer—pretreatment detection, staging, and surveillance. J Am
Coll Radiol 2013;10(2):83–92.

50. Yacoub JH, Verma S, Moulton JS, et al. Imaging-
guided prostate biopsy: conventional and emerging
techniques. Radiographics 2012;32(3):819–37.

51. Mai KT, Belanger EC, Al-Maghrabi HM, et al. Primary
prostatic central zone adenocarcinoma. Pathol Res
Pract 2008;204(4):251–8.

52. Wasserman NF, Spilseth B, Golzarian J, et al. Use of
MRI for lobar classification of benign prostatic hyperplasia: potential phenotypic biomarkers for
research on treatment strategies. Am J Roentgenol
2015;205(3):564–71.

53. Guneyli S, Ward E, Thomas S, et al. Magnetic resonance imaging of benign prostatic hyperplasia. Diagn Interv Radiol 2016;22(3):215–9.

54. Jenkins LC, Nogueira M, Wilding GE, et al. Median
lobe in robot-assisted radical prostatectomy: evaluation and management. Urology 2008;71(5):810–3.

55. Huang AC, Kowalczyk KJ, Hevelone ND, et al. The
impact of prostate size, median lobe, and prior
benign prostatic hyperplasia intervention on robot-
assisted laparoscopic prostatectomy: technique
and outcomes. Eur Urol 2011;59(4):595–603.

56. Jeong CW, Lee S, Oh JJ, et al. Quantification of median lobe protrusion and its impact on the base
surgical margin status during robot-assisted laparoscopic prostatectomy. World J Urol 2014;32(2):
419–23.

Technique of Multiparametric MR Imaging of the Prostate

Andrei S. Purysko, MD[a],*, Andrew B. Rosenkrantz, MD[b]

KEYWORDS

- MR imaging • Prostate cancer • Diffusion-weighted imaging

KEY POINTS

- The prostate imaging reporting and data system version 2 defines minimum acceptable technical parameters for multiparametric MR imaging of the prostate.
- All prostate MR imaging studies should include T2-weighted, T1-weighted, diffusion-weighted, and dynamic contrast-enhanced images.
- Diffusion-weighted images with high b-values ($\geq$1400 s/mm^2) can be calculated from the images with lower b-values (50–1000 s/mm^2) or acquired separately.
- Prostate MR imaging can be adequately performed on 1.5-T or 3-T systems with a pelvic phased array coil and optionally combined with an endorectal coil.
- Eliminating gas and stool from the rectum before the examination is important to minimize artifacts that negatively affect image quality.

 Video content accompanies this article at http://www.radiologic.theclinics.com

INTRODUCTION

Since the use of MR imaging of the prostate was first reported in the early 1980s, this imaging modality has become an established noninvasive tool for the assessment of prostate cancer (PCa).[1,2] Advances in hardware and software have since led to faster acquisition of images, improvements in image quality, and the development of pulse sequences that have the ability to probe tissue properties, such as cellularity and perfusion, thus improving the ability of MR imaging to distinguish between benign and malignant tissues. These improvements, coupled with the evolution of MR imaging–targeted biopsy, have facilitated the use of MR imaging in the detection of PCa,

assessment of tumor aggressiveness, disease staging, treatment planning, follow-up of patients on active surveillance, and follow-up after treatment in patients with biochemical recurrence.[2]

Despite these advances, significant variations in imaging acquisition, interpretation, and reporting across institutions have resulted in heterogeneous performance of prostate MR imaging and have limited the widespread adoption and acceptance of this method.[3] As a first step toward the standardization of prostate MR imaging, in 2012, the European Society of Urogenital Radiology developed consensus-based guidelines aiming to establish minimum acceptable technical parameters for prostate MR imaging, along with a structured category assessment system known as the

Disclosures: A.S. Purysko has no conflicts of interest to disclose. A.B. Rosenkrantz receives royalties from Thieme Medical Publishers.
[a] Section of Abdominal Imaging, Imaging Institute, Cleveland Clinic, 9500 Euclid Avenue, Mail Code JB-3, Cleveland, OH 44195, USA; [b] Department of Radiology, New York University Langone Medical Center, 660 First Avenue, New York, NY 10016, USA
* Corresponding author:
E-mail address: puryska@ccf.org

Radiol Clin N Am 56 (2018) 211–222
https://doi.org/10.1016/j.rcl.2017.10.004

Prostate Imaging and Reporting and Data System (PI-RADS) version 1 (PI-RADS v1).[4] In collaboration with the American College of Radiology through the PI-RADS Steering Committee, the second iteration of the guidelines (PI-RADS v2) was released in December of 2014, bringing important changes to the system.[5]

This review discusses the techniques that are used in state-of-the-art MR imaging of the prostate, including imaging protocols, hardware considerations, and important aspects of patient preparation, with an emphasis on the recommendations provided in the PI-RADS v2 guidelines.

SEQUENCES

PI-RADS v2 recommends the inclusion of T2-weighted imaging (T2-WI), T1-weighted imaging (T1-WI), diffusion-weighted imaging (DWI), and dynamic contrast-enhanced (DCE) pulse sequences for all prostate MR imaging studies. A set of minimal technical parameters for each of these pulse sequences is provided in the guidelines (Box 1). Because sequence acquisition is influenced by equipment availability and capability, centers are encouraged to optimize imaging protocols in order to obtain the best and most consistent image quality.

One change introduced in PI-RADS v2 was the exclusion of findings from magnetic resonance spectroscopic imaging (MRSI) in lesion assessment. This technique requires special expertise and is time consuming; thus, it is considered impractical for widespread use.

T2-Weighted Imaging

T2-WI offers excellent soft tissue contrast and detailed depiction of the zonal anatomy of the prostate, the seminal vesicles, and the neurovascular bundles (NVBs). High-quality T2-WI is considered critical for local staging of PCa, because this method helps to identify the presence of extraprostatic extension (EPE) of tumors and involvement of the seminal vesicles and NVBs.[6,7] According to PI-RADS v2, T2-WI should also be the dominant parameter used to assess lesions in the transition zone (TZ).

Two-dimensional (2D) fast-spin-echo (FSE) or turbo-spin-echo (TSE) T2-WI pulse sequences provide images with high signal-to-noise ratio (SNR) and high spatial resolution. These images are acquired in the true sagittal and oblique axial and oblique coronal planes (Fig. 1). Sagittal T2-WI can be obtained first to help define the range of coverage and orientation of the axial and coronal T2-WI. Axial T2-WI should be obtained in a perpendicular fashion through the

---

Box 1

Summary of technical specifications described in Prostate Imaging Reporting and Data System version 2

T2-weighted images
- Pulse sequence: 2D fast spin-echo or turbo spin-echo (3D can be used as an adjunct to 2D)
- Imaging planes: Sagittal and oblique axial and coronal planes
- Field of view (FOV): 12 to 20 cm (to cover entire prostate gland and seminal vesicles)
- Slice thickness: $\leq$3 mm, no gap
- In-plane dimension: $\leq$0.7 mm (phase) $\times$ $\leq$0.4 mm (frequency)

Diffusion-weighted images (DWI)
- Pulse sequence: Spin-echo echo-planar imaging (EPI) DWI (free-breathing with fat saturation)
- Imaging planes: Same as axial T2-weighted images
- FOV: 16 to 22 cm
- Slice thickness: $\leq$4 mm, no gap
- TE $\leq$90 ms; TR $\leq$3000 ms
- In plane dimension: $\leq$2.5-mm phase and frequency
- b-values: Minimum of 2 for ADC map creation (lower b-value 50–100 s/mm^2, higher value 800–1000 s/mm^2); additional high b-values image ($\geq$1400 s/mm^2) should be acquired separately or calculated from images obtained with b-values <1000 s/mm^2

Dynamic contrast-enhanced images
- Pulse sequence: 2D or 3D T1-weighted gradient echo (3D preferred)
- Fat-suppression technique or subtraction should be considered
- Imaging plane: Same as axial T2-WI
- Contrast injection rate: 2 to 3 mL/s
- FOV: Encompass the entire prostate gland and seminal vesicles
- Slice thickness: $\leq$3 mm, no gap
- TE <5 ms; TR <100 ms
- In plane dimension: $\leq$2.0-mm phase and frequency
- Temporal resolution $\leq$10 s ($\leq$7 s is preferred)
- Acquisition time $\geq$2 min

Abbreviations: TE, echo time; TR, repetition time.

---

long axis of the prostate. Axial T1-WI, DWI, and DCE images should be obtained in the same plane as axial T2-WI to facilitate the precise correlation of findings observed with these pulse sequences.

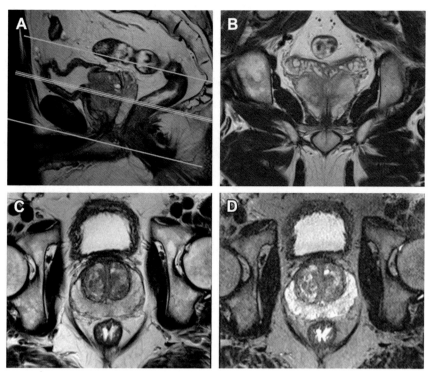

Fig. 1. Multiplanar 2D TSE T2-WI of the prostate obtained in the sagittal (*A*), coronal (*B*), and axial (*C*) planes. The sagittal T2-WI of the prostate can be used to define the scan range (in between the parallel *orange lines*, *A*) and the orientation of the axial T2-WI, diffusion-weighted, and DCE T1-WI images (*green lines* perpendicular through the long axis of the prostate, *A*). (*D*) Axial high-resolution 3D T2-WI can optionally be obtained in the same plane.

In PI-RADS v2, high-resolution 3-dimensional (3D) FSE T2-WI is described as an adjunct to 2D acquisitions. Currently available 3D T2-WI pulse sequences use various acceleration techniques that allow for the acquisition of images with isotropic voxels and have 2 main potential advantages.[7] First, by reducing volume-averaging artifacts, these images can be used to help assess certain characteristics of lesions (eg, the presence of a capsule around a nodule in the TZ, which favors a diagnosis of benign prostatic hyperplasia nodule) and to assess the integrity of the prostate capsule (**Fig. 2**). Second, the volumetric data set acquired with isotropic voxels can be used to reconstruct images in all 3 planes, which in turn may shorten the examination time by reducing the number of T2-WI sequences that need to be obtained. However, these images may have lower soft tissue contrast and in-plane resolution compared with 2D images. Furthermore, motion artifacts during the long 3D acquisition could result in distortion of the entire data set.

T1-Weighted Imaging

T1-WI is useful in detecting postbiopsy changes that can affect the interpretation of other pulse sequences (**Fig. 3**). In general, using spin-echo or gradient-echo sequences with or without fat suppression, T1-WI obtained immediately before intravenous contrast administration can be used to identify such changes. In addition, after DCE images are acquired, T1-WI with a large field of view can be obtained below the level of the aortic bifurcation for evaluation of the lymph nodes and osseous lesions (**Fig. 4**).

Diffusion-Weighted Imaging/Apparent Diffusion Coefficient Maps

DWI assesses the degree of tissue cellularity by measuring the mobility or diffusion of water molecules within tissues. In prostate tissue that has an increased fraction of epithelium in comparison with other tissue compartments, such as in high-grade PCa, water diffusion is impeded or restricted. The first reports of the successful application of DWI echo-planar imaging pulse sequences for evaluation of the prostate occurred in the early 2000s.[8] Since then, numerous studies have demonstrated the value of DWI in detecting and characterizing PCa.[9–11]

DWI plays a key role in the PI-RADS v2 guidelines and is currently considered the dominant

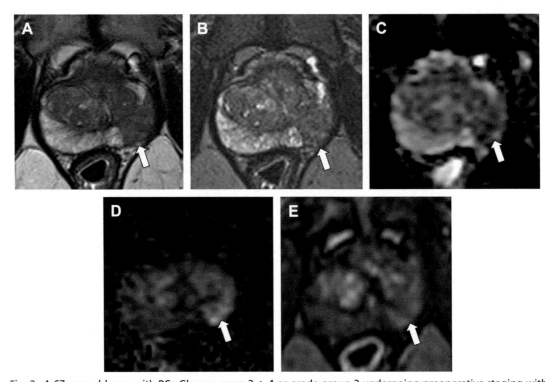

Fig. 2. A 67-year-old man with PCa Gleason score 3 + 4 or grade group 2 undergoing preoperative staging with MR imaging. (*A*) Axial 2D TSE T2-WI shows a 1.6-cm lesion in the right posterolateral PZ with low signal intensity and broad (>1-cm) capsular contact (*arrow, A*), which raises concern for EPE (T2-WI PI-RADS score: 5). (*B*) On axial 3D TSE T2-WI, in addition to broad capsular contact, there is irregularity and discontinuity of the capsule (*arrow, B*). (*C, D*) The lesion demonstrates markedly hypointense signal on the axial ADC map (*arrow, C*) and markedly hyperintense signal on the axial calculated high b-value (1500 s/mm^2) DWI (*arrow, D*) (ADC/DWI PI-RADS score: 5). (*E*) The lesion demonstrates early arterial enhancement on axial DCE T1-WI (*arrow, E*) (DCE: positive). Because the findings are compatible with extraprostatic extension, the lesion's PI-RADS assessment category is 5. The patient underwent radical prostatectomy, which confirmed the presence of extraprostatic extension.

parameter for the evaluation of lesions in the peripheral zone (PZ). DWI also plays an important but secondary role in the assessment of lesions in the TZ, because there is significant overlap between cancer and benign prostatic hyperplasia nodules rich in stromal elements.[12]

An important technical parameter for DWI is the selection of b-values. These values are impacted by the magnitude and duration of the gradient applied in the tissue during image acquisition. A monoexponential model of signal decay with increasing b-values is applied to calculate the apparent diffusion coefficient (ADC) values (measured in squared millimeters per second), and the values of each voxel are then displayed in an image that is known as the ADC map. ADC maps are interpreted in conjunction with DWI to qualitatively determine the presence of diffusion restriction. ADC maps can also be used to obtain a quantitative assessment of lesions by measuring their ADC values. Although an inverse correlation between ADC values and PCa grade has been

demonstrated in several studies,[11,13] the clinical adoption of a quantitative assessment is limited by many factors, including a significant overlap between benign and pathologic conditions and the variability in ADC values depending on the selection of different sets of b-values, the magnetic field strength, and MR imaging scanner vendor.

PI-RADS v2 provides specific recommendations regarding the selection of b-values. For the creation of ADC maps, DWI should be acquired with at least 2 b-values, with the lowest b-values set at 50 to 100 s/mm^2 and the highest set at 800 to 1000 s/mm^2. In addition, DWI images with high b-values ($\geq$1400 s/mm^2) are also required. The high b-value images tend to improve tumor conspicuity, distinguishing between PCa and normal tissue or benign conditions (**Fig. 5**).[14] This high b-value DWI can be obtained in 1 of 2 ways.[15] On some MR imaging systems or third-party software, high b-value DWI can be extrapolated or calculated from the DWI data set obtained with lower b-values to

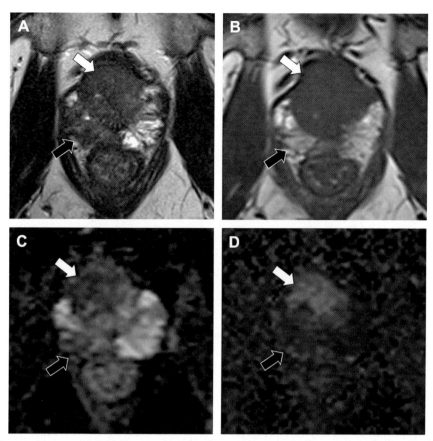

Fig. 3. A 59-year-old man with PCa Gleason score 3 + 4 or grade group 2 diagnosed on TRUS-guided biopsy performed 7 weeks before the staging MR imaging. (A) Axial T2-WI shows a focal lesion with low signal intensity in the right posterolateral, posteromedial, and anterior PZ at the midgland associated with capsule irregularity mimicking an aggressive PCa lesion with extraprostatic extension (*black arrow, A*). In addition, there is a 1.6-cm focal lesion in the right anterior TZ with homogenous low signal intensity and ill-defined margins (*white arrow, A*) (T2-WI PI-RADS score 5). (B) Axial T1-WI shows diffuse increased signal intensity in the PZ, including in the area with signal abnormality on T2-WI (*black arrow, B*) consistent with postbiopsy hemorrhage. The anterior TZ lesion demonstrates low signal intensity and is spared from the postbiopsy changes (*white arrow, B*). (C–D) On the axial ADC map, there is markedly low signal intensity in the right PZ (*black arrow, C*), but without corresponding high signal intensity in the axial calculated high b-value (1500 s/mm^2) DWI (*black arrow, D*); conversely, the right anterior TZ lesion demonstrates markedly low signal intensity on the ADC map (*white arrow, C*) and markedly high signal intensity on DWI (*white arrow, D*) (ADC/DWI PI-RADS score: 5). Because there is high signal intensity on T1-WI, the right PZ lesion is highly unlike to represent clinically significant PCa (PI-RADS assessment category 1). Because the T2-WI score is the dominant score for TZ lesions, the PI-RADS assessment category of the right anterior TZ lesion is 5. The patient underwent radical prostatectomy, which confirmed the absence of cancer in the PZ and revealed a Gleason score 4 + 3 or grade group 3 in the TZ.

generate the ADC map. If this is not possible, the high b-value DWI is advised to be obtained in a separate acquisition from the standard b-values used in ADC map calculation, because the high b-value DWI can affect the appearance of the ADC map. Generating the high b-value DWI from the lower b-value data set is advantageous in that it does not require additional scanning time and is less prone to artifacts; acquiring the high b-value DWI separately may require longer echo times to accommodate the strong gradient pulses needed.

Diffusion kurtosis imaging (DKI) and restriction spectrum imaging (RSI) are extensions of DWI with additional requirements regarding the DWI acquisition and specialized postprocessing. DKI works on the assumption that water diffusion is non-Gaussian in behavior, a property that may help assess tissue with microstructural complexity.[16] RSI is a multiple b-value, multidirectional diffusion technique. By obtaining an extended spectrum of diffusion images, this technique is able to focus on signal arising from intracellular water and potentially more effectively

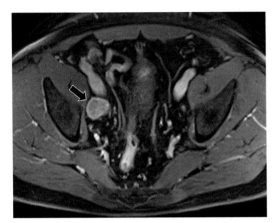

Fig. 4. A 68-year-old man with PCa Gleason score 4 + 5 or grade group 5 detected by TRUS-guided biopsy undergoing preoperative staging with MR imaging. Large field-of-view T1-WI obtained after intravenous administration of gadolinium chelate contrast media demonstrates an enlarged right external iliac lymph node (*black arrow*). Metastatic involvement by PCa was confirmed on pelvic lymph node dissection performed along with radical prostatectomy.

evaluate tissue cellularity; highly cellular tumors are thus highlighted by this method.[17] The application of DKI and RSI techniques in prostate imaging has gained attention in recent years because initial studies have shown potential for better distinction of PCa from normal tissue and better discrimination between low-grade and high-grade PCa with these methods.[16,17] RSI and DKI are not included in the PI-RADS v2 recommendations, but these, or other advanced diffusion methods, could be incorporated into future versions if validated in larger and more robust studies.

Dynamic Contrast-Enhanced Imaging

DCE imaging enables noninvasive imaging characterization of tissue vascularity. Angiogenesis in PCa is associated with an increased number or density of poorly organized and poorly formed vessels with increased capillary permeability, which leads to faster and greater enhancement of cancerous lesions relative to the normal surrounding tissues.[18]

DCE consists of a series of T1-WI scans acquired before, during, and after the rapid intravenous administration of a bolus of a low-molecular-weight gadolinium-based contrast agent (Video 1). 3D T1-WI spoiled gradient-recalled echo sequences are used to repeatedly image the prostate over several minutes to assess the enhancement characteristics; a 3D sequence is preferred for this purpose. These images are

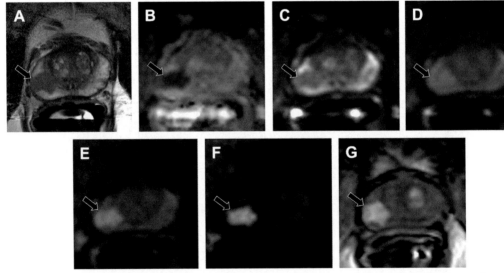

Fig. 5. A 62-year-old man with PCa Gleason score 4 + 3 or grade group 3 undergoing preoperative staging with MR imaging. (*A*) Axial T2-WI shows a well-circumscribed, low-signal-intensity nodule in the right posterolateral and anterior PZ at the midgland and base (*black arrow, A*) (T2-WI PI-RADS score: 5). (*B*) The lesion measures 1.6 cm and shows markedly low signal intensity on the ADC map (*arrow, B*). (*C–F*) Axial DWIs obtained with b-values of 50 (*C*), 400 (*D*), 900 (*E*), and 2000 (*F*) s/mm² demonstrate progressive decrease of the signal intensity of the prostate and surrounding tissues, and progressive increase of the signal intensity of the lesion in the right PZ (*arrows, C–F*) that is most conspicuous and markedly hyperintense on the 2000 s/mm² b-value image (ADC/DWI PI-RADS score: 5). (*G*) Axial DCE T1-WI shows early enhancement by the lesion (*black arrow, G*) that matches the area of signal abnormalities identified on T2-WI and ADC/DWI (DCE: positive). Because ADC/DWI is the dominant parameter for PZ abnormalities, this focal lesion was assigned a PI-RADS assessment category 5. The patient underwent radical prostatectomy that revealed a PCa Gleason score 4 + 4 or grade group 4.

obtained with a high temporal resolution (faster than at least 10 seconds and preferably than at least 7 seconds, per PI-RADS v2) so as to demonstrate early enhancing lesions. In addition, PI-RADS only requires a DCE acquisition duration of at least 2 minutes. Fat suppression techniques or the creation of imaging data sets from the subtraction of precontrast from postcontrast images is recommended to facilitate the visual assessment of these enhancement characteristics.

Because of the significant variability in enhancement patterns of cancerous lesions and the overlap with enhancement patterns of benign conditions (namely prostatitis and benign prostatic hyperplasia), DCE has a relatively limited role in the characterization of PCa lesions when compared with T2-WI and DWI.[19,20] Because of these limitations, and to simplify the interpretation of DCE images, the assessment of DCE in PI-RADS v2 is based exclusively on qualitative visual assessment of the individual time points of DCE images. A lesion is considered to be DCE "positive" if it demonstrates early arterial enhancement and has a corresponding signal abnormality on DWI or T2-WI (Fig. 6). The presence of delayed "washout" is no longer included as a diagnostic imaging feature. PI-RADS v2 does not require the use of a semi-quantitative method for the evaluation of enhancement kinetic curves that plot the signal intensity of a lesion as a function of time (as described in PI-RADS v1), nor more sophisticated quantitative methods, because of insufficient evidence to support their use. Furthermore, these methods require specific software for postprocessing of the images that typically is not available in standard picture archiving and communication systems.

HARDWARE
Magnetic Field Strength

At present, it is generally accepted that multiparametric MR imaging (mpMR imaging) can be

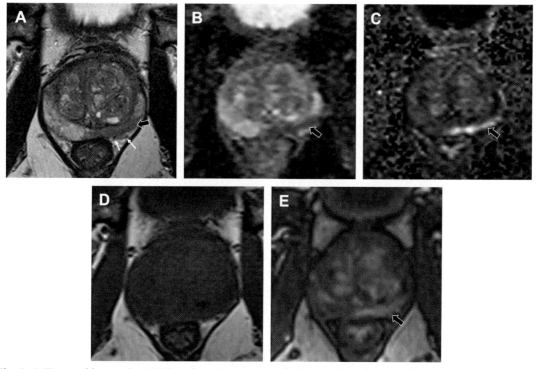

Fig. 6. A 63-year-old man who initially deferred treatment or follow-up biopsy for a PCa Gleason score 3 + 3 or grade group 1 diagnosed 4 years ago and currently presents with increasing prostate-specific antigen (PSA) level (11.4 ng/mL). (*A*) Axial T2-WI shows a lesion with low signal intensity in the left posteromedial and posterolateral PZ (*black arrow, A*) with extraprostatic extension and asymmetric thickening of the ipsilateral NVB fibers (*white arrows, A*) concerning for NVB invasion (T2-WI PI-RADS score 5). (*B–C*) The lesion measures 1.5 cm and demonstrates markedly low signal intensity on axial ADC map (*arrow, B*) and markedly high signal intensity on the axial calculated high b-value (1500 s/mm^2) DWI (*arrow, C*) (ADC/DWI PI-RADS score: 5). (*D–E*) Axial DCE T1-WIs obtained before (*D*) and at the peak arterial enhancement (*E*) show a focal enhancing lesion (*arrow, E*) in the area corresponding to the lesion seen on T2-WI and ADC/DWI (DCE: positive). Because ADC/DWI is the dominant parameter in the PZ, the PI-RADS assessment category is 5. MR/TRUS fusion-guided biopsy of the lesion was performed revealing PCa Gleason score 4 + 3 or grade group 3.

adequately performed on 1.5-T or 3-T systems.[5,21] Scanner platforms with field strengths lower than 1.5 T are generally not optimized to obtain pulse sequences with the parameters recommended in the PI-RADS v2 guidelines. Furthermore, the current literature validating the clinical utility of MR imaging in PCa detection and staging is based on images obtained on 1.5-T or 3-T scanners.[9,22]

An increase in magnetic field strength brings certain limitations, such as increased chemical shift and susceptibility artifacts, increased dielectric resonance effects, and increased radiofrequency energy deposition in tissues. Despite these limitations, 3-T MR imaging has clear advantages compared with 1.5-T MR imaging, including a nearly 2-fold increase in SNR, improved spatial resolution, and shortened acquisition times.[23] Thus, although MR imaging examinations can be adequately performed on 1.5-T systems, 3-T systems should be used when available.

Receiver Frequency Coils

MR imaging examinations are performed with a pelvic phased-array coil (PPAC), preferably with a relatively high number of external phased array coil elements and radiofrequency channels (ie, $\geq$16), with or without an endorectal coil (ERC). The ERC model most commonly used is equipped with a balloon that, when filled, fixes the coil to the rectum. Perfluorocarbon fluid or barium sulfate mixtures are frequently used to fill the balloon; this helps to reduce the susceptibility artifacts and spatial distortions that can affect DWI and MRSI.

The development of an ERC several years after prostate MR imaging was initially introduced represented a major advance that was needed to compensate for the low field strengths available at that time, because the addition of an ERC to MR imaging greatly improves SNR.[24] An ERC was also considered essential to the performance of prostate MRSI.[25] However, using an ERC during MR imaging has significant disadvantages. The addition of an ERC increases the cost and examination time and causes significant patient discomfort. The use of an ERC also leads to deformity of the prostate contour and shape, and this anatomic distortion can potentially hamper the pathology correlation and fusion with other imaging methods that are used for treatment planning.[26,27]

Because of these disadvantages, and because MRSI is no longer recommended in PI-RADS v2, there is an ongoing debate regarding whether the use of an ERC can be avoided, at least for studies performed on 3-T scanners. In fact, investigators have demonstrated that using 3-T scanners without an ERC may achieve image quality, PCa detection rates, and staging accuracy at least comparable to what is achieved with 1.5-T scanners with an ERC.[22,28] Studies comparing images obtained on 3-T scanners with and without an ERC have demonstrated some advantage for PCa detection with the use of an ERC.[29–31] For example, Costa and colleagues[30] showed that using both an ERC and a PPAC provides superior sensitivity for the detection of PCa when compared with not using an ERC, although in this study, overall accuracy was not significantly different when the images obtained with an ERC were compared with those obtained without an ERC but obtained with an increased number of signal averages. This finding suggests that optimization of the images may help to decrease the performance gap between examinations performed with and without an ERC. For MR imaging studies used to stage PCa, a meta-analysis demonstrated that the addition of an ERC appeared to improve the detection of EPE in scans performed at 1.5 T and in scans that used T2-WI as the only parameter. However, when 3-T field strength or additional functional techniques (eg, DWI and DCE images) were used, scans with an ERC showed lower sensitivity than scans without an ERC.[22]

Based on these results, the use of an ERC is not currently considered by PI-RADS v2 an absolute requirement on 1.5-T or 3-T scanners.[5]

PATIENT PREPARATION

There is no general consensus regarding patient preparation for prostate MR imaging. Several measures are commonly used to address factors that may negatively affect image quality, although scientific evidence to support some of these measures is scarce.

Interval Between Transrectal Ultrasound–Guided Biopsy and mpMR Imaging

MR imaging is commonly performed in men who have previously undergone transrectal ultrasound-guided (TRUS) biopsy. Of note, current statements from major national organizations support the use of MR imaging in men with prior negative TRUS biopsy and in men with biopsy-proven PCa who are undergoing preoperative staging.[32–34] TRUS biopsy causes hemorrhage and inflammation of the prostate gland. The resultant changes on imaging are most evident in the PZ and may persist for many weeks or months. These postbiopsy changes can obscure tumor or misleadingly suggest the presence of EPE of the tumor.[35] Although the optimal time interval between TRUS biopsy and MR imaging to minimize the effect of these changes on imaging interpretation has not been defined, an interval of at least 6 weeks is commonly recommended, especially when MR imaging is performed for disease staging. However, this interval may be modified based on individual circumstances, because studies have shown that mpMR imaging, when properly interpreted, has adequate accuracy for disease detection and staging even in the presence of postbiopsy changes.[35,36] Careful evaluation of DWI and of ADC, in correlation with T1-WI in which postbiopsy changes manifest as areas with intermediate to high signal intensity, may help to prevent confusion.[37]

Bowel Preparation

Patients should be encouraged to evacuate the bowel before the examination to try to eliminate as much stool and gas from the rectum as possible.

Stool interferes with the placement of the ERC, and gas can cause distortion of DWI, particularly in examinations performed without an ERC.[38] At some institutions, men are instructed to self-administer a cleansing enema before the examination, although this measure has not been shown to significantly improve image quality or reduce artifacts in prostate MR imaging.[39] If an enema is used, it should not be administered immediately before the examination, because doing so may stimulate bowel peristalsis. Alternative methods can be used if gas-related artifacts are encountered during an examination performed without an ERC. These methods include performing the examination with the patient in the prone position, decompressing the rectum using suction through a small catheter, and introducing ultrasound gel into the rectum (**Fig. 7**).[5,38,39]

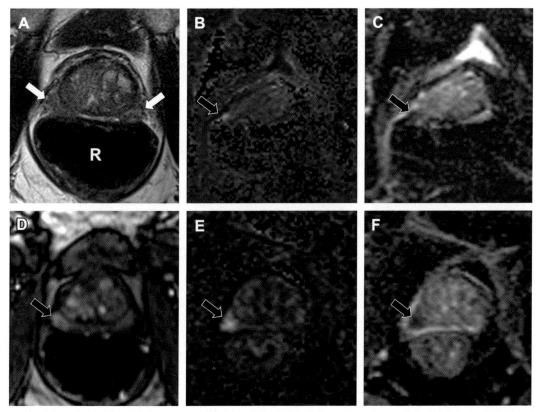

Fig. 7. A 72-year-old man with elevated PSA level (5.5 ng/mL) and previous negative TRUS-guided biopsy. (*A*) Axial T2-WI shows diffuse decreased signal intensity of the PZ (*white arrows, A*) (PI-RADS score 2). There is also significant distension of the rectum (R) with gas. (*B, C*) Axial calculated high b-value (1500 s/mm²) DWI and ADC map shows significant distortion of the prostate due to artifacts from rectal gas. There is an equivocal focal lesion with high signal intensity on DWI (*arrow, B*) and low signal intensity on ADC map (*arrow, C*). (*D*) Axial DCE T1-WI demonstrates a focal lesion with early arterial enhancement (*black arrow, D*) in the same location with equivocal finding on DWI/ADC map (DCE positive). (*E, F*) Axial calculated high b-value (1500 s/mm²) DWI and ADC map obtained after the rectal gas was removed with a tube demonstrate a significant improvement of the image quality and confirmed the presence of a 0.8-cm focal lesion with markedly increased signal intensity on DWI (*black arrow, E*) and markedly low signal intensity on ADC map (*black arrow, F*) in the right posterolateral PZ at the midgland (DWI/ADC score 4). Because DWI/ADC is the dominant sequence in the PZ, the PI-RADS assessment category was 4. MR/ultrasound fusion-guided biopsy of the lesion identified PCa Gleason score 3 + 4 or grade group 2. The patient was treated with radical prostatectomy.

Antiperistaltic Agents

Patients undergoing MR imaging of the pelvis are often given an antiperistaltic agent such as glucagon or butylscopolamine to reduce artifacts induced by bowel motion, mainly from the small bowel.[40] In prostate MR imaging, the improvement in image quality with an antiperistaltic agent has not been shown to be significant for examinations performed either with or without an ERC.[41,42] The lack of a significant benefit is likely related to the distance between the prostate and the small bowel.[42] Furthermore, the use of these agents increases the cost of the examination and can be associated with side effects.[41] Thus, although the use of an antiperistaltic agent may be helpful in some patients, routine use is not formally recommended.

Abstinence from Ejaculation

The effect of abstinence from ejaculation on PCa detection and staging has not been demonstrated and is therefore not recommended in PI-RADS v2. After ejaculation, T2-WI and ADC values are decreased in the PZ, which in theory could affect PCa detection.[43] In addition, after ejaculation, the seminal vesicles may become collapsed, which can impair assessment. Kabakus and colleagues[44] found that abstinence from ejaculation for 3 or more days before MR imaging improved the assessment of the seminal vesicles in men aged more than 60 years, but this study did not evaluate the effect of this finding on the accuracy of PCa staging.

SUMMARY

MR imaging provides detailed anatomic assessment of the prostate as well as information that allows the detection and characterization of PCa. To obtain high-quality MR imaging of the prostate, radiologists must understand sequence optimization to overcome commonly encountered technical challenges; they must also be aware of the various hardware considerations and important aspects of patient preparation. The use of minimum parameters provided in the PI-RADS v2 guidelines should help to standardize MR imaging protocols. Institutions should strive to optimize imaging protocols in order to obtain the best and most consistent image quality possible with the equipment available.

SUPPLEMENTARY DATA

Supplementary data related to this article can be found online at https://doi.org/10.1016/j.rcl.2017.10.004.

REFERENCES

1. Steyn JH, Smith FW. Nuclear magnetic resonance imaging of the prostate. Br J Urol 1982;54:726–8.
2. Muthigi A, Sidana A, George AK, et al. Current beliefs and practice patterns among urologists regarding prostate magnetic resonance imaging and magnetic resonance-targeted biopsy. Urol Oncol 2017;35:32.e1-7.
3. Heidenreich A. Consensus criteria for the use of magnetic resonance imaging in the diagnosis and staging of prostate cancer: not ready for routine use. Eur Urol 2011;59:495–7.
4. Barentsz JO, Richenberg J, Clements R, et al. European Society of Urogenital Radiology. ESUR prostate MR guidelines 2012. Eur Radiol 2012;22:746–57.
5. Weinreb JC, Barentsz JO, Choyke PL, et al. PI-RADS prostate imaging–reporting and data system: 2015, version 2. Eur Urol 2016;69(1):16–40.
6. Hricak H, Dooms GC, McNeal JE, et al. MR imaging of the prostate gland: normal anatomy. AJR Am J Roentgenol 1987;148:51–8.
7. Rosenkrantz AB, Neil J, Kong X, et al. Prostate cancer: comparison of 3D T2-weighted with conventional 2D T2-weighted imaging for image quality and tumor detection. AJR Am J Roentgenol 2010;194:446–52.
8. Gibbs P, Tozer DJ, Liney GP, et al. Comparison of quantitative T2 mapping and diffusion-weighted imaging in the normal and pathologic prostate. Magn Reson Med 2001;46:1054–8.
9. de Rooij M, Hamoen EHJ, Futterer JJ, et al. Accuracy of multiparametric MRI for prostate cancer detection: a meta-analysis. AJR Am J Roentgenol 2014;202:343–51.
10. Turkbey B, Shah VP, Pang Y, et al. Is apparent diffusion coefficient associated with clinical risk scores for prostate cancers that are visible on 3-T MR images? Radiology 2011;258(2):488–95.
11. Hambrock T, Somford DM, Huisman HJ, et al. Relationship between apparent diffusion coefficients at 3.0-T MR imaging and Gleason grade in peripheral zone prostate cancer. Radiology 2011;259(2):453–61.
12. Delongchamps NB, Rouanne M, Flam T, et al. Multiparametric magnetic resonance imaging for the detection and localization of prostate cancer: combination of T2-weighted, dynamic contrast-enhanced and diffusion-weighted imaging. BJU Int 2011;107(9):1411–8.
13. Vargas HA, Akin O, Franiel T, et al. Diffusion-weighted endorectal MR imaging at 3 T for prostate cancer: tumor detection and assessment of aggressiveness. Radiology 2011;259(3):775–84.
14. Godley KC, Syer TJ, Toms AP, et al. Accuracy of high b-value diffusion-weighted MRI for prostate

cancer detection: a meta-analysis. Acta Radiol 2017. https://doi.org/10.1177/0284185117702181.

15. Bittencourt LK, Attenberger UI, Lima D, et al. Feasibility study of computed vs measured high b-value (1400 s/mm²) diffusion-weighted MR images of the prostate. World J Radiol 2014;6(6):374–80.

16. Rosenkrantz AB, Padhani AR, Chenevert TL, et al. Body diffusion kurtosis imaging: basic principles, applications, and considerations for clinical practice. J Magn Reson Imaging 2015;42:1190–202.

17. McCammack KC, Kane CJ, Parsons JK, et al. In vivo prostate cancer detection and grading using restriction spectrum imaging-MRI. Prostate Cancer Prostatic Dis 2016;19:168–73.

18. Alonzi R, Padhani AR, Allen C. Dynamic contrast enhanced MRI in prostate cancer. Eur J Radiol 2007;63:335–50.

19. Stanzione A, Imbriaco M, Cocozza S, et al. Biparametric 3T magnetic resonance imaging for prostatic cancer detection in a biopsy-naïve patient population: a further improvement of PI-RADS v2? Eur J Radiol 2016;85(12):2269–74.

20. Hoeks CM, Hambrock T, Yakar D, et al. Transition zone prostate cancer: detection and localization with 3-T multiparametric MR imaging. Radiology 2013;266:207–17.

21. Ullrich T, Quentin M, Oelers C, et al. Magnetic resonance imaging of the prostate at 1.5 versus 3.0 T: a prospective comparison study of image quality. Eur J Radiol 2017;90:192–7.

22. de Rooij M, Hamoen EH, Witjes JA, et al. Accuracy of magnetic resonance imaging for local staging of prostate cancer: a diagnostic meta-analysis. Eur Urol 2016;70:233–45.

23. Rouviere O, Hartman RP, Lyonnet D. Prostate MR imaging at high-field strength: evolution or revolution? Eur Radiol 2006;16:276–84.

24. Schnall MD, Lenkinski RE, Pollack HM, et al. Prostate: MR imaging with an endorectal surface coil. Radiology 1989;172:570–4.

25. Rajesh A, Coakley FV. MR imaging and MR spectroscopic imaging of prostate cancer. Magn Reson Imaging Clin N Am 2004;12:557–79.

26. Heijmink SW, Scheenen TW, van Lin EN, et al. Changes in prostate shape and volume and their implications for radiotherapy after introduction of endorectal balloon as determined by MRI at 3T. Int J Radiat Oncol Biol Phys 2009;73:1446–53.

27. Vilanova JC, Barcelo J. Prostate cancer detection: magnetic resonance (MR) spectroscopic imaging. Abdom Imaging 2007;32:253–61.

28. Shah ZK, Elias SN, Abaza R, et al. Performance comparison of 1.5-T endorectal coil MRI with 3.0-T nonendorectal coil MRI in patients with prostate cancer. Acad Radiol 2015;22:467–74.

29. Turkbey B, Merino MJ, Gallardo EC, et al. Comparison of endorectal coil and nonendorectal coil T2W and diffusion-weighted MRI at 3 Tesla for localizing prostate cancer: correlation with whole-mount histopathology. J Magn Reson Imaging 2014;39:1443–8.

30. Costa DN, Yuan Q, Xi Y, et al. Comparison of prostate cancer detection at 3-T MRI with and without an endorectal coil: a prospective, paired-patient study. Urol Oncol 2016;34:255.e7-13.

31. Heijmink SW, Futterer JJ, Hambrock T, et al. Prostate cancer: body-array versus endorectal coil MR imaging at 3T – comparison of image quality, localization, and staging performance. Radiology 2007;244:184–95.

32. Eberhardt SC, Carter S, Casalino DD, et al. ACR Appropriateness Criteria prostate cancer-pretreatment detection, staging, and surveillance. J Am Coll Radiol 2013;10:83–92.

33. Carroll PR, Parsons JK, Andriole G, et al. NCCN guidelines insights. Prostate cancer early detection, version 2.2016. Featured updates to the NCCN guidelines. J Natl Compr Canc Netw 2016;14:509–19.

34. Rosenkrantz AB, Verma S, Choyke P, et al. Prostate magnetic resonance imaging and magnetic resonance imaging targeted biopsy in patients with a prior negative biopsy: a consensus statement by AUA and SAR. J Urol 2016;196(6):1613–8.

35. Tamada T, Sone T, Jo Y, et al. Prostate cancer: relationships between postbiopsy hemorrhage and tumor detectability at MR diagnosis. Radiology 2008;248:531–9.

36. Sharif-Afshar AR, Feng T, Koopman S, et al. Impact of post prostate biopsy hemorrhage on multiparametric magnetic resonance imaging. Can J Urol 2015;22:7698–702.

37. Barrett T, Vargas HA, Akin O, et al. Value of the hemorrhage exclusion sign on T1-weighted prostate MR images for the detection of prostate cancer. Radiology 2012;263:751–7.

38. Caglic I, Hansen NL, Slough RA, et al. Evaluating the effect of rectal distension on prostate multiparametric MRI image quality. Eur J Radiol 2017;90:174–80.

39. Lim C, Quon J, McInnes M, et al. Does a cleansing enema improve image quality of 3T surface coil multiparametric prostate MRI? J Magn Reson Imaging 2015;42:689–97.

40. Zand KR, Reinhold C, Haider MA, et al. Artifacts and pitfalls in MR imaging of the pelvis. J Magn Reson Imaging 2007;26:480–97.

41. Wagner M, Rief M, Busch J, et al. Effect of butylscopolamine on image quality in MRI of the prostate. Clin Radiol 2010;65:460–4.

42. Roethke MC, Kuru TH, Radbruch A, et al. Prostate magnetic resonance imaging at 3 Tesla: is administration of hyoscine-N-butyl-bromide mandatory? World J Radiol 2013;5:259–63.

43. Medved M, Sammet S, Yousuf A, et al. MR imaging of the prostate and adjacent anatomic structures before, during, and after ejaculation: qualitative and quantitative evaluation. Radiology 2014;271:452–60.

44. Kabakus IM, Borofsky S, Mertan FV, et al. Does abstinence from ejaculation before prostate MRI improve evaluation of the seminal vesicles? AJR Am J Roentgenol 2016;207:1205–9.

Multiparametric MR imaging of the Prostate
Interpretation Including Prostate Imaging Reporting and Data System Version 2

Alessandro Furlan, MD[a], Amir A. Borhani, MD[a],
Antonio C. Westphalen, MD, PhD[b,c,*]

KEYWORDS

- Prostate cancer • Multiparametric MR imaging • PI-RADS

KEY POINTS

- The key sequences of a prostate mp-MRI scan are high-resolution T2-weighted, high b-value diffusion-weighted, and dynamic contrast-enhanced imaging.
- PI-RADS standardizes interpretation of mp-MRI, resulting in moderate-to-high accuracy for the diagnosis of clinically significant prostate cancer.
- A quantitative approach to functional imaging of the prostate has the potential to further improve diagnostic accuracy of mp-MRI and to provide insights into tumor aggressiveness and prognosis.

INTRODUCTION

Radiologists in the United States are experiencing a significant growth of volume of prostate MR imaging studies.[1] This mirrors an increasing interest from the urology community in the application of this technique for the management of patients with, or at risk for, prostate cancer, particularly for biopsy guidance. The technological developments experienced in the last two decades culminated in a mp-MRI approach that combines anatomic and functional imaging. However, the greater complexity of this technique, along with an increasing demand, brought new challenges to imaging interpretation. The Prostate Imaging Reporting and Data System (PI-RADS), first proposed in 2011 by the European Society of Uroradiology, is an effort to address these challenges through a standardized approach to the interpretation of prostate mp-MRI.[2] The second version of PI-RADS (PI-RADS v2) was released in 2015 with many simplifications and improvements.[3]

The first part of this article is focused on interpretation of the pulse sequences recommended in the PI-RADS v2 guidelines, including useful tips based on the authors' experiences at two large academic institutions. In the second part, we review advanced quantitative imaging tools and discuss future directions.

[a] Department of Radiology, University of Pittsburgh, UPMC Presbyterian Campus, Radiology Suite 200 East Wing, 200 Lothrop Street, Pittsburgh, PA 15213, USA; [b] Department of Radiology and Biomedical Imaging, University of California San Francisco, 505 Parnassus Avenue, M392, Box 0628, San Francisco, CA 94143, USA; [c] Department of Urology, University of California San Francisco, 1825 4th Street, 4th Floor, Box 1711, San Francisco, CA 94143, USA
* Corresponding author. Department of Radiology and Biomedical Imaging, University of California San Francisco, 505 Parnassus Avenue, M392, Box 0628, San Francisco, CA 94143.
E-mail address: AntonioCarlos.Westphalen@ucsf.edu

Radiol Clin N Am 56 (2018) 223–238
https://doi.org/10.1016/j.rcl.2017.10.005
0033-8389/18/© 2017 Elsevier Inc. All rights reserved.

INTERPRETATION OF MULTIPARAMETRIC MR IMAGING: PULSE SEQUENCES INCLUDED IN PROSTATE IMAGING REPORTING AND DATA SYSTEM VERSION 2

An mp-MRI of the prostate is an examination comprised of multiple pulse sequences, including anatomic and functional images. The key pulse sequences recommended in the PI-RADS v2 guidelines are three-plane high-resolution axial T2-weighted images (T2WI), high b-value axial diffusion-weighted images (DWI), apparent diffusion coefficient (ADC) map, and axial dynamic contrast-enhanced (DCE) images.[3] The high-resolution coronal and sagittal T2WI help to better define the morphology and spatial relationship of a finding already identified on the axial images. A practical approach to review this large data set is to organize the key pulse sequences and display them simultaneously on the viewing monitors, allowing the radiologist to link and quickly correlate the findings detected on anatomic and functional images. According to the PI-RADS v2 guidelines, each prostatic finding should be assigned a score between 1 and 5 based on its appearance on T2WI, DWI, and DCE MR imaging. A score of 5 indicates very high probability of clinically significant prostate cancer, defined as Gleason score greater than or equal to 7, and/or volume greater than or equal to 0.5 mL, and/or extraprostatic extension (EPE).[3]

Anatomic Imaging

T2-weighted images: peripheral zone
Multiplanar high-resolution T2WI is the hallmark sequence for anatomic evaluation of the prostate. In contrast to the normal peripheral zone (PZ), which has high signal intensity (SI) on T2WI because of its large water content, most tumors exhibit low SI.[4] Moreover, tumors with higher Gleason scores tend to have lower SI than less aggressive cancers.[5,6] This is because tumor grade increase represents a progressive loss of the normal glandular anatomy and continuing dedifferentiation and clustering of cancer cells.[7] Three other important anatomic features depicted on T2WI are shape, borders, and size of lesions. Prostate cancer tends to present as a focal round or crescent abnormality on imaging, whereas benign lesions are more often indistinct or have a linear or triangular shape.[8] Although there is an overlap between the features of benign and low-to-intermediate grade prostate cancers, tumors with high Gleason score are usually more noticeable lesions.[6] Lastly, lesion size has been positively correlated with chance of malignancy and Gleason score, that is, larger lesions are more likely to represent high-grade prostate cancer than smaller ones.[8,9] Furthermore, there is also a positive correlation between tumor size and the probability of EPE and seminal vesicle invasion.[9]

It is not surprising, therefore, that the T2WI PI-RADS v2 categories are based on these four features (Table 1).[3] Lesions with high probability of representing a clinically significant prostate cancer are focal masslike, circumscribed, and have homogeneous moderately low SI (score 4 or 5) (Fig. 1). The distinction between a score 4 and 5 is based on the presence of definite EPE or size, where the lesions greater than or equal to 1.5 cm are assigned a score 5. On the other end of the spectrum are lesions that are likely benign (score 2). Those lesions are linear, wedge-shaped, or present as areas of mildly low SI with indistinct borders (Fig. 2). Lesions that have moderately low SI, but are heterogeneous or noncircumscribed are considered indeterminate and receive a score of 3 (Fig. 3). T2WI is only moderately accurate for the detection of cancer, although its performance improves when the goal is to identify high-grade disease. Mucinous adenocarcinomas of the prostate, for example, may have a predominantly high SI resulting in false-negative based on T2WI score.[10] However, many nontumoral lesions, such as inflammation, fibrosis, and hemorrhage, can mimic cancer on T2WI.[11]

T2-weighted images: transition zone
The accurate identification and characterization of prostate cancer within the transition zone (TZ) likely represents the greatest challenge of mp-MRI interpretation. The difficulty arises with the development of benign prostatic hyperplasia (BPH), which affects virtually all middle age or older men, the same population at risk for prostate cancer. BPH affects glandular and stromal tissues and it is characterized by the growth of multiple nodules and intervening hyperplastic stroma, depicted on T2WI as a large, distorted, and markedly heterogeneous TZ, an appearance described as "organized chaos."[12] Differentiating the intertwined hyperplastic stroma or stroma-rich nodule from cancer is problematic because both entities present with low SI on T2WI, and the random appearance of BPH allows prostate cancer to blend within the nodular TZ.[12,13] Hence, detection of these tumors requires a careful analysis of the lesion morphology on high-resolution T2WI (see Table 1). Well circumscribed and encapsulated nodules with low or heterogeneous T2 SI are typically benign (PI-RADS v2 score 2) (Fig. 4). High-grade tumors, however, characteristically present as lenticular or indistinct foci of homogenous moderately low SI (PI-RADS v2

Table 1
T2 score for peripheral and transition zone according to PI-RADS v2

Score	Signal Intensity	Shape	Size - EPE
Peripheral zone			
1 (normal)	• High • Homogeneous	• N/A	N/A
2	• Low	• Linear/wedge-shaped • Diffuse (homogeneous) • Indistinct	Any size EPE absent
3[a]	• Low (moderate) • Heterogeneous	• Round/noncircumscribed • Diffuse	Any size EPE absent
4	• Moderate-to-low • Homogeneous	• Focus/mass • Circumscribed	<1.5 cm EPE absent
5	• Moderate-to-low • Homogeneous	• Focus/mass • Circumscribed	≥1.5 cm and/or EPE definitely present
Transition zone			
1 (normal)	• Intermediate • Homogeneous	• N/A	N/A
2	• Low/high • Heterogeneous • Homogeneous	• Circumscribed nodule	Any size EPE absent
3[a]	• Heterogeneous	• Obscured margins	Any size EPE absent
4	• Moderate-to-low • Homogeneous	• Lenticular • Noncircumscribed	<1.5 cm EPE absent
5	• Moderate-to-low • Homogeneous	• Lenticular • Noncircumscribed	≥1.5 cm and/or EPE definitely present

Abbreviation: NA, not applicable.
[a] Score 3 also includes lesions that do not fit in categories 2, 3, 4, and 5.

score 4 or 5) (**Fig. 5**). The identification of a heterogeneous lesion, however, is not as definitive for the diagnosis of cancer; these may represent stromal-rich BPH associated with cystic ectasia and hyperplastic glandular components that are seen on T2WI as foci of high SI.[14] As for lesions in the PZ, the distinction between PI-RADS v2 scores 4 and 5 is based on the lesion size and/or the presence of definite EPE. Lesions that do not meet the criteria for the benign or high-grade lesions are assigned a score 3, denoting an indeterminate finding with equivocal likelihood for clinically significant cancer.

T1-weighted images

Unenhanced T1-weighted images (T1WI) have a limited role in the assessment of prostate cancer and are mainly used for detection of postbiopsy hemorrhage, which appears as focal or diffuse areas of high SI compared with the background gland. Identification of postbiopsy hemorrhage is relevant because it may present as focal or diffuse areas of low SI on T2WI and ADC map, thus mimicking cancer.[15,16] Previous studies, however, showed that tumors have significantly lower T2 SI and lower ADC values compared with areas of hemorrhage.[16] Additionally, the interpretation of raw DCE images could be confounded by the inherent high T1 SI on baseline precontrast images. Misinterpretation can, however, be avoided with the use of subtraction images. Accordingly, when hemorrhage is detected on T1WI, the additional sequences should be evaluated with higher scrutiny to avoid overestimation of tumor presence or size.

The normal prostatic tissue has a greater concentration of citrate than foci that harbor prostate cancer. Because citrate has an anticoagulant effect, postbiopsy hemorrhage tends to resolve faster within the tumor compared with the surrounding tissue.[17,18] This phenomenon can result in the "hemorrhage exclusion" or "halo" sign, which is defined as presence of a well-defined iso-intense mass surrounded by hyperintense area on T1WI (**Fig. 6**).[19] When interpreted in conjunction with T2WI and DWI, the sign is highly specific for the detection of cancer and helps to better determine the tumor size.[2]

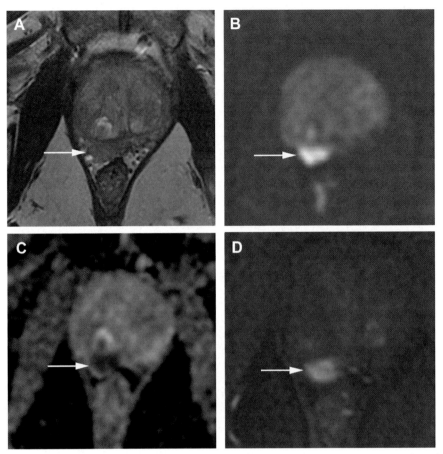

Fig. 1. A 67-year-old man in active surveillance for a Gleason score 6 prostate adenocarcinoma undergoing mp-MRI because of increasing prostate-specific antigen (PSA) value (PSA = 12.6 ng/mL; PSA density = 0.12 ng/mL^2). (*A*) Axial T2WI shows a 1.2-cm hypointense mass in the right peripheral zone of the midgland with extraprostatic extension and invasion of neurovascular bundle (*arrow*). The lesion appears markedly hyperintense on high b-value (b = 1500 s/mm^2) axial DWI (*arrow, B*) and markedly hypointense (mean value = 600 × 10^{-3} mm^2/s) on the ADC map (*arrow, C*) corresponding to a PI-RADS category 5 lesion. The lesion shows avid early enhancement on the axial contrast-enhanced T1WI gradient-recalled echo (GRE) (*arrow, D*).

T1WI can also be used for detection of lymphadenopathy. The conventional size criteria for characterization of abnormal pelvic lymph nodes have low diagnostic accuracy, however, with a reported pooled sensitivity and specificity of 0.39 and 0.82, respectively.[20] Different thresholds, ranging from 8 mm to 15 mm, have been proposed[21] and PI-RADS v2 classifies lymph nodes larger than 8 mm in short axis as suspicious.[3] Inclusion of lymph node shape, border, enhancement, and ADC values may improve the diagnostic performance of MR imaging.[22]

Functional Imaging

Diffusion-weighted imaging and apparent diffusion coefficient map

Among the functional techniques that comprise a mp-MRI scan of the prostate, DWI plays a key role. Several studies in the last decade have proven that the addition of DWI to T2WI significantly increases the sensitivity and specificity of the technique for the detection of prostate cancer.[23–25] Briefly, DWI depicts the random motion of water molecules within a voxel. The SI on DWI depends on the molecules' motion and the diffusion weighting, which is affected by the imaging acquisition technique (eg, b-value). Generally, the sensitivity of DWI improves when high b-values are used, but this happens at the expense of signal-to-noise ratio. Trace DWI images are, however, diffusion- and T2-weighted. So, lesions with a long T2 value may appear bright on DWI but not restrict diffusion, a phenomenon known as T2 shine-through. Findings on the high-b-value DWI should, therefore, always be correlated with and interpreted in conjunction with the ADC map. Although the

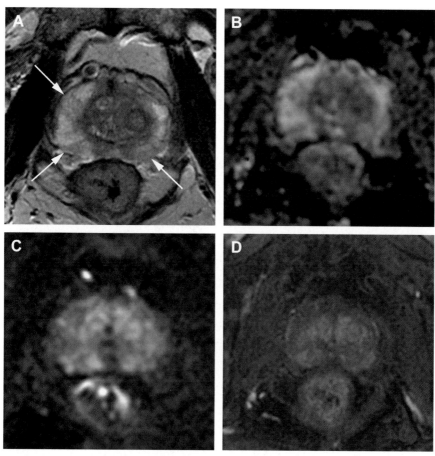

Fig. 2. A 71-year-old man undergoing mp-MRI because of a new diagnosis of prostate adenocarcinoma (Gleason score 3 + 3 = 6) at systematic prostate biopsy. (*A*) Axial T2WI shows multiple and bilateral triangular-shaped areas of mildly low signal intensity (*arrows*) in the peripheral zone of the midgland. (*B*) ADC map at the same level shows indistinct area of low signal intensity. Axial high b-value (b = 1500 s/mm²) DWI (*C*) and axial early contrast-enhanced T1WI GRE (*D*) show no focal abnormality corresponding to a PI-RADS category 2 lesion. The repeated biopsy toward the triangular-shaped foci seen on the images revealed normal prostatic tissue.

normal PZ demonstrates homogenous low SI on DWI and high SI on ADC map, the more restricted environment of cancer, secondary to the higher cellular density compared with the surrounding glandular tissue, leads to high SI on DWI and low SI on the ADC map.[26,27]

Per PI-RADS v2, each lesion receives a DWI/ADC score that ranges from 1 to 5 based on SI, size, and presence of EPE. The criteria are applicable to lesions located in the PZ or TZ (**Table 2**). A score of 1 denotes normal tissue and absence of abnormalities. A score of 2 is defined as an indistinct area of low SI on the ADC map. A focal abnormality receives a score of 3 or greater, depending on its SI on DWI and ADC map. Lesions highly concerning for prostate cancer (score 4 and 5) show markedly elevated SI on the high b-value DWI and marked low SI on the ADC map (see **Figs. 1** and **5**). A size threshold of 1.5 cm and/or EPE are again used to assign a score 4 or 5. DWI/ADC is the dominant sequence for characterization of a lesion in the PZ. In the TZ, the sequence plays a secondary role to T2WI because of its lower specificity. Stromal-rich nodules may show restricted diffusion, thus mimicking cancer (**Fig. 7**).[28] Nevertheless, the sensitivity of DWI for detection of cancer in the TZ is high[29] and the technique is used to identify suspicious foci. Once foci with marked restricted diffusion are detected on DWI/ADC, they are characterized based on their appearance on T2WI. DWI/ADC is particularly helpful to detect lesions that are very anterior along the anterior fibromuscular stroma.[30]

Dynamic contrast-enhanced MR imaging
DCE MR imaging consists of multiple series of T1WI, typically three-dimensional gradient-echo images, performed sequentially through the

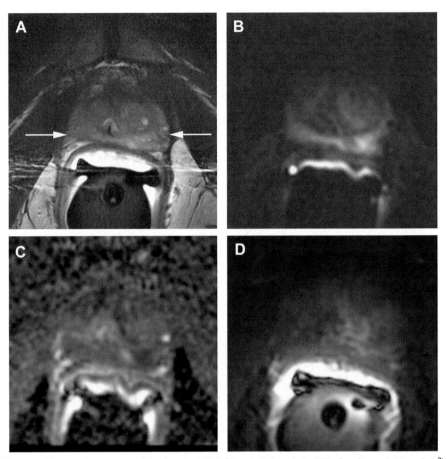

Fig. 3. A 57-year-old man presenting with elevated PSA (PSA = 7.9 ng/mL; PSA density = 0.11 ng/mL^2). (*A*) Axial T2WI shows heterogeneous and moderately low signal intensity in the peripheral zone of the apex (*arrows*). The same area shows heterogeneous mildly high signal intensity on the high b-value (b = 1500 s/mm^2) DWI (*B*) and moderately low (mean = 900 × 10^{-3} mm^2/s) signal intensity on the ADC map (*C*). The DCE study (*D*) is negative for focal early enhancement. The lesion is compatible with a PI-RADS category 3 lesion. Target biopsy of the left posteroapical area showed chronic inflammation.

prostate before, during, and after the intravenous injection of a gadolinium-based contrast agent.[31] The goal of this technique is to assess the tissue perfusion kinetics with high temporal resolution to detect prostate cancer based on the presence of neovascularity and increased vascular permeability.[32] In general, prostate cancer shows earlier and more intense enhancement than the surrounding normal gland.[33]

DCE MR imaging is perhaps the most controversial of all mp-MRI sequences. It has been shown that the technique increases the diagnostic accuracy for cancer detection when added to the anatomic sequences[34,35] and that it is helpful to differentiate tumors located in the anterior gland from the normal anterior fibromuscular stroma because of their earlier enhancement.[30] Unfortunately, DCE MR imaging lacks specificity because multiple other conditions can lead to increased

vascularity and early enhancement, including inflammation in the PZ and some BPH nodules in the TZ.[31] Moreover, lack of standardization of the technique leads to inconsistent results across institutions. Finally, recent publications have documented a limited added value of DCE MR imaging for the detection of prostate cancer when compared with a biparametric approach including T2WI and DWI.[36,37]

Because of these controversies, the role of DCE MR imaging in PI-RADS v2 is limited to the characterization of a PZ lesion considered indeterminate based on DWI. The PI-RADS v2 guidelines recommend a qualitative interpretation of DCE MR imaging, that is, a visual assessment of changes in SI over multiple time points after contrast injection, and a binary description of the pattern of enhancement.[3] If the lesion demonstrates focal and early or contemporaneous

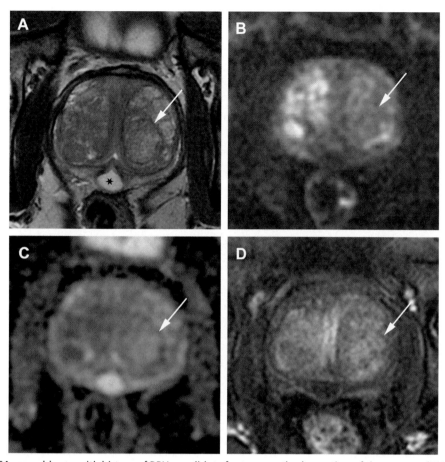

Fig. 4. A 64-year-old man with history of BPH, candidate for transurethral resection of the prostate (PSA = 6.5 ng/mL; prostate volume = 120 mL; PSA density = 0.05 ng/mL^2). (*A*) Axial T2WI shows an enlarged transition zone replaced by innumerable nodules, compatible with BPH. A benign BPH nodule (PI-RADS category 2) is circumscribed with complete hypointense rim on T2WI (*arrow, A*), isointense on high b-value (b = 1500 s/mm^2) DWI (*arrow, B*) and ADC map (*arrow, C*), and shows no early enhancement on the contrast-enhanced T1WI GRE (*arrow, D*). Note a benign utricle cyst (*black star, A*).

enhancement compared with the surrounding normal prostatic parenchyma, DCE MR imaging is considered positive (see **Figs. 1** and **5**). Any other finding on DCE MR imaging denotes a negative result.

Prostate Imaging Reporting and Data System Version 2 Overall Assessment

After each lesion (up to four, according to the guidelines) is assigned an individual score based on its T2WI, DWI/ADC, and DCE MR imaging features, a simple algorithm is applied to determine the final PI-RADS category (**Fig. 8**).[3] Lesions are grouped into five categories of risk for clinically significant cancer as follows:

- PI-RADS 1: Very low risk
- PI-RADS 2: Low risk
- PI-RADS 3: Intermediate risk
- PI-RADS 4: High risk
- PI-RADS 5: Very high risk

PI-RADS v2 uses the concept of a dominant sequence, that is, the sequence most affecting the final assessment. Lesions in the PZ are mainly categorized based on their appearance on DWI and ADC map. The indeterminate lesions, that is, score 3, are upgraded to a category 4 if DCE MR imaging is positive. TZ lesions, however, are classified mostly based on their appearance on T2WI. In the TZ, indeterminate lesions are upgraded to a category 4 if their DWI/ADC map score is 5.

Prostate Imaging Reporting and Data System Version 2: Diagnostic Accuracy and Main Limitations

Several retrospective studies reported moderate to high accuracy of PI-RADS v2 for the detection

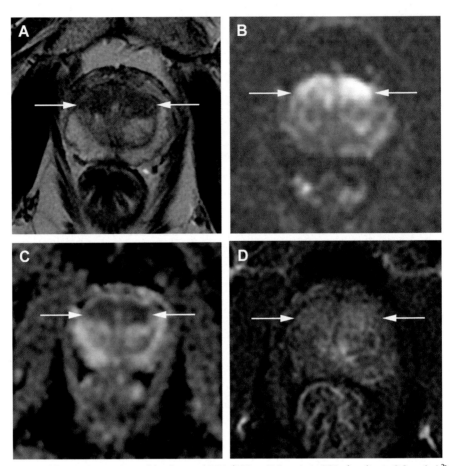

Fig. 5. A 64-year-old man presenting with elevated PSA (PSA = 5.7 ng/mL; PSA density = 0.2 ng/mL^2) and prior negative prostate biopsies. (A) Axial T2WI shows a lenticular, noncircumscribed mass with low signal intensity in the anterior midgland (*arrows*) compatible with a PI-RADS category 5 lesion. The mass shows markedly high signal intensity on high b-value (b = 1500 s/mm^2) DWI (*arrows, B*), markedly low signal intensity on ADC map (*arrows, C*), and early enhancement on contrast-enhanced T1WI GRE (*arrows, D*). Target biopsy revealed invasive prostatic adenocarcinoma, Gleason score 3 + 4 = 7.

of clinically significant prostate cancer, with areas under the receiver operating characteristic curve ranging from 0.66 to 0.87.[38–40] A recent meta-analysis showed pooled sensitivity and specificity of 89% and 73% for detection of prostate cancer Gleason 3 + 3 or higher using PI-RADS v2 criteria.[41] A recent prospective analysis found that among patients undergoing targeted MR imaging/TRUS fusion biopsy, 78% of lesions categorized as PI-RADS v2 5 represented were cancer.[42] However, PI-RADS v2 scores 4 and 3 were associated with a significantly lower cancer detection rate of 30% and 16%, respectively, suggesting a need for refinement of the current criteria. Another reason for further development of the system comes from interobserver variability studies that report only moderate agreement.[40,43] Additionally, no data are available on the performance of the system by less experienced radiologists in a nonacademic setting. Finally, the current recommendations are based on qualitative assessment of images, but, as described in the next section, quantitative data from functional images may provide additional information that characterizes tumor biology.

ADVANCED AND QUANTITATIVE IMAGING ANALYSIS OF MULTIPARAMETRIC MR IMAGING OF THE PROSTATE
Diffusion-Weighted Imaging: Apparent Diffusion Coefficient Values

Multiple studies have shown that the measurement of ADC values may improve the characterization of tumor aggressiveness. The ADC values of prostate cancer have an inverse correlation with the Gleason score and the D'Amico clinical risk classification,[26,44–48] and higher degrees of

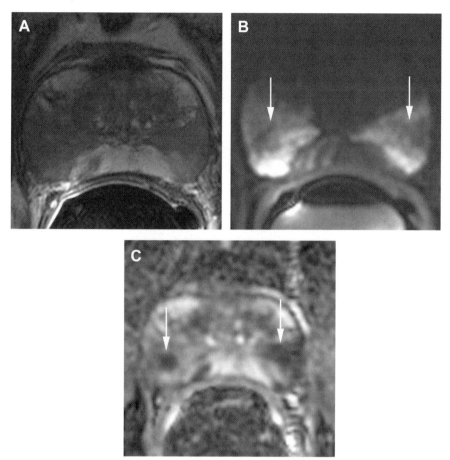

Fig. 6. A 62-year-old man with history of bilateral prostate cancer detected on a systematic biopsy performed 3 weeks before mp-MRI (Gleason score not available; PSA = 4.7 ng/mL). (*A*) Axial T2WI shows extensive areas of hypointensity in posterolateral aspect of midgland peripheral zone on both sides. (*B*) Corresponding precontrast axial T1WI shows diffuse T1 hyperintensity compatible with postbiopsy hemorrhage. Two areas in peripheral zone (*arrows*), however, are spared from hemorrhage (halo sign). (*C*) Corresponding ADC map shows marked restricted diffusion in those areas (*arrows*). Hemorrhage exclusion or halo sign is highly specific for the detection of cancer.

Table 2
DWI score for peripheral and transition zone according to PI-RADS v2

Score	Signal Intensity High b-Value DWI	Signal Intensity ADC Map	Size - EPE
Peripheral and transition zone			
1 (normal)	• Homogeneous • No focal abnormality	• Homogeneous • No focal abnormality	N/A
2	• No focal abnormality	• Indistinct • Low	Any size EPE absent
3	• Focal • Iso-to-mildly high	• Focal • Mildly-to-moderately low	Any size EPE absent
4	• Focal • Markedly high	• Focal • Markedly low	<1.5 cm EPE absent
5	• Focal • Markedly high	• Focal • Markedly low	≥1.5 cm and/or EPE definitely present

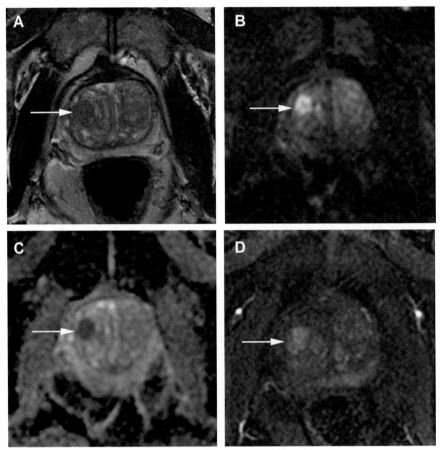

Fig. 7. A 65-year-old man with elevated PSA (PSA = 15.1 ng/mL) and history of chronic prostatitis. (*A*) Axial T2WI of the prostate midgland shows a 1.2-cm circumscribed hypointense nodule (*arrow*) in the enlarged right transition zone. The nodule is hyperintense on high b-value DWI (*arrow*, *B*), hypointense (mean ADC value = 720×10^{-3} mm^2/s) on ADC map (*arrow*, *C*), and shows early enhancement on the axial contrast-enhanced T1WI GRE (*arrow*, *D*). Target biopsy revealed normal prostatic tissue.

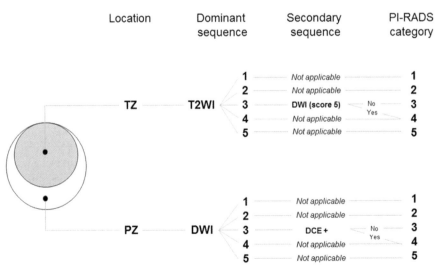

Fig. 8. Diagram is a representation of the algorithm used in PI-RADS v2 to determine the final category of risk for clinically significant risk based on the imaging appearance on mp-MRI.

restricted diffusion, characterized by lower ADC values, have been associated with a greater probability of EPE.[49] The main limitation of a quantitative interpretation of DWI is the variability of ADC values across institutions, because these are dependent of multiple technical variables and patient features.[45,50] Although a particular threshold cannot be recommended, it is generally accepted that clinically significant tumors have an ADC value lower than approximately 1000×10^{-6} mm^2/s. It is important, however, to determine the range ADC values seen at one's institution, if these will be used to further characterize lesions identified on DWI and ADC maps.

Although the most commonly used method to generate an ADC map from the source DWI is a monoexponential model (based on a Gaussian [ie, random] diffusion behavior), other more sophisticated options are available and promise to capture additional biologic information. These methods are based on the fact that the diffusion signal tends to depart from a monoexponential decay at low (eg, <200) and high (eg, >1000) b-values,[51,52] but to exploit these differences, images need to be obtained with a large number and range of b-values. According to the intravoxel incoherent motion theory, the signal decay is made of perfusion (fast component: water moving within the capillaries) and diffusion (slow component).[53] When low b-value data are acquired, a bi-exponential model is used to take into account these two components.[54] Although the intravoxel incoherent motion–derived parameter molecular diffusion coefficient (D) and perfusion fraction (f) have been shown to be lower in prostate cancer compared with normal parenchyma,[55] the added value of the technique for tumor detection is yet unclear.[56] On the opposite end of the spectrum, when high b-values (>1000) are used, a diffusion kurtosis model can be obtained, based on a non-Gaussian diffusion assumption.[52] The diffusion kurtosis–derived parameter k (apparent diffusional kurtosis) has been shown to be significantly higher in prostate cancer compared with benign tissue.[57] However, the added value of this technique compared with a monoexponential calculation of ADC is also not yet defined.[58,59]

Dynamic Contrast-Enhanced Imaging: Semiquantitative Analysis of Curves of Enhancement and Pharmacokinetic Modeling

Although the current PI-RADS v2 guidelines recommend a qualitative interpretation of the DCE MR imaging, the data can be processed and analyzed semiquantitatively or quantitatively to improve diagnostic accuracy and to extract prognostic imaging biomarkers.[31]

Enhancement curves (semiquantitative analysis)

The SI on DCE MR imaging are plotted against time to create curves of enhancement. Curves are typically classified into three types: type 1, progressive enhancement; type 2, initial upslope followed by plateau; and type 3, decline after initial upslope (wash-in and wash-out) (Fig. 9).[31] Type 3 curves are considered the most specific of the curves for the diagnosis of prostate cancer. Although this semiquantitative approach has been advocated by several authors and included in the initial version of PI-RADS,[2] it has been found to have limited effectiveness in differentiating malignant from benign prostatic tissue, particularly in the TZ, and therefore is not included in the updated version of the guidelines.[60] The curves of enhancement can also be processed to extract multiple other parameters, including maximal contrast enhancement, time to peak enhancement, speed of contrast uptake (wash-in), and clearance rate of contrast agent (wash-out).[61] The wash-in parameter has been shown to be the most useful for detecting tumor and discriminating it from benign tissue.[61] Lack of standardization remains the main limitation for a wider application of these semiquantitative tools.

Pharmacokinetic modeling (quantitative analysis)

Changes in concentration of contrast medium over time are quantified using pharmacokinetic modeling.[62] A detailed review of the pharmacokinetic modeling is beyond the purpose of this article. Interested readers are invited to review the excellent papers by Verma and colleagues[31] and Sourbron and Buckley.[62] Commercially available software allows the calculation and display (ie, color-coded parametric maps) of the following parameters, which are particularly relevant for prostate cancer (Fig. 10):

- K^{trans} [min^{-1}]: (forward) volume transfer constant or influx (from vascular to extracellular space) rate constant
- k_{ep} [min^{-1}]: reverse reflux rate constant or efflux (from extracellular space to the vascular space) rate constant
- Ve [mL/100 mL]: interstitial volume = K^{trans}/k_{ep}
- Vp [mL/100 mL]: plasma volume

K^{trans} and k_{ep} increase in prostate cancer because of increased cellular and microvascular

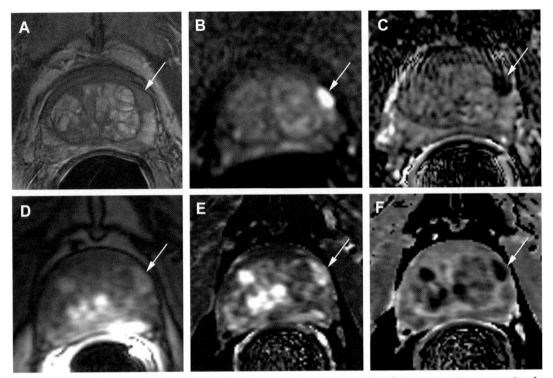

Fig. 9. A 75-year-old man with elevated PSA (8.3 ng/mL) undergoing mp-MRI of the prostate in preparation for fusion biopsy. Axial T2WI (*A*) of the prostate midgland shows a 1.0-cm well-defined T2-hypointense lesion in the left peripheral zone (*arrow*) that appears markedly hyperintense on high b-value (b = 1350 s/mm^2) DWI (*arrow, B*) and markedly hypointense on the ADC map (*arrow, C*) compatible with PI-RADS category 5. The lesion shows focal early enhancement on the axial contrast-enhanced T1WI GRE (*arrow, D*), early wash-in (*arrow on E,* grayscale wash-in map), and early washout (*arrow on F,* grayscale wash-out map).

density with decreased extracellular space, and correlate with tumor aggressiveness.[63,64] Despite the promising results as prognostic biomarker, the adoption of these metrics in the daily evaluation of mp-MRI of the prostate adds complexity to the examination.

Magnetic Resonance Spectroscopy Imaging

MR spectroscopic imaging provides information that is used to characterize the metabolic profile of the prostatic tissue. Increased cellular density and cell membrane turnover in tumor, along with disruption of the normal glandular tissue, lead to higher levels of choline and lower levels of citrate compared with the normal gland.[65] The results of the postprocessing of data are usually visualized as multiple spectra on a grid that is overlaid on the corresponding axial T2WI. For a quantitative analysis, the choline-plus-creatine-to-citrate ratio is calculated: a choline-plus-creatine-to-citrate ratio of at least three standard deviations greater than the mean normal value (0.22 ± 0.013) is highly suggestive of cancer.[66] Despite the results of several studies showing the usefulness of MR

spectroscopic imaging for cancer detection, assessment of tumor aggressiveness and response to treatment,[67] recent evidence shows no added value of MR spectroscopic imaging for tumor detection when compared with a combination of anatomic and functional (ie, DWI, DCE) imaging.[68,69] In addition, this technique requires a high level of expertise for acquisition and analysis, markedly limiting its widespread use.

FUTURE DIRECTIONS

Preliminary works on texture analysis, a mathematical postprocessing algorithm to quantify the spatial distribution and randomness of pixel intensities, have shown promising results for the assessment of tumor biology. A recent study suggested differences between T2WI MR imaging–derived textural parameters of prostate cancers Gleason score 4 + 3 and 3 + 4.[70] Finally, recent efforts toward the development of dedicated computer-aided diagnostic systems for mp-MRI have the potential of improving interobserver and/or intraobserver variability and diagnostic accuracy.[71]

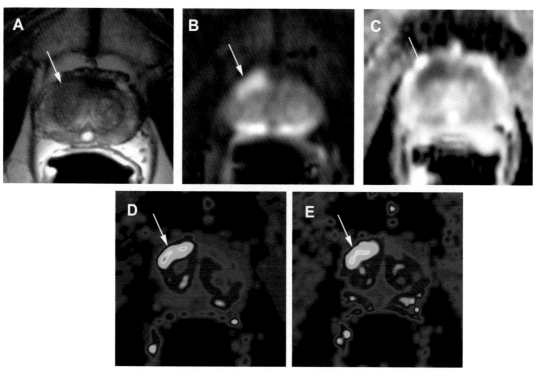

Fig. 10. Role of DCE for the detection of anterior gland prostate cancer. A tumor in the anterior gland shows lenticular shape and ill-defined margins on T2WI (*arrow, A*), markedly high signal intensity on high b-value DWI (*arrow, B*), and markedly low signal intensity on ADC map (*arrow, C*) compatible with a PI-RADS category 5 lesion. Color-encoded K^{trans} forward volume transfer constant (*D*) and k_{ep} reverse reflux rate constant map (*E*) delineate the tumor (*arrow*) against the surrounding gland. (*Courtesy of* Dr Daniel Margolis, Weill Cornell Medicine, New York, NY.)

SUMMARY

mp-MRI of the prostate is a complex imaging study comprising anatomic and functional sequences. The use of the PI-RADS v2 system results in a more standardized interpretation scheme with higher diagnostic accuracy. Further developments, however, are required to overcome the current shortcomings.

REFERENCES

1. Oberlin DT, Casalino DD, Miller FH, et al. Dramatic increase in the utilization of multiparametric magnetic resonance imaging for detection and management of prostate cancer. Abdom Radiol (NY) 2017; 42:1255–8.
2. Barentsz JO, Richenberg J, Clements R, et al. ESUR prostate MR guidelines 2012. Eur Radiol 2012;22: 746–57.
3. Weinreb JC, Barentsz JO, Choyke PL, et al. PI-RADS prostate imaging - reporting and data system: 2015, version 2. Eur Urol 2016;69:16–40.
4. Roethke MC, Lichy MP, Jurgschat L, et al. Tumorsize dependent detection rate of endorectal MRI of prostate cancer: a histopathologic correlation with whole-mount sections in 70 patients with prostate cancer. Eur J Radiol 2011;79:189–95.
5. Ikonen S, Karkkainen P, Kivisaari L, et al. Magnetic resonance imaging of prostatic cancer: does detection vary between high and low Gleason score tumors? Prostate 2000;43:43–8.
6. Wang L, Mazaheri Y, Zhang J, et al. Assessment of biologic aggressiveness of prostate cancer: correlation of MR signal intensity with Gleason grade after radical prostatectomy. Radiology 2008;246: 168–76.
7. Gleason DF, Mellinger GT. Prediction of prognosis for prostatic adenocarcinoma by combined histological grading and clinical staging. J Urol 1974;111:58–64.
8. Cruz M, Tsuda K, Narumi Y, et al. Characterization of low-intensity lesions in the peripheral zone of prostate on pre-biopsy endorectal coil MR imaging. Eur Radiol 2002;12:357–65.
9. Mizuno R, Nakashima J, Mukai M, et al. Maximum tumor diameter is a simple and valuable index associated with the local extent of disease in clinically localized prostate cancer. Int J Urol 2006;13:951–5.
10. Westphalen AC, Coakley FV, Kurhanewicz J, et al. Mucinous adenocarcinoma of the prostate: MRI

and MR spectroscopy features. AJR Am J Roentgenol 2009;193:W238–43.

11. Sciarra A, Barentsz J, Bjartell A, et al. Advances in magnetic resonance imaging: how they are changing the management of prostate cancer. Eur Urol 2011;59:962–77.

12. Ishida J, Sugimura K, Okizuka H, et al. Benign prostatic hyperplasia: value of MR imaging for determining histologic type. Radiology 1994;190:329–31.

13. Moosavi B, Flood TA, Al-Dandan O, et al. Multiparametric MRI of the anterior prostate gland: clinical-radiological-histopathological correlation. Clin Radiol 2016;71:405–17.

14. Guneyli S, Ward E, Thomas S, et al. Magnetic resonance imaging of benign prostatic hyperplasia. Diagn Interv Radiol 2016;22:215–9.

15. White S, Hricak H, Forstner R, et al. Prostate cancer: effect of postbiopsy hemorrhage on interpretation of MR images. Radiology 1995;195:385–90.

16. Rosenkrantz AB, Kopec M, Kong X, et al. Prostate cancer vs. post-biopsy hemorrhage: diagnosis with T2- and diffusion-weighted imaging. J Magn Reson Imaging 2010;31:1387–94.

17. Janssen MJ, Huijgens PC, Bouman AA, et al. Citrate versus heparin anticoagulation in chronic haemodialysis patients. Nephrol Dial Transplant 1993;8:1228–33.

18. Zakian KL, Shukla-Dave A, Ackerstaff E, et al. 1H magnetic resonance spectroscopy of prostate cancer: biomarkers for tumor characterization. Cancer Biomark 2008;4:263–76.

19. Katz S, Rosen M. MR imaging and MR spectroscopy in prostate cancer management. Radiol Clin North Am 2006;44:723–34, viii.

20. Hovels AM, Heesakkers RA, Adang EM, et al. The diagnostic accuracy of CT and MRI in the staging of pelvic lymph nodes in patients with prostate cancer: a meta-analysis. Clin Radiol 2008;63:387–95.

21. Sankineni S, Brown AM, Fascelli M, et al. Lymph node staging in prostate cancer. Curr Urol Rep 2015;16:30.

22. Thoeny HC, Froehlich JM, Triantafyllou M, et al. Metastases in normal-sized pelvic lymph nodes: detection with diffusion-weighted MR imaging. Radiology 2014;273:125–35.

23. Wu LM, Xu JR, Ye YQ, et al. The clinical value of diffusion-weighted imaging in combination with T2-weighted imaging in diagnosing prostate carcinoma: a systematic review and meta-analysis. AJR Am J Roentgenol 2012;199:103–10.

24. Kitajima K, Kaji Y, Fukabori Y, et al. Prostate cancer detection with 3 T MRI: comparison of diffusion-weighted imaging and dynamic contrast-enhanced MRI in combination with T2-weighted imaging. J Magn Reson Imaging 2010;31:625–31.

25. Haider MA, van der Kwast TH, Tanguay J, et al. Combined T2-weighted and diffusion-weighted MRI for localization of prostate cancer. AJR Am J Roentgenol 2007;189:323–8.

26. Gibbs P, Liney GP, Pickles MD, et al. Correlation of ADC and T2 measurements with cell density in prostate cancer at 3.0 Tesla. Invest Radiol 2009;44:572–6.

27. Zelhof B, Pickles M, Liney G, et al. Correlation of diffusion-weighted magnetic resonance data with cellularity in prostate cancer. BJU Int 2009;103:883–8.

28. Oto A, Kayhan A, Jiang Y, et al. Prostate cancer: differentiation of central gland cancer from benign prostatic hyperplasia by using diffusion-weighted and dynamic contrast-enhanced MR imaging. Radiology 2010;257:715–23.

29. Rosenkrantz AB, Kim S, Campbell N, et al. Transition zone prostate cancer: revisiting the role of multiparametric MRI at 3 T. AJR Am J Roentgenol 2015;204:W266–72.

30. Ward E, Baad M, Peng Y, et al. Multi-parametric MR imaging of the anterior fibromuscular stroma and its differentiation from prostate cancer. Abdom Radiol (NY) 2017;42:926–34.

31. Verma S, Turkbey B, Muradyan N, et al. Overview of dynamic contrast-enhanced MRI in prostate cancer diagnosis and management. AJR Am J Roentgenol 2012;198:1277–88.

32. Russo G, Mischi M, Scheepens W, et al. Angiogenesis in prostate cancer: onset, progression and imaging. BJU Int 2012;110:E794–808.

33. Engelbrecht MR, Huisman HJ, Laheij RJ, et al. Discrimination of prostate cancer from normal peripheral zone and central gland tissue by using dynamic contrast-enhanced MR imaging. Radiology 2003;229:248–54.

34. Turkbey B, Pinto PA, Mani H, et al. Prostate cancer: value of multiparametric MR imaging at 3 T for detection–histopathologic correlation. Radiology 2010;255:89–99.

35. Tan CH, Hobbs BP, Wei W, et al. Dynamic contrast-enhanced MRI for the detection of prostate cancer: meta-analysis. AJR Am J Roentgenol 2015;204:W439–48.

36. Vargas HA, Hotker AM, Goldman DA, et al. Updated prostate imaging reporting and data system (PIRADS v2) recommendations for the detection of clinically significant prostate cancer using multiparametric MRI: critical evaluation using whole-mount pathology as standard of reference. Eur Radiol 2016;26:1606–12.

37. De Visschere P, Lumen N, Ost P, et al. Dynamic contrast-enhanced imaging has limited added value over T2-weighted imaging and diffusion-weighted imaging when using PI-RADSv2 for diagnosis of clinically significant prostate cancer in patients with elevated PSA. Clin Radiol 2017;72:23–32.

38. Lin WC, Muglia VF, Silva GE, et al. Multiparametric MRI of the prostate: diagnostic performance and

interreader agreement of two scoring systems. Br J Radiol 2016;89:20151056.

39. Lin WC, Westphalen AC, Silva GE, et al. Comparison of PI-RADS 2, ADC histogram-derived parameters, and their combination for the diagnosis of peripheral zone prostate cancer. Abdom Radiol (NY) 2016;41: 2209–17.

40. Muller BG, Shih JH, Sankineni S, et al. Prostate cancer: interobserver agreement and accuracy with the revised prostate imaging reporting and data system at multiparametric MR imaging. Radiology 2015; 277(3):741–50.

41. Woo S, Suh CH, Kim SY, et al. Diagnostic performance of prostate imaging reporting and data system version 2 for detection of prostate cancer: a systematic review and diagnostic meta-analysis. Eur Urol 2017;72(2):177–88.

42. Mertan FV, Greer MD, Shih JH, et al. Prospective evaluation of the prostate imaging reporting and data system version 2 for prostate cancer detection. J Urol 2016;196:690–6.

43. Rosenkrantz AB, Ginocchio LA, Cornfeld D, et al. Interobserver reproducibility of the PI-RADS version 2 lexicon: a multicenter study of six experienced prostate radiologists. Radiology 2016;280:793–804.

44. deSouza NM, Riches SF, Vanas NJ, et al. Diffusion-weighted magnetic resonance imaging: a potential non-invasive marker of tumour aggressiveness in localized prostate cancer. Clin Radiol 2008;63: 774–82.

45. Tamada T, Sone T, Jo Y, et al. Apparent diffusion coefficient values in peripheral and transition zones of the prostate: comparison between normal and malignant prostatic tissues and correlation with histologic grade. J Magn Reson Imaging 2008;28:720–6.

46. Nagarajan R, Margolis D, Raman S, et al. Correlation of Gleason scores with diffusion-weighted imaging findings of prostate cancer. Adv Urol 2012;2012: 374805.

47. Vargas HA, Akin O, Franiel T, et al. Diffusion-weighted endorectal MR imaging at 3 T for prostate cancer: tumor detection and assessment of aggressiveness. Radiology 2011;259:775–84.

48. Turkbey B, Shah VP, Pang Y, et al. Is apparent diffusion coefficient associated with clinical risk scores for prostate cancers that are visible on 3-T MR images? Radiology 2011;258:488–95.

49. Kim CK, Park SY, Park JJ, et al. Diffusion-weighted MRI as a predictor of extracapsular extension in prostate cancer. AJR Am J Roentgenol 2014;202: W270–6.

50. Kim CK, Park BK, Kim B. Diffusion-weighted MRI at 3 T for the evaluation of prostate cancer. AJR Am J Roentgenol 2010;194:1461–9.

51. Jambor I, Merisaari H, Taimen P, et al. Evaluation of different mathematical models for diffusion-weighted imaging of normal prostate and prostate cancer

using high b-values: a repeatability study. Magn Reson Med 2015;73:1988–98.

52. Rosenkrantz AB, Padhani AR, Chenevert TL, et al. Body diffusion kurtosis imaging: basic principles, applications, and considerations for clinical practice. J Magn Reson Imaging 2015;42:1190–202.

53. Le Bihan D, Breton E, Lallemand D, et al. Separation of diffusion and perfusion in intravoxel incoherent motion MR imaging. Radiology 1988;168:497–505.

54. Shinmoto H, Oshio K, Tanimoto A, et al. Biexponential apparent diffusion coefficients in prostate cancer. Magn Reson Imaging 2009;27:355–9.

55. Shinmoto H, Tamura C, Soga S, et al. An intravoxel incoherent motion diffusion-weighted imaging study of prostate cancer. AJR Am J Roentgenol 2012;199: W496–500.

56. Kuru TH, Roethke MC, Stieltjes B, et al. Intravoxel incoherent motion (IVIM) diffusion imaging in prostate cancer: what does it add? J Comput Assist Tomogr 2014;38:558–64.

57. Rosenkrantz AB, Sigmund EE, Johnson G, et al. Prostate cancer: feasibility and preliminary experience of a diffusional kurtosis model for detection and assessment of aggressiveness of peripheral zone cancer. Radiology 2012;264:126–35.

58. Roethke MC, Kuder TA, Kuru TH, et al. Evaluation of diffusion kurtosis imaging versus standard diffusion imaging for detection and grading of peripheral zone prostate cancer. Invest Radiol 2015;50:483–9.

59. Tamada T, Prabhu V, Li J, et al. Prostate cancer: diffusion-weighted MR imaging for detection and assessment of aggressiveness-comparison between conventional and kurtosis models. Radiology 2017;284(1):100–8.

60. Hansford BG, Peng Y, Jiang Y, et al. Dynamic contrast-enhanced MR imaging curve-type analysis: is it helpful in the differentiation of prostate cancer from healthy peripheral zone? Radiology 2015;275:448–57.

61. Isebaert S, De Keyzer F, Haustermans K, et al. Evaluation of semi-quantitative dynamic contrast-enhanced MRI parameters for prostate cancer in correlation to whole-mount histopathology. Eur J Radiol 2012;81:e217–22.

62. Sourbron SP, Buckley DL. Classic models for dynamic contrast-enhanced MRI. NMR Biomed 2013; 26:1004–27.

63. Vos EK, Litjens GJ, Kobus T, et al. Assessment of prostate cancer aggressiveness using dynamic contrast-enhanced magnetic resonance imaging at 3 T. Eur Urol 2013;64:448–55.

64. Langer DL, van der Kwast TH, Evans AJ, et al. Prostate tissue composition and MR measurements: investigating the relationships between ADC, T2, K(trans), v(e), and corresponding histologic features. Radiology 2010;255:485–94.

65. Starobinets O, Korn N, Iqbal S, et al. Practical aspects of prostate MRI: hardware and software

considerations, protocols, and patient preparation. Abdom Radiol (NY) 2016;41:817–30.

66. Jung JA, Coakley FV, Vigneron DB, et al. Prostate depiction at endorectal MR spectroscopic imaging: investigation of a standardized evaluation system. Radiology 2004;233:701–8.

67. Kurhanewicz J, Vigneron DB. Advances in MR spectroscopy of the prostate. Magn Reson Imaging Clin N Am 2008;16:697–710, ix–x.

68. Polanec SH, Pinker-Domenig K, Brader P, et al. Multiparametric MRI of the prostate at 3 T: limited value of 3D (1)H-MR spectroscopy as a fourth parameter. World J Urol 2016;34:649–56.

69. Platzek I, Borkowetz A, Toma M, et al. Multiparametric prostate magnetic resonance imaging at 3 T: failure of magnetic resonance spectroscopy to provide added value. J Comput Assist Tomogr 2015;39(5): 674–80.

70. Nketiah G, Elschot M, Kim E, et al. T2-weighted MRI-derived textural features reflect prostate cancer aggressiveness: preliminary results. Eur Radiol 2016;27(7):3050–9.

71. Litjens GJ, Barentsz JO, Karssemeijer N, et al. Clinical evaluation of a computer-aided diagnosis system for determining cancer aggressiveness in prostate MRI. Eur Radiol 2015;25(11):3187–99.

Multiparametric Prostate MR Imaging: Impact on Clinical Staging and Decision Making

Petar Duvnjak, MD[a,b], Ariel A. Schulman, MD[c],
Jamie N. Holtz, MD[a], Jiaoti Huang, MD, PhD[d,e],
Thomas J. Polascik, MD[c,e], Rajan T. Gupta, MD[a,c,e,*]

KEYWORDS

- Prostate cancer • Multiparametric MR imaging (mpMRI) • Staging

KEY POINTS

- The current paradigm for prostate cancer staging is changing with increased incorporation of multi-parametric MR imaging (mpMRI) into clinical decision making.
- MpMRI has proved useful in differentiating organ-confined disease (stage $\leq$T2) from locally advanced (stage $\geq$T3) disease due to the high sensitivity and specificity for the detection of extraprostatic extension (EPE) and seminal vesicle invasion (SVI).
- Much work on mpMRI is forthcoming regarding the use of mpMRI in preoperative volumetric tumor assessment, improving biopsy targeting of transrectal ultrasound (TRUS)-negative tumors, and selection and follow-up of men on active surveillance.

INTRODUCTION

Prostate cancer is the most common noncutaneous malignancy and second leading cause of cancer-related deaths in men in the United States, with an estimated 180,890 new cases and 26,120 deaths in 2016.[1] The overall 5-year survival rate is relatively high and has increased from 83% in the 1980s to 99% from 2005 to 2011, in part due to earlier detection and earlier aggressive therapy for high-risk disease. Despite the overall high 5-year survival rate, outcomes are variable, ranging from near 100% survival in organ-confined disease to as low as 28% survival

This project was performed at the Departments of Radiology, Pathology, and Surgery at Duke University Medical Center.

There is no external or internal funding for this project. This article is not under consideration elsewhere.

Financial Disclosures/Conflicts of Interest relevant to this submitted work: Dr R.T. Gupta has no financial disclosures or conflicts of interest related to this work. Dr R.T. Gupta does serve as a consultant to Bayer Pharma AG and Invivo Corp. Dr R.T. Gupta also serves on the Speakers Bureau for Bayer Pharma AG. Dr P. Duvnjak, Dr A.A. Schulman, Dr J.N. Holtz, Dr J. Huang, and Dr T.J. Polascik have no conflicts of interest.

[a] Department of Radiology, Duke University Medical Center, DUMC Box 3808, Durham, NC 27710, USA; [b] Department of Radiology, Medical College of Wisconsin, 9200 West Wisconsin Avenue, Milwaukee, WI 53226, USA; [c] Division of Urologic Surgery, Department of Surgery, Duke Prostate Center, Duke University Medical Center, DUMC Box 2804, Durham, NC 27710, USA; [d] Department of Pathology, Duke University Medical Center, DUMC Box 3712, Durham, NC 27710, USA; [e] Duke Cancer Institute, DUMC Box 3917, Durham, NC 27710, USA

* Corresponding author. Department of Radiology, Duke University Medical Center, DUMC Box 3808, Durham, NC 27710.

E-mail address: rajan.gupta@duke.edu

in more advanced stages.[2] Studies have shown that many men with low-risk disease in the United States are overtreated, resulting in significant economic impact and individual morbidity associated with aggressive therapy.[3]

In the past decade, there have been meaningful changes in the approach to the diagnosis, characterization, and management of clinically localized prostate cancer. These have become increasingly defined by more selective population screening, integration of novel diagnostic tools, and increased acceptance of active surveillance and partial ablative strategies as viable management strategies.[4] These trends have driven demand for optimized prostate imaging. The need for accurate pretherapy staging is, therefore, paramount for risk stratification with the ultimate goals of preventing overtreatment of low-risk disease in favor of active surveillance and selection of the optimal early aggressive intervention in high-risk disease. The aim of this article is to review the current and changing paradigm in prostate cancer staging with specific emphasis on the evolving role of multiparametric MR imaging (mpMRI) and how it is being integrated into clinical decision making.

OVERVIEW OF PROSTATE CANCER STAGING AND CLINICAL NOMOGRAMS

Clinical and pathologic staging is most widely performed according to the American Joint Committee on Cancer (AJCC) 2010 TNM classification system, which incorporates clinical T stage (based on digital rectal examination [DRE]) and, if available, serum prostate-specific antigen (PSA) and Gleason score.[5] The AJCC Cancer Staging Manual, eighth edition, recently released, incorporates several important changes to the current prostate cancer staging paradigm. Notably, the eighth edition includes the prostate prognostic group grade to histopathologic assessment, which is to be reported along with the Gleason score. Additionally, pathologic staging no longer subcategorizes pT2 due to increased emphasis placed on tumor volume over laterality, because this has been shown to have more practical and prognostic significance.[6]

Numerous clinical nomograms have been developed over the years that take into account various parameters to predict pathologic stage at radical prostatectomy.[7] One of the most widely used clinical nomograms are the Partin tables, which factor in a patient's clinical T stage, serum PSA, and Gleason score.[8,9] The Memorial Sloan Kettering nomogram includes percent positive cores from transrectal ultrasound (TRUS)-guided biopsy and

the University of California, San Francisco, Cancer of the Prostate Risk Assessment scoring system also includes the patient age.[10,11]

The current paradigm for prostate cancer diagnosis centers on performing systematic 12-core TRUS-guided biopsy in men with elevated PSA or positive DRE. Aside from issues related to the morbidity of the procedure, there are several well documented limitations to this approach.[12] On one hand, undersampling can occur and has been shown to lead to false-negative biopsy results in up to 30% of cases, particularly in men with larger glands or those with anterior prostate cancers.[13] Undersampling can also lead to inaccurate risk stratification in some men. For example, a 2010 prospective study of 1565 patients showed that 47% of men classified as low-risk (≤Gleason 6) who may have been potential candidates for active surveillance were actually upgraded to Gleason 7 or greater after prostatectomy.[14] Attempts to overcome undersampling errors by increasing the number of core samples by performing serial biopsies have been shown to increase the overall cancer detection rate; however, in 1 study, a majority of these cases were classified as clinically insignificant (75 of 119 cases).[15]

INTEGRATION OF MULTIPARAMETRIC MR IMAGING INTO CLINICAL ALGORITHMS AND STAGING SYSTEMS
Detection and Characterization of Prostate Cancer with Multiparametric MR Imaging

mpMRI has the potential to overcome many of the shortcomings associated with TRUS biopsy systems and has proved valuable for improving the detection of higher-grade disease (histologic Gleason score) and higher-stage disease (extraprostatic extension [EPE] and tumor volume), thereby offering a more complete clinical picture for clinical decision making. In some studies, mpMRI has been shown to increase cancer detection rates and lead to pathologic upgrading in up to 38% of cases in men with persistent clinical suspicion of prostate cancer despite prior negative biopsy.[16] A recent prospective National Institutes of Health study on 1003 men with elevated PSA or positive DRE who underwent mpMRI compared random TRUS biopsy and magnetic resonance (MR) fusion–guided biopsy. They demonstrated a 30% increase in the diagnosis of high-risk disease and a 17% decrease in the detection of low-risk disease in the targeted MR-biopsy group. For men in the series who underwent radical prostatectomy, targeted biopsy alone was the best discriminator between low-risk and intermediate/high-risk disease.[17] Radtke and colleagues[18] also found that integration of MR fusion biopsy decreases the detection of clinically insignificant disease (Gleason score 3 + 3).

mpMRI also has a growing role in the initial evaluation of men without a histologic diagnosis of cancer. Although the utility of mpMRI in men with an elevated PSA but negative TRUS biopsy is well established, there is particular recent interest in mpMRI before biopsy.[19] As noted in the Prostate MR Imaging Study (PROMIS), Ahmed and colleagues[20] demonstrated the potential benefit of mpMRI in the prebiopsy setting with markedly better sensitivity and negative predictive value compared with TRUS biopsy. The investigators found that using mpMRI to select men for biopsy could decrease primary biopsies by 27% and reduce detection of clinically insignificant cancer by 5% and suggested that men with a negative mpMRI can forgo biopsy. It must be recognized, however, that of the 158 nonsuspicious mpMRIs in the study, 17 men (10.8%) harbored clinically significant cancer. Thus, although an increasingly important role of mpMRI before biopsy is recognized, the authors believe that current evidence supports the need for additional systematic TRUS biopsies as well as any targeted biopsies to maximize detection of clinically significant, MR imaging–negative cancers. Yin and colleagues[21] recently proposed a diagnostic algorithm that integrates prebiopsy mpMRI, TRUS biopsy, and targeted biopsy for MR-suspicious lesions and the use of molecular markers to improve risk stratification.

Role of Multiparametric MR Imaging in Clinical Staging

With the emerging role of mpMRI, the current paradigm of prostate cancer staging is shifting, with increased emphasis placed on incorporating mpMRI into clinical staging nomograms. mpMRI-specific staging systems have been developed, one of which is summarized in **Table 1**.[22] There has been a rapidly growing body of literature over the past several years demonstrating the potential utility of mpMRI in prostate cancer staging. For example, a 2012 retrospective study of 388 men with clinically low-risk prostate cancer showed that mpMRI obtained with endorectal coils (ERCs) at 1.5T and 3T could help predict findings on confirmatory biopsy, therefore aiding in stratifying patients eligible for active surveillance versus definitive treatment.[23] There have also been several recent studies that show the benefit of mpMRI compared with clinical staging nomograms in predicting organ-confined disease. For example, work done by the authors' group demonstrated that the predictive accuracy of mpMRI was significantly greater than the Partin tables in predicting organ-confined disease, with a positive predictive value of 91.2% and negative predictive value of 89.7%.[22] Similar studies have shown that the addition of preoperative mpMRI to clinical nomograms improves the predictive accuracy for detection of EPE compared with clinical nomograms alone.[24–26] A more recent study of 158 patients by the authors' group validated mpMRI staging as a valuable stand-alone test for predicting organ-confined disease (area under the curve [AUC] 0.88) compared with Partin tables (AUC 0.70).[27]

MR Imaging Stage	Stage Description
	Table 1 **Multiparametric MR imaging staging for prostate cancer**
T1	No lesions considered suspicious for cancer
T2a	Unilateral lesion(s) highly suspicious for cancer, occupying <50% of the affected side of the gland
T2b	Unilateral lesion(s) highly suspicious for cancer, occupying >50% of the affected side of the gland
T2c	Bilateral lesion(s) highly suspicious for cancer
T3a	High degree of suspicion for extracapsular extension (unilateral or bilateral) without invasion of seminal vesicles
T3b	High degree of suspicion of SVI(s) without involvement of adjacent structures
T4	Tumor invades adjacent structures other than the seminal vesicles, such as the external sphincter, rectum, bladder, levator muscles, and pelvic wall

Adapted from Gupta RT, Faridi KF, Singh AA, et al. Comparing 3-T multiparametric MR Imaging and the Partin tables to predict organ-confined prostate cancer after radical prostatectomy. Urol Oncol 2014;32(8):1293; with permission.

mpMRI also improves tumor staging with better assessment of the anterior gland, detection of non–organ-confined disease, and estimates of tumor volume. Kongnyuy and colleagues[28] showed the value of mpMRI in detecting anterior lesions classically missed by TRUS biopsy, which in most cases represented the highest-grade tumor in a respective gland (**Fig. 1**). mpMRI also offers a novel way to estimate tumor volume more accurately than conventional staging. Bratan and colleagues[29] examined a cohort of 202 men who underwent mpMRI before prostatectomy and showed that mpMRI volume estimates were most accurate for tumors with the highest Likert suspicion scores and Gleason score greater than or equal to 7.

Multiparametric MR imaging in detecting T3 disease

One of the most important decision points in the management of prostate cancer is the detection of locally advanced (T3) versus organ-confined (T2 or lower) disease. Detection of EPE, seminal vesicle invasion (SVI), and neurovascular bundle involvement not only affects outcome but also can alter the surgical approach. A 2012 prospective study on 104 patients undergoing prostatectomy showed that preoperative mpMRI altered the initial surgical plan with respect to neurovascular bundle sparing 27% of the time, switching to nerve-sparing technique in 17 of 104 patients and to non–nerve-sparing in 11 patients, demonstrating the ability of mpMRI to accurately predict neurovascular bundle involvement prospectively.[30] Similarly, a more recent study of 122 men receiving mpMRI with ERC at 3T showed that management decisions were changed in a risk-dependent manner. In this study, treatment decisions were altered 18% of the time after mpMRI, occurring in 9%, 18%, and 33% of low-risk, intermediate-risk, and high-risk patients, respectively.[31] The data regarding the accuracy of mpMRI for detection of locally advanced disease has been heterogeneous, largely in part due

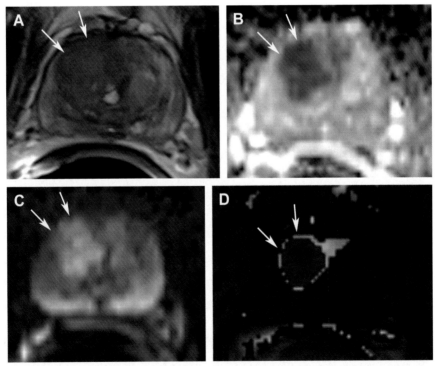

Fig. 1. A 73-year-old man with a serum PSA level of 12.2 ng/mL and negative TRUS-guided biopsy was referred for mpMRI with ERC to assess for prostate cancer due to rising PSA. (*A*) Axial T2WI shows a large region of decreased T2 signal with poorly defined margins in the right anterior midtransition zone (TZ) (*arrows*). This lesion does not demonstrate gross EPE but there is broad-based contact with the anterior fibromuscular stroma and prostate margin. (*B*) Axial apparent diffusion coefficient (ADC) map and (*C*) axial high *b*-value DWIs (*b* = 1400 s/mm^2) demonstrate corresponding marked restricted diffusion (*arrows*). (*D*) Colored perfusion map created using postprocessing software from dynamic contrast-enhanced MR imaging acquisition demonstrates suspicious perfusion kinetics for prostate cancer (*arrows*), corresponding to the findings seen on T2WI and ADC/DWI. PI-RADS score is 5. The patient underwent radical prostatectomy revealing Gleason 4 + 3 = 7 cancer in right anterior TZ with focal EPE.

to differences in MR imaging technique (ie, use of an ERC or varying field strengths) and variable reader experience. A recent meta-analysis of 75 studies, incorporating 9796 patients, reported sensitivities in the high 50% range and specificities in the 90% range for detection of EPE and SVI.[32] Similar results were achieved in a more recent systematic review of 62 studies for the detection of EPE or SVI, although the significant heterogeneity among studies within these analyses potentially limits generalizability.[33]

One of the major hurdles that needs to be addressed as it pertains to mpMRI's role in prostate cancer staging is the great variability between the experienced and nonexperienced prostate MR imaging reader. Although prostate MR imaging has been around for approximately 3 decades, recent advances in research and technology have led to a boom in prostate MR imaging interest, and in turn, a high demand for high-quality mpMRI. There is a substantial learning curve associated with this imaging technique and the lack of experience can lead to some of the discrepancies between dedicated readers who have received training and nonexperienced prostate MR imaging readers. A recent retrospective study of 133 patients at a single community hospital who underwent radical prostatectomy demonstrated sensitivity and specificity for the detection of EPE of 12.5% and 93%, respectively.[34] Similarly, Tay and colleagues[26] showed that the addition of a mpMRI standard read did not significantly improve the detection of EPE over clinical nomograms; however, the addition of a second, subspecialized read improved specificity of organ confined status from 44% to 81%. More recent studies from experienced readers at 3T have demonstrated higher performance for the detection of EPE, with sensitivities and specificities as high as 95% and 100%, respectively.[35–37] A 2014 study by Otto and colleagues[38] showed that mpMRI performed at 3T has an accuracy of 97% and sensitivity/specificity near 100% for the detection of SVI and approximately 80% accuracy for the detection of EPE.

Some of this heterogeneity in reader performance can be mitigated by implementing a standardized reporting system, such as the Prostate Imaging—Reporting and Data System (PI-RADS). This system has proved a helpful tool in standardizing prostate MR imaging interpretations and reducing variability among readers with varying levels of experience. Currently in its second iteration, PI-RADS continues to evolve to facilitate the integration of mpMRI into clinical practice.[39] Another factor that can reduce reader heterogeneity is dedicated training programs. The effect of having a dedicated education program has also been shown to significantly increase the diagnostic accuracy for detection of dominant index cancers, anterior cancers, Gleason grade and reader confidence.[40] To harness the full potential of mpMRI, the continuing need for education is paramount and many additional training resources, in the form of hands-on courses and workshops, among other methods of self-study, are available to those with interest.[41]

Extraprostatic Extension

The International Society of Urological Pathology (ISUP) defines EPE as "the presence of tumor beyond the confines of the prostate."[42] Although a seemingly straightforward definition, EPE can be extremely difficult to diagnose both on mpMRI and on pathologic specimens because the prostate lacks a true "capsule" and determining the border between prostate parenchyma and periprostatic soft tissue is somewhat arbitrary. Pathologically, EPE upstages the tumor to pT3a (EPE or microscopic invasion of the bladder neck) or pT3b (SVI).[5] In comparison to stage pT3b disease, detection of subtle pT3a disease in the form of microscopic invasion/EPE on mpMRI is less reliable, with some reported sensitivities as low as 43% in academic centers and 12.5% in community practice.[34] This is largely due to the fact that SVI occurs in aggressive or advanced-stage tumors whereas less aggressive tumors may only show subtle signs of EPE. For mpMRI to be valuable in staging of disease, it is critical for mpMRI to be able to reliably detect EPE and thereby differentiate non–organ-confined T3 disease from organ-confined disease.

At a 2009 ISUP consensus meeting, the most reliable histologic feature for EPE in the posterior and posterolateral gland is the presence of tumor admixed with periprostatic fat. Diagnosis of EPE in the anterior gland and apex is much more difficult and there is less consensus among pathologists given the lack of periprostatic fat and the fact that prostate stroma blends in with the bladder smooth muscle.[42] Imaging criteria for assessing EPE on mpMRI take advantage of the high anatomic and spatial resolution of T2-weighted MR imaging (T2WI). Detection of EPE on T2WI centers on alterations in morphologic features of the normal prostatic capsule, including asymmetry and contour changes, anatomic narrowing of the rectoprostatic angle, and altered morphology of the neurovascular bundles with loss of surrounding fat planes (**Fig. 2**). Further discussion of the criteria for EPE can be referenced in the latest PI-RADS, Version 2 document.[43] The

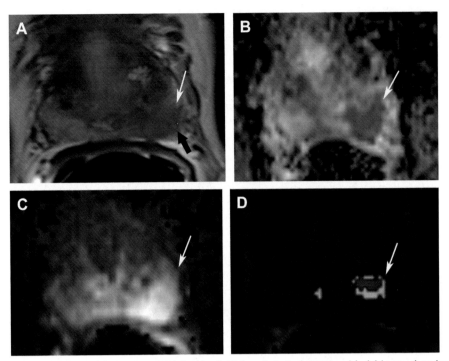

Fig. 2. A 57-year-old man with a serum PSA level of 10.3 ng/mL and TRUS-guided biopsy showing Gleason 4 + 3 = 7 cancer (4/8 cores, 60%–90% each) throughout the left gland. (A) Axial T2WI shows a large area of decreased T2 signal intensity in the left base and midlateral peripheral zone (PZ) (*white arrow*). There is associated irregularity and spiculation of the periprostatic fat (*black solid arrow*). (B) Axial ADC map and (C) axial high b-value DWI (b = 1400 s/mm²) demonstrate corresponding marked restricted diffusion (*arrows*). (D) Suspicious enhancement kinetics are shown, corresponding to the findings on T2WI and DWI (*arrow*). PI-RADS score is 5 with evidence of gross EPE. The patient underwent radical prostatectomy revealing Gleason 4 + 3 = 7 cancer in the left PZ with EPE at the left base.

length of capsular contact on T2WI has recently been shown one of the most sensitive criteria for detection of EPE with reduced inter-reader variability compared with subjective interpretations using threshold lengths of 10 mm for gross EPE and 6 mm for focal EPE.[44] A similar study showed that tumor contact length (with a threshold value of 12.5 mm) was an independent predictor for EPE (AUC 0.71) (Fig. 3).[45]

With regard to EPE detection, a multiparametric MR imaging approach has been shown to increase accuracy. For example, a 2007 study by Bloch and colleagues[46] reported a significant increase in sensitivity (>25%) with an accuracy of 95% for the detection of EPE when using a multiparametric approach compared with T2WI alone. Diffusion-weighted imaging (DWI) has also been shown to be an independent marker for side-specific assessment of EPE with a comparable accuracy to T2WI and better inter-reader agreement and sensitivity for subtle (<2 mm) EPE.[47] More recently, a study of 117 patients by Woo and colleagues[48] demonstrated that DWI adds incremental value in detecting EPE when there is low suspicion on

T2WI. Dynamic contrast-enhanced MR imaging has not been shown as effective in assessing EPE as DWI when combined with T2WI.[49]

Seminal Vesicle Invasion

The detection of SVI on mpMRI is one of the most reliable markers for EPE and easier to diagnose compared with T3a disease given the high spatial resolution of T2WI and aggressive nature of stage T3b tumors. The incidence of SVI in high-risk prostate cancer is relatively low, reported at 7% in some surgical series,[50] but this diagnosis is critical to make on mpMRI because the presence of SVI can preclude surgical intervention in some cases. In general, mpMRI has been shown highly specific for the detection of SVI; however, the data regarding sensitivity of SVI detection are mixed, with some studies reporting sensitivities as low as 44%.[51] A recent meta-analysis by de Rooij and colleagues[32] reported overall sensitivities for SVI of 51% and 59% without and with the use an ERC. Furthermore, they reported increased sensitivity for SVI when using a multiparametric

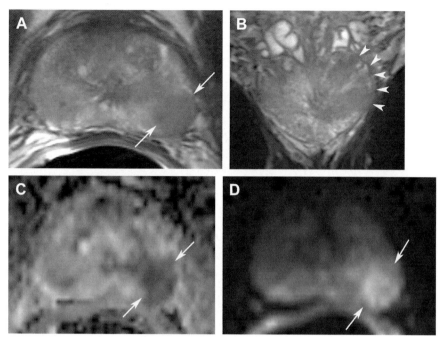

Fig. 3. A 51-year-old man with a serum PSA of 8 ng/nL and TRUS-guided biopsy showing Gleason 4 + 3 = 7 cancer (8/12 cores, 35%–100% each). (*A*) Axial T2WI shows a large area of decreased T2 signal intensity in the left posterolateral peripheral zone at the level of the base to midgland (*arrows*). (*B*) Coronal T2WI shows the large area of decreased T2 signal intensity in the left posterolateral peripheral zone at the level of the base to midgland with broad-based capsular contact (>1 cm) without gross evidence of EPE (*arrowheads*). (*C*) Axial ADC map and (*D*) axial high *b*-value DWI (*b* = 1400 s/mm²) demonstrate corresponding marked restricted diffusion (*arrows*). PI-RADS score is 5 based on lesion size with no evidence of gross EPE but the presence of broad-based capsular contact is suspicious for microscopic EPE. The patient underwent radical prostatectomy revealing Gleason 3 + 4 = 7 cancer in the left PZ with microscopic EPE in the midgland and base.

approach compared with T2WI alone, with sensitivities increasing from 53% to 64%. They also showed that there was no overall significant difference between field strength (1.5T vs 3T); however, sensitivity at 1.5 T was highest with the use of an ERC (62% vs 37%). The reported sensitivity at 3T was higher without the use of an ERC (65% vs 45%), potentially due to the increasing susceptibility effects at higher field strengths. The highest overall sensitivity for SVI detection was found when combing 3T with a multiparametric approach (73% sensitivity and 95% specificity).[32] Criteria for SVI can be found in the latest PI-RADS, Version 2 document and include direct extension of low T2WI signal tumor directly into the seminal vesicles with associated restricted diffusion (**Fig. 4**).[43]

Nodal and Metastatic Staging

The current staging and management algorithms for patients with newly diagnosed prostate cancer are complex, taking into account numerous clinical factors, the T stage, and various nomograms to predict the probability of nodal or distant metastatic disease.[52] Stage N1 disease is defined as involvement of 1 or more regional pelvic nodes, whereas stage M1a is considered involvement of nonregional nodes (ie, common iliac or retroperitoneal nodes). The presence of osseous metastasis denotes stage M1b whereas involvement of other distant sites defines M1c.[5] Nodal staging may be performed with preoperative imaging or at the time of prostatectomy in the form of pelvic lymph node dissection. If performed preoperatively, patients who are high risk (≥T3) or are low risk, with a greater than 10% probability for nodal metastasis based on nomograms, are candidates to undergo pelvic MR imaging or CT to assess for suspicious nodes and receive biopsy if indicated.[52] According to PI-RADS, Version 2, nodes that are enlarged (>8-mm short axis diameter), morphologically abnormal (ie, rounded or spiculated), or hyperenhancing are considered suspicious for metastatic disease.[43] Although the major focus of prostate mpMRI has been on the detection and characterization of disease within and immediately around the prostate, it has been

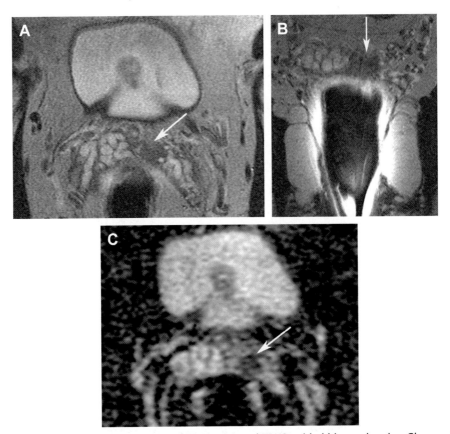

Fig. 4. A 58-year-old man with a serum PSA of 39.1 ng/nL and TRUS-guided biopsy showing Gleason 4 + 3 = 7 throughout the left gland with Gleason 4 + 4 = 8 tumor in the left lateral base. (*A*) Axial and (*B*) coronal T2WIs show a focal region of marked decreased T2 signal in the left seminal vesicles with loss of normal seminal vesicle morphology (*arrows*). (*C*) Axial ADC map demonstrates marked corresponding restricted diffusion at this location (*arrow*). The patient underwent radical prostatectomy revealing Gleason 4 + 3 = 7 cancer in 70% of the gland (left > right) with extensive SVI.

shown that mpMRI may be helpful in the setting of detection of lymph node involvement as well. For instance, a 2015 study showed a low sensitivity (55%) but a high specificity of mpMRI for nodal metastases (90%) in patients with intermediate or high-risk cancer who underwent preoperative node staging with 3T mpMRI and received subsequent extended pelvic lymph node dissection.[53]

With regard to distant metastatic disease staging, the most common site of disease is the skeleton, specifically, the lumbar spine, pelvis, femoral heads, and ribs. Solid organ metastases, on the other hand, are comparatively rare.[54] The current staging algorithms recommend that high-risk patients receive a bone scan and/or CT of the chest, abdomen, and pelvis to evaluate for distant metastatic disease.[52] Given that the bony pelvis, proximal femurs, and lumbar spine are such frequent sites of osseous metastatic disease and are included in the typical field of view in mpMRI, these findings can be depicted on these

staging mpMRI examinations. Vargas and colleagues[55] recently looked at 3765 patients receiving preoperative mpMRI and showed that although a majority of patients (approximately 70%) had incidental bone lesions, the incidence of osseous metastasis was only 1.5%. Furthermore, there were no cases of bone metastases in any of the low-risk patients. As such, the investigators recommended against expanding standard mpMRI protocols to include larger field of views than currently performed to evaluate for distant sites of osseous metastatic lesions.

IMAGING PITFALLS AND LIMITATIONS OF MULTIPARAMETRIC MR IMAGING STAGING

A variety of imaging pitfalls of mpMRI have been previously described, including normal anatomic structures and benign entities that mimic prostate tumors as well as various technical limitations.[56–58] This topic is discussed in further detail later in this issue; however, it is important to recognize that postbiopsy hemorrhage, susceptibility artifact from hip prostheses, and misinterpretation of the normal periprostatic venous plexus and neurovascular bundles all may lead to overestimation of index tumor size or an incorrect diagnosis of EPE.[56,57] As it pertains to postbiopsy hemorrhage, the presence of blood products may mask underlying tumor, and the "MR imaging exclusion sign" has been described, which aids in detection of tumor in the presence of background hemorrhage.[59]

Although suspicious mpMRI findings improve risk stratification, potential limitations of mpMRI must also be recognized. As it pertains to estimation of tumor volume, Priester and colleagues[60] compared mpMRI visible lesions to whole-mount prostatectomy specimens in 114 men and found that the median tumor had a 13.5-mm maximal extent beyond the MR imaging contour and 80% of cancer volume from matched tumors was outside region of interest boundaries. Le Nobin and colleagues[61] similarly demonstrated MR volumetric underestimation and noted that it was more likely to occur in lesions with an imaging suspicion score greater than or equal to 4 or histologic Gleason score greater than or equal to 7. Truong and colleagues[62] reviewed 22 prostatectomy specimens and found that the architectural variations of Gleason score 4 lesions greater than or equal to 0.5 cm had an impact on MR visibility, specifically that only 5/14 (36%) of Gleason 4 cribriform lesions were seen on mpMRI. Thus, the authors advocate both targeted biopsy of MR suspicious lesions and systematic biopsy of the remaining gland to minimize underdetection, undergrading, or understaging of disease.

It is also important to recognize that the pretest probability of adverse pathology reflected by D'Amico risk has an impact on the predictive utility of mpMRI. Somford and colleagues[63] examined a risk-mixed cohort of 183 men who underwent mpMRI followed by radical prostatectomy and found that the positive predictive value of mpMRI for detecting EPE was highest in high-risk men (88.8%) whereas the negative predictive value was greatest in low-risk men (87.7%).

IMPACT OF MULTIPARAMETRIC MR IMAGING ON CLINICAL DECISION MAKING AND FUTURE DIRECTIONS

In recent years, mpMRI has assumed an increasingly important role in multiple aspects of the initial diagnosis, staging, and management of prostate cancer. As the use of mpMRI expands, communication between the treating physician and interpreting radiologist has become increasingly important to continually optimize the collaborative process and highlight the most clinically relevant aspects of a particular case. As management of localized prostate cancer has become more nuanced, mpMRI findings have become increasingly useful in initiating and maintaining appropriate men on active surveillance, planning partial gland ablation, and informing surgical decisions. Several recent studies have demonstrated the utility of mpMRI in confirming candidacy for active surveillance, improving biopsy targeting of occult higher-grade disease missed by TRUS biopsy, and follow-up of men on active surveillance.[64–66] mpMRI may also play a central role in the growing practice of partial gland ablation with particular recent growth in focal cryotherapy and high-intensity focused ultrasound.[67,68] For men with higher-risk disease undergoing surgery or radiation therapy, mpMRI improves staging of non–organ-confined disease and may optimize the degree of margin sparing in surgery and modulate radiation therapy.[69,70]

Ultimately, mpMRI provides the highest clinical value when it is used as part of a multidisciplinary collaboration between the treating physician and interpreting radiologist. Distinct clinical scenarios have an impact on both the accuracy of information provided by mpMRI and those areas of the study that require special attention. As the use of mpMRI expands, it is critical that the information that it can provide is used while also continuing to identify and address clinical limitations of mpMRI that are particularly important for men on active surveillance or considering partial gland ablation.

REFERENCES

1. Siegel RL, Miller KD, Jemal A. Cancer statistics, 2016. CA Cancer J Clin 2016;66(1):7–30.
2. Miller KD, Siegel RL, Lin CC, et al. Cancer treatment and survivorship statistics, 2016. CA Cancer J Clin 2016;66(4):271–89.
3. Aizer AA, Gu X, Chen MH, et al. Cost implications and complications of overtreatment of low-risk prostate cancer in the United States. J Natl Compr Canc Netw 2015;13(1):61–8.
4. Lavery HJ, Cooperberg MR. Clinically localized prostate cancer in 2017: a review of comparative effectiveness. Urol Oncol 2017;35(2):40–1.
5. Edge SB, Compton CC. The American Joint Committee on Cancer: the 7th edition of the AJCC cancer staging manual and the future of TNM. Ann Surg Oncol 2010;17(6):1471–4.
6. Buyyounouski MK, Choyke PL, McKenney JK, et al. Prostate cancer - major changes in the American Joint Committee on Cancer eighth

edition cancer staging manual. CA Cancer J Clin 2017;67(3):245–53.

7. Ross PL, Scardino PT, Kattan MW. A catalog of prostate cancer nomograms. J Urol 2001;165(5):1562–8.

8. Partin AW, Mangold LA, Lamm DM, et al. Contemporary update of prostate cancer staging nomograms (Partin tables) for the new millennium. Urology 2001;58(6):843–8.

9. Eifler JB, Feng Z, Lin BM, et al. An updated prostate cancer staging nomogram (Partin tables) based on cases from 2006 to 2011. BJU Int 2013;111(1):22–9.

10. Cooperberg MR, Pasta DJ, Elkin EP, et al. The University of California, San Francisco Cancer of the Prostate Risk Assessment score: a straightforward and reliable preoperative predictor of disease recurrence after radical prostatectomy. J Urol 2005; 173(6):1938–42.

11. Ohori M, Kattan MW, Koh H, et al. Predicting the presence and side of extracapsular extension: a nomogram for staging prostate cancer. J Urol 2004;171(5):1844–9 [discussion: 1849].

12. Bjurlin MA, Carter HB, Schellhammer P, et al. Optimization of initial prostate biopsy in clinical practice: sampling, labeling and specimen processing. J Urol 2013;189(6):2039–46.

13. Serefoglu EC, Altinova S, Ugras NS, et al. How reliable is 12-core prostate biopsy procedure in the detection of prostate cancer? Can Urol Assoc J 2013;7(5–6):E293–8.

14. Mufarrij P, Sankin A, Godoy G, et al. Pathologic outcomes of candidates for active surveillance undergoing radical prostatectomy. Urology 2010;76(3): 689–92.

15. Zaytoun OM, Stephenson AJ, Fareed K, et al. When serial prostate biopsy is recommended: most cancers detected are clinically insignificant. BJU Int 2012;110(7):987–92.

16. Bjurlin MA, Meng X, Le Nobin J, et al. Optimization of prostate biopsy: the role of magnetic resonance imaging targeted biopsy in detection, localization and risk assessment. J Urol 2014;192(3):648–58.

17. Siddiqui MM, Rais-Bahrami S, Turkbey B, et al. Comparison of MR/ultrasound fusion-guided biopsy with ultrasound-guided biopsy for the diagnosis of prostate cancer. JAMA 2015;313(4):390–7.

18. Radtke JP, Kuru TH, Boxler S, et al. Comparative analysis of transperineal template saturation prostate biopsy versus magnetic resonance imaging targeted biopsy with magnetic resonance imaging-ultrasound fusion guidance. J Urol 2015;193(1): 87–94.

19. Mendhiratta N, Rosenkrantz AB, Meng X, et al. Magnetic resonance imaging-ultrasound fusion targeted prostate biopsy in a consecutive cohort of men with no previous biopsy: reduction of over detection through improved risk stratification. J Urol 2015; 194(6):1601–6.

20. Ahmed HU, El-Shater Bosaily A, Brown LC, et al. Diagnostic accuracy of multi-parametric MRI and TRUS biopsy in prostate cancer (PROMIS): a paired validating confirmatory study. Lancet 2017; 389(10071):815–22.

21. Yin Y, Zhang Q, Zhang H, et al. Molecular signature to risk-stratify prostate cancer of intermediate risk. Clin Cancer Res 2017;23(1):6–8.

22. Gupta RT, Faridi KF, Singh AA, et al. Comparing 3-T multiparametric MRI and the Partin tables to predict organ-confined prostate cancer after radical prostatectomy. Urol Oncol 2014;32(8):1292–9.

23. Vargas HA, Akin O, Afaq A, et al. Magnetic resonance imaging for predicting prostate biopsy findings in patients considered for active surveillance of clinically low risk prostate cancer. J Urol 2012; 188(5):1732–8.

24. Feng TS, Sharif-Afshar AR, Wu J, et al. Multiparametric MRI improves accuracy of clinical nomograms for predicting extracapsular extension of prostate cancer. Urology 2015;86(2):332–7.

25. Morlacco A, Sharma V, Viers BR, et al. The incremental role of magnetic resonance imaging for prostate cancer staging before radical prostatectomy. Eur Urol 2017;71(5):701–4.

26. Tay KJ, Gupta RT, Brown AF, et al. Defining the incremental utility of prostate multiparametric magnetic resonance imaging at standard and specialized read in predicting extracapsular extension of prostate cancer. Eur Urol 2016;70(2):211–3.

27. Gupta RT, Brown AF, Silverman RK, et al. Can Radiologic staging with multiparametric MRI enhance the accuracy of the Partin tables in predicting organ-confined prostate cancer? AJR Am J Roentgenol 2016;207(1):87–95.

28. Kongnyuy M, Sidana A, George AK, et al. The significance of anterior prostate lesions on multiparametric magnetic resonance imaging in African-American men. Urol Oncol 2016;34(6):254.e15-21.

29. Bratan F, Melodelima C, Souchon R, et al. How accurate is multiparametric MR imaging in evaluation of prostate cancer volume? Radiology 2015;275(1): 144–54.

30. McClure TD, Margolis DJ, Reiter RE, et al. Use of MR imaging to determine preservation of the neurovascular bundles at robotic-assisted laparoscopic prostatectomy. Radiology 2012;262(3):874–83.

31. Liauw SL, Kropp LM, Dess RT, et al. Endorectal MRI for risk classification of localized prostate cancer: radiographic findings and influence on treatment decisions. Urol Oncol 2016;34(9):416.e15-21.

32. de Rooij M, Hamoen EH, Witjes JA, et al. Accuracy of magnetic resonance imaging for local staging of prostate cancer: a diagnostic meta-analysis. Eur Urol 2016;70(2):233–45.

33. Salerno J, Finelli A, Morash C, et al. Multiparametric magnetic resonance imaging for pre-treatment local

staging of prostate cancer: a cancer care Ontario clinical practice guideline. Can Urol Assoc J 2016; 10(9–10):E332–9.

34. Davis R, Salmasi A, Koprowski C, et al. Accuracy of multiparametric magnetic resonance imaging for extracapsular extension of prostate cancer in community practice. Clin Genitourin Cancer 2016;14(6): e617–22.

35. Augustin H, Fritz GA, Ehammer T, et al. Accuracy of 3-Tesla magnetic resonance imaging for the staging of prostate cancer in comparison to the Partin tables. Acta Radiol 2009;50(5):562–9.

36. Cerantola Y, Valerio M, Kawkabani Marchini A, et al. Can 3T multiparametric magnetic resonance imaging accurately detect prostate cancer extracapsular extension? Can Urol Assoc J 2013;7(11–12):E699–703.

37. Xylinas E, Yates DR, Renard-Penna R, et al. Role of pelvic phased array magnetic resonance imaging in staging of prostate cancer specifically in patients diagnosed with clinically locally advanced tumours by digital rectal examination. World J Urol 2013; 31(4):881–6.

38. Otto J, Thormer G, Seiwerts M, et al. Value of endorectal magnetic resonance imaging at 3T for the local staging of prostate cancer. Rofo 2014;186(8): 795–802.

39. Rosenkrantz AB, Oto A, Turkbey B, et al. Prostate imaging reporting and data system (PI-RADS), version 2: a critical look. AJR Am J Roentgenol 2016;206(6):1179–83.

40. Garcia-Reyes K, Passoni NM, Palmeri ML, et al. Detection of prostate cancer with multiparametric MRI (mpMRI): effect of dedicated reader education on accuracy and confidence of index and anterior cancer diagnosis. Abdom Imaging 2015;40(1):134–42.

41. Gupta RT, Spilseth B, Froemming AT. How and why a generation of radiologists must be trained to accurately interpret prostate mpMRI. Abdom Radiol (NY) 2016;41(5):803–4.

42. Magi-Galluzzi C, Evans AJ, Delahunt B, et al. International Society of Urological Pathology (ISUP) consensus conference on handling and staging of radical prostatectomy specimens. Working group 3: extraprostatic extension, lymphovascular invasion and locally advanced disease. Mod Pathol 2011; 24(1):26–38.

43. Weinreb JC, Barentsz JO, Choyke PL, et al. PI-RADS Prostate imaging - reporting and data system: 2015, version 2. Eur Urol 2016;69(1):16–40.

44. Rosenkrantz AB, Shanbhogue AK, Wang A, et al. Length of capsular contact for diagnosing extraprostatic extension on prostate MRI: Assessment at an optimal threshold. J Magn Reson Imaging 2016; 43(4):990–7.

45. Kongnyuy M, Sidana A, George AK, et al. Tumor contact with prostate capsule on magnetic resonance imaging: a potential biomarker for staging and prognosis. Urol Oncol 2017;35(1): 30.e1–8.

46. Bloch BN, Furman-Haran E, Helbich TH, et al. Prostate cancer: accurate determination of extracapsular extension with high-spatial-resolution dynamic contrast-enhanced and T2-weighted MR imaging– initial results. Radiology 2007;245(1):176–85.

47. Rosenkrantz AB, Chandarana H, Gilet A, et al. Prostate cancer: utility of diffusion-weighted imaging as a marker of side-specific risk of extracapsular extension. J Magn Reson Imaging 2013;38(2):312–9.

48. Woo S, Cho JY, Kim SY, et al. Extracapsular extension in prostate cancer: added value of diffusion-weighted MRI in patients with equivocal findings on T2-weighted imaging. AJR Am J Roentgenol 2015;204(2):W168–75.

49. Tan CH, Wei W, Johnson V, et al. Diffusion-weighted MRI in the detection of prostate cancer: meta-analysis. AJR Am J Roentgenol 2012;199(4):822–9.

50. Meeks JJ, Walker M, Bernstein M, et al. Seminal vesicle involvement at salvage radical prostatectomy. BJU Int 2013;111(8):E342–7.

51. Lee H, Kim CK, Park BK, et al. Accuracy of preoperative multiparametric magnetic resonance imaging for prediction of unfavorable pathology in patients with localized prostate cancer undergoing radical prostatectomy. World J Urol 2017;35(6):929–34.

52. Mohler JL, Armstrong AJ, Bahnson RR, et al. Prostate cancer, version 1.2016. J Natl Compr Canc Netw 2016;14(1):19–30.

53. von Below C, Daouacher G, Wassberg C, et al. Validation of 3 T MRI including diffusion-weighted imaging for nodal staging of newly diagnosed intermediate- and high-risk prostate cancer. Clin Radiol 2016;71(4):328–34.

54. Kundra V, Silverman PM, Matin SF, et al. Imaging in oncology from the University of Texas M. D. Anderson Cancer Center: diagnosis, staging, and surveillance of prostate cancer. AJR Am J Roentgenol 2007;189(4):830–44.

55. Vargas HA, Schor-Bardach R, Long N, et al. Prostate cancer bone metastases on staging prostate MRI: prevalence and clinical features associated with their diagnosis. Abdom Radiol (NY) 2017;42(1): 271–7.

56. Rosenkrantz AB, Taneja SS. Radiologist, be aware: ten pitfalls that confound the interpretation of multiparametric prostate MRI. AJR Am J Roentgenol 2014;202(1):109–20.

57. Panebianco V, Barchetti F, Barentsz J, et al. Pitfalls in interpreting mp-MRI of the prostate: a pictorial review with pathologic correlation. Insights Imaging 2015;6(6):611–30.

58. Kitzing YX, Prando A, Varol C, et al. Benign conditions that mimic prostate carcinoma: MR imaging features with histopathologic correlation. Radiographics 2016;36(1):162–75.

59. Purysko AS, Herts BR. Prostate MRI: the hemorrhage exclusion sign. J Urol 2012;188(5):1946–7.

60. Priester A, Natarajan S, Khoshnoodi P, et al. Magnetic resonance imaging underestimation of prostate cancer geometry: use of patient specific molds to correlate images with whole mount pathology. J Urol 2017;197(2):320–6.

61. Le Nobin J, Rosenkrantz AB, Villers A, et al. Image guided focal therapy for magnetic resonance imaging visible prostate cancer: defining a 3-dimensional treatment margin based on magnetic resonance imaging histology co-registration analysis. J Urol 2015; 194(2):364–70.

62. Truong M, Hollenberg G, Weinberg E, et al. Impact of Gleason subtype on prostate cancer detection using multiparametric Magnetic Resonance Imaging: correlation with final histopathology. J Urol 2017. [Epub ahead of print].

63. Somford DM, Hamoen EH, Futterer JJ, et al. The predictive value of endorectal 3 Tesla multiparametric magnetic resonance imaging for extraprostatic extension in patients with low, intermediate and high risk prostate cancer. J Urol 2013;190(5): 1728–34.

64. Radtke JP, Kuru TH, Bonekamp D, et al. Further reduction of disqualification rates by additional MRI-targeted biopsy with transperineal saturation biopsy compared with standard 12-core systematic biopsies for the selection of prostate cancer patients for active surveillance. Prostate Cancer Prostatic Dis 2016;19(3):283–91.

65. Schoots IG, Petrides N, Giganti F, et al. Magnetic resonance imaging in active surveillance of prostate cancer: a systematic review. Eur Urol 2015;67(4): 627–36.

66. Nassiri N, Margolis DJ, Natarajan S, et al. Targeted biopsy to detect gleason score upgrading during active surveillance for men with low versus intermediate risk prostate cancer. J Urol 2017;197(3 Pt 1): 632–9.

67. Schulman AA, Tay KJ, Robertson CN, et al. High-intensity focused ultrasound for focal therapy: reality or pitfall? Curr Opin Urol 2017;27(2):138–48.

68. Valerio M, Shah TT, Shah P, et al. Magnetic resonance imaging-transrectal ultrasound fusion focal cryotherapy of the prostate: a prospective development study. Urol Oncol 2017;35(4):150.e1–7.

69. Pullini S, Signor MA, Pancot M, et al. Impact of multiparametric magnetic resonance imaging on risk group assessment of patients with prostate cancer addressed to external beam radiation therapy. Eur J Radiol 2016;85(4):764–70.

70. Radtke JP, Hadaschik BA, Wolf MB, et al. The impact of magnetic resonance imaging on prediction of extraprostatic extension and prostatectomy outcome in patients with low-, intermediate- and high-risk prostate cancer: try to find a standard. J Endourol 2015;29(12):1396–405.

MR Imaging for Prostate Cancer Screening and Active Surveillance

Sasha C. Druskin, MD[a], Katarzyna J. Macura, MD, PhD[a,b],*

KEYWORDS

- Prostate cancer • MR imaging • Biopsy • Active surveillance • Cancer screening

KEY POINTS

- The risk that an MR imaging–detected prostate lesion represents cancer is highly dependent on the setting (diagnostic, confirmatory, active surveillance) in which the MR imaging is conducted. In the active surveillance setting, even high Prostate Imaging Reporting and Data System score lesions are rarely aggressive cancer.
- In the prostate cancer screening setting, the use of MR imaging for men with elevated prostate-specific antigen may reduce overdiagnosis.
- Men considering active surveillance likely benefit from MR imaging at the time of enrollment, because at least half may be made ineligible based on the MR imaging results.

INTRODUCTION

Prostate Cancer Screening

The screen-diagnose-treat paradigm of prostate cancer (PCa) management has been criticized in recent years for contributing to the overdiagnosis and overtreatment of the disease,[1] leading the US Preventative Services Task Force to recommend against prostate-specific antigen (PSA) screening for PCa.[2] Despite this criticism, screening for PCa has been shown in multiple large trials, namely the Göteborg[3] and European Randomized Study of Screening for Prostate Cancer[4] trials, to contribute to decreased rates of PCa-specific mortality (PCSM). Nonetheless, with numbers needed to screen (NNS) and diagnose in order to prevent one PCa death ranging from 293 to 781 and 12 to 27, respectively, in those 2 studies, clearly, an improved strategy to diagnose and treat PCa is warranted. The high NNS is in part due to the low specificity and sensitivity of PSA for PCa,[5,6] whereby it can be abnormally elevated in men who do not have PCa or in the normal range for men with PCa. It is also due to the fact that most PCa detected by screening is low-risk disease,[7] which is unlikely to be clinically significant during a man's lifetime.[8] In order to address deficits in screening, multiple urine and serum markers, including percentage of free-to-total PSA,[5] PSA density,[5] prostate health index (PHI)[9] and PHI density,[10] 4K score (OPKO Lab, Nashville, TN),[11] and PCA3,[11] have become available and may help more precisely select patients for prostate biopsy. Another approach to screening is the use of multiparametric prostate MR imaging (mpMRI). mpMRI has been shown to have good performance for the detection of clinically significant PCa[12–14] and has been used to decide on whether or not to biopsy and to help target lesions during initial biopsy.[13,15–18]

Financial Disclosures: Research grant from Profound Medical Corp (K.J. Macura).
a James Buchanan Brady Urological Institute, Johns Hopkins University School of Medicine, 600 North Wolfe Street, Marburg 134, Baltimore, MD 21287, USA; b Department of Radiology and Radiological Science, Johns Hopkins University School of Medicine, 600 North Wolfe Street, Sheikh Zayed Tower, Baltimore, MD 21287, USA
* Corresponding author.
E-mail address: kmacura@jhmi.edu

Active Surveillance for Prostate Cancer

In order to address overtreatment of PCa, which is the case when disease that is unlikely to affect a man's well-being during his lifetime is nonetheless treated, active surveillance (AS) has taken an increasing role in the management of PCa.[19] AS is generally chosen as a management strategy for men with favorable-risk disease.[19] The premise of AS is that instead of treating PCa at the time of diagnosis, a patient is monitored at frequent intervals for signs of disease progression, at which point the plan is to treat the cancer with definitive curative therapy.[19] Cancer progression is usually monitored with a combination of PSA, digital rectal examination (DRE), and systematic transrectal ultrasound-guided (TRUS) biopsy (SB).[19] Progression on AS is generally regarded as upgrading (so-called grade-reclassification), or an increase in PCa volume (usually seen as an increase in the number of positive biopsy cores or percentage of a core that is positive for cancer, so-called volume-reclassification).[19] In general, progression of disease out of AS eligibility is the trigger for urologists to recommend definitive treatment (generally radical prostatectomy [RP] or radiation therapy for localized disease).[19] There are multiple institutions throughout the world that have been leaders in studying AS, and each has its own specific eligibility criteria[19]; however, most require National Comprehensive Cancer Network (NCCN) very-low-risk (T1c, Gleason ≤6, PSA <10 ng/mL, <3 positive biopsy cores, ≤50% of each core with cancer, PSA density <0.15 ng/mL/g) or low-risk (T1-2a, Gleason ≤6, PSA <10 ng/mL) disease,[20] and a few allow for NCCN low-intermediate-risk disease (low-volume Gleason score 3 + 4) for men with limited life expectancy.[19]

The 2016 NCCN guidelines[20] on PCa provide AS as a management option for men with low- or very-low-risk disease and ≥10 years of life expectancy. Under the 2016 European Association of Urology guidelines,[21] qualifying for AS requires that a man have greater than 10 years of life expectancy and a cancer profile that is similar to NCCN very-low-risk criteria, except that T2 disease also qualifies, and there is no PSA density cutoff.

In general, oncologic outcomes have been excellent, with rates of metastatic disease ranging from 0.1% to 2.8%, overall PCSM ranging from 0% to 1.5%, 15-year PCSM ranging from 0.1% to 5.7%, and rates of secondary definitive treatment ranging from 24% to 40% at 5 years and 36% to 55% at 10 years.[19] Despite these successes, AS is not without its difficulties, which include a laborious monitoring program (with frequent PSA checks and prostate biopsies every 1–2 years[19–21]) and the occasional inaccurate risk-classification of a patient that results in cancer-related morbidity and mortality. As with screening, biomarkers and MR imaging are being investigated in the AS realm[22] in order to improve patient risk classification.

In AS, MR imaging has had multiple roles. The first is in identifying potential disease that was missed on SB, in order to evaluate a patient's eligibility for AS.[23–30] SB generally samples only the posterior prostate, with limited sampling of the apex of the prostate[31]; indeed, in patients going on to RP, Gleason score is upgraded from SB to RP in 36.3%, according to one large study.[32] MR imaging can potentially identify an apical (**Fig. 1**) or anterior cancer (**Fig. 2**) missed on SB that could be sampled with targeted biopsy (TB).[33] Using this approach, a patient eligible for AS based on the pathology on their SB could be reassured that they likely do not have more extensive disease (given a negative MR imaging),[18] or made ineligible for AS (with a lesion on MR imaging that is found to be higher-grade cancer on TB) (see **Fig. 1**). The second role for MR imaging in AS is in monitoring during AS (**Fig. 3**).[12,34–36] In this article, the authors review the current literature on MR imaging in the screening and AS realms.

LITERATURE REVIEW
MR Imaging Diagnostic Performance

The ability of MR imaging to detect clinically significant prostate cancer

The ability of MR imaging to detect clinically significant PCa is dependent on the clinical setting. Ma and colleagues[12] showed in a study of MR imaging–TRUS fusion biopsy that the pathologies of lesions seen on MR imaging are very different for patients in the diagnostic setting versus the AS setting, with more aggressive cancer being detected and a higher incidence of cancer detection in the former. Those rates in the confirmatory biopsy setting, which is a surveillance biopsy within 1 year of AS enrollment, were in between those of the diagnostic and AS settings.

In the diagnostic setting, there are multiple ways that lesions on MR imaging can be compared with biopsy pathology. Looking at RP specimens[37] would be the definitive reference standard, but that limits the cohort to patients with a diagnosis of cancer and a diagnosis of aggressive enough cancer that treatment is warranted. Another strategy is to use MR imaging–TRUS fusion TB,[12] which can include patients with and without cancer (ie, the diagnostic setting). With that strategy, there is the risk for inaccurate targeting[37] and

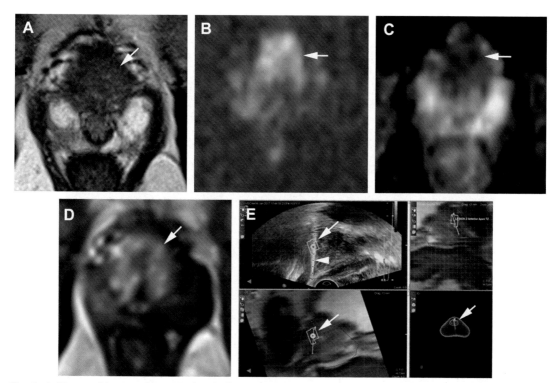

Fig. 1. A 66-year-old man with a PSA level of 10.8 ng/mL, increasing over 4 years from 4.1 ng/mL; 2 prior TRUS-guided biopsies of the prostate with benign results; prostate volume 50 mL, prostate–specific antigen density (PSAD) 0.2. Multiparametric MRI of the prostate at 3 T performed without endorectal coil shows a discrete nodule in the anterior apex transition zone that measures 1.8 cm and has homogeneously hypointense signal on T2-weighted imaging (*A, arrow*), hyperintense signal on high b-value diffusion-weighted imaging (*B, arrow*), a corresponding low signal on ADC map imaging (*C, arrow*), and early contrast enhancement on dynamic contrast-enhanced MR imaging (*D, arrow*); PIRADS 5. Patient had a follow-up MR-TRUS fusion biopsy (*E*) that targeted the anterior apex nodule (*arrow*) revealing prostatic adenocarcinoma Gleason score 3 + 4 = 7 (grade group 2: intermediate risk cancer) involving three cores. Note the biopsy needle (*arrowhead*) directed to the target nodule. Systematic biopsies during the same procedure showed only two small foci of low-grade PCa Gleason score 3 + 3 = 6 involving less than 5% of two cores and high-grade prostatic intraepithelial neoplasia, as well as a separate focus of atypical glands. Based on the pathology result from the MR-guided biopsy of the index nodule in the anterior apex, the patient was offered external beam radiation with six months of androgen deprivation therapy for his unfavorable (PSA >10) intermediate-risk PCa.

tumor heterogeneity. Another technique is the use of a saturation biopsy as a reference.[13] That technique is normally done via a perineal approach using a template, with biopsies separated by 5 mm.[13] In a recent landmark trial, Ahmed and colleagues,[13] using templated saturation biopsy as the reference, showed that in the biopsy-naïve setting, 1.5-T mpMRI had an 88% sensitivity and 45% specificity for Gleason score ≥3 + 4 PCa. The corresponding sensitivity and specificity for TRUS SB was 48% and 99%, respectively. A recent systematic review[14] of 12 studies found that mpMRI detected clinically significant (defined heterogeneously across studies, but most used Gleason score ≥7) PCa with a sensitivity and specificity of 58% to 96% and 23% to 87%, respectively. The reference standard to which mpMRI was compared was widely

heterogeneous, including the RP specimen, MR imaging–TRUS fusion biopsy, and saturation biopsy.

The ability of MR imaging to detect prostate cancer organ confinement

In a recent meta-analysis of 75 studies assessing the ability of mpMRI to locally stage PCa across a range of PCa risk levels, de Rooij and colleagues[38] found mpMRI to have a sensitivity and specificity of 57% and 91% for extracapsular extension and 58% and 96% for seminal vesicle invasion. In an earlier study, Somford and colleagues[39] found that 3.0-T mpMRI with an endorectal coil had a sensitivity/specificity/positive predictive value (PPV)/negative predictive value (NPV) (%) of 33.3/86.7/33.3/86.7 for detecting extracapsular extension in a subset of patients

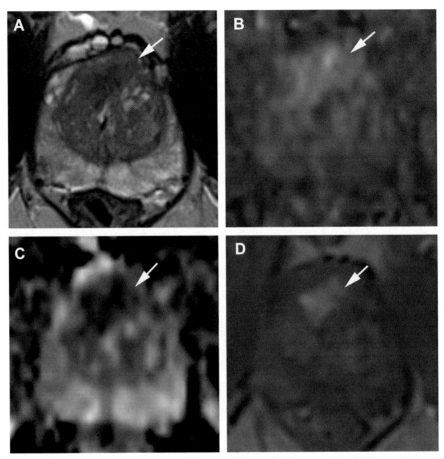

Fig. 2. A 70-year-old man was followed for PSA elevation (from 2.3 rising to 6.6 ng/mL) over 8 years in AS; prostate volume 90 mL; PSAD 0.07. He had a negative TRUS biopsy 8 years before prostate MR imaging. Multiparametric MRI of the prostate was performed at 3 T without an endorectal coil and showed a 2-cm nodule in the anterior transition zone with a homogeneously low signal on T2-weighted imaging (A, arrow), focally restricted diffusion with high signal on high b-value diffusion-weighted imaging (B, arrow), a corresponding low signal on ADC map imaging (C, arrow), as well as early intense enhancement on dynamic contrast-enhanced MR imaging (D, arrow); PIRADS 5. Following MR imaging, the patient had a targeted MR-TRUS fusion prostate biopsy that revealed prostate adenocarcinoma Gleason score 3 + 4 = 7 (grade group 2: intermediate risk cancer) in three cores from the target nodule as well as in one core from the SB of the right apex. The patient underwent open radical retropubic prostatectomy with final pathology showing a dominant nodule with Gleason score 3 + 4 = 7 (grade group 2), which was the same risk cancer as predicted by MR-guided prostate biopsy. Cancer was organ confined.

with low-volume, low-risk PCa. Sensitivity and PPV appeared to increase, and NPV appeared to decrease, as cancer risk level increased, up to sensitivity/specificity/PPV/NPV (%) of 64.9/ 72.7/88.9/38.1 for high-risk disease. Thus, it appears that in low-risk patients, where T3 disease is rare, mpMRI is useful in ruling out T3 disease; this is a useful attribute when it comes to selecting patients appropriate for AS. In high-risk patients, in whom T3 disease is more common, mpMRI is more useful in ruling in T3 disease. In addition, in a largely intermediate-risk cohort going on to RP, mpMRI was found to be superior to clinicopathologic variables (via the Partin tables) in predicting cancer organ confinement.[40] That study had a 91.2% PPV for organ-confined disease and an 89.7% NPV for extracapsular extension.

Prostate Cancer Screening Incorporating MR Imaging

Currently, the diagnostic paradigm for PCa screening is to biopsy patients with elevated PSA and/or abnormal DRE.[41] Using MR imaging as a screening tool for PCa can take 2 general

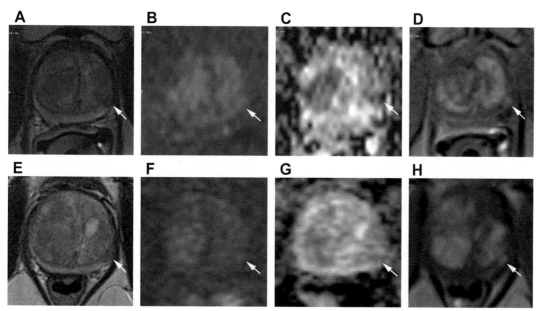

Fig. 3. A 71-year-old man with T1c adenocarcinoma of the prostate Gleason score 3 + 3 = 6 (grade group 1) that has been managed with AS for greater than 11 years; PSA 3.7 ng/mL; prostate volume 64 mL; PSAD 0.06. While in the AS program, the patient underwent mpMRI at the seventh and then at the eleventh year. Initial MR imaging examination was performed at 3 T with an endorectal coil and showed a single 8-mm nodule in the left mid peripheral zone, which had well-defined circumscribed margins on T2-weighted imaging (A, arrow), an isointense signal on high b-value diffusion-weighted imaging (B, arrow), and focally hypointense signal on ADC map imaging (C, arrow). There was early focal enhancement in the nodule on the dynamic contrast-enhanced (DCE) MR imaging (D, arrow). Morphologically, this nodule had the appearance of an extruded benign prostatic hyperplasia nodule (PIRADS 2). On the follow-up MR imaging examination performed four years later at 3 T without endorectal coil, there was no change in size or appearance of the left peripheral zone nodule on T2-weighted imaging (E, arrow) or diffusion-weighted imaging (F, arrow). The nodule became isointense on ADC map imaging (G, arrow) and continued to show early enhancement on DCE MR imaging (H, arrow). With stability of the MR imaging findings, along with negative DRE, as well as low PSA density, the patient continues expectant management.

forms: (a) patients with low clinical suspicion of PCa (based on PSA, DRE, or other indices) are screened using a *qualifying* approach, whereby MR imaging is used in order to steer them toward biopsy (given a concerning MR imaging), and (b) patients with moderate clinical suspicion of PCa are screened using a *disqualifying* approach, whereby MR imaging is used in order to steer them away from biopsy (given a reassuring MR imaging). Literature on each of these approaches is discussed below.

Prostate cancer screening incorporating MR imaging: the qualifying approach

Grenabo Bergdahl and colleagues[15] reported the results of a pilot study undertaken with patients from the Göteborg cohort, in which 124 men with PSA ≥1.8 ng/mL had an mpMRI before any biopsy. Biopsy was recommended to the men with PSA ≥3.0 ng/mL or lesions of Prostate Imaging Reporting and Data System (PIRADS) score ≥3 on MR imaging. Such lesions underwent "cognitive" TB in addition to SB. The investigators considered the targeted biopsies separately from the systematic biopsies and found that compared with performing SB on everyone with PSA ≥3.0 ng/mL, performing TB (without SB) in everyone with PSA ≥1.8 ng/mL and a PIRADS ≥3 lesion on MR imaging was more sensitive and specific for PCa and increased the detection of clinically significant PCa by nearly 50%.

Prostate cancer screening incorporating MR imaging: the disqualifying approach

The publication by Ahmed and colleagues[13] discussed above included 576 biopsy-naïve men with PSA ≤15 ng/mL. They report a mean PSA of 7.1 ng/mL and a standard deviation of 2.9 ng/mL, so it would be expected that 84% of patients would have had a PSA ≥4.2 ng/mL, assuming a normal distribution. Thus, this cohort was largely of moderate risk for PCa, based on the well-accepted PSA biopsy threshold of 3 to 4 ng/mL. Each patient had 1.5-T mpMRI, TRUS SB, and perineal saturation biopsy, the latter of which was the reference standard. They examined the pathologies of the TRUS SBs and the saturation biopsies and correlated those pathologies with the lesions observed on mpMRI. In total, 158/576 (27%) of the men had a negative MR imaging, but 38 of those men (24%) had Gleason score ≥3 + 4 disease. Thus, if MR imaging were used to decide on biopsy in this cohort, 27% of the entire cohort would have avoided biopsy, but 38/158 (24%) of those patients would have had a missed diagnosis of clinically significant cancer. Thus, this study argues against the *disqualifying* approach to MR imaging screening for PCa.

In another study, Thompson and colleagues[16] reported 150 men with abnormal PSA and/or DRE. No specific definition of abnormal PSA was provided, but median PSA was 5.6 ng/mL (interquartile range [IQR] 4.5–7.5) and 29.3% had an abnormal DRE. In total, 88% of men were biopsy naïve. All men had 1.5- or 3.0-T mpMRI graded with PIRADS v1, transperineal templated biopsy with 30 cores, and additional MR imaging–directed cores for regions of interest (ROIs) outside the template area. They found that forgoing biopsy in men with PIRADS ≤2 on MR imaging would avoid biopsy in 50% of men without significant cancer, decrease the diagnosis of low-risk cancer by 34%, and miss Gleason score 3 + 4 in 1% of patients, without missing any higher-grade cancer.

Pokorny and colleagues[17] reported 223 biopsy-naïve men with elevated PSA, all of whom underwent mpMR imaging with MR imaging–guided biopsy (if targetable lesions were present) and separate TRUS biopsy by a urologist blinded to the MR imaging. The investigators found that using mpMRI and MR imaging–guided TB for equivocal or concerning lesions, without TRUS SB, would reduce the number of patients needing biopsy by 51%. Compared with TRUS SB, that strategy would be associated with an 89.4% lower rate of diagnosing low-risk disease, and a 17.7% higher rate of diagnosing intermediate- or high-risk disease. The NPV of mpMRI for the diagnosis of intermediate- or high-risk disease was 97%.

Similarly, in a study of 29 biopsy-naïve men with a median PSA of 3.7 ng/mL (IQR 2.9–4.9), Wysock and colleagues[18] showed that TRUS SB after a negative 3-T mpMRI found pathologic grade group ≥2 cancer in none of the patients, giving an NPV of 100%.

Prostate cancer screening incorporating MR imaging: cost-effectiveness

Literature in this area is sparse. A cost analysis by the National Collaborating Centre for Cancer in the United Kingdom[42] found that the cost-effectiveness of mpMRI depended on the method used for lesion targeting and at which phase of diagnosis it was used. They found that when MR imaging–TRUS fusion TB was used to target lesions on MR imaging in the diagnostic setting, there was increased detection of PCa and earlier time to diagnosis, which led to an increase in quality-adjusted life-years (QALY). Given a cost-effectiveness threshold of £20,000/QALY, they estimated that systematic TRUS biopsy had a 94% chance of being cost-effective, whereas SB with MR imaging–TRUS fusion TB had a 6% chance of being cost-effective. They were not able to make any conclusions about using MR imaging to rule out patients of needing biopsy, but speculated that that approach might be cost-effective in the future, once it is shown that the strategy is safe and effective.

MR Imaging in Prostate Cancer Active Surveillance

MR imaging in prostate cancer active surveillance: determining patient eligibility for active surveillance

A systematic review by Schoots and colleagues[23] published in 2015 found that two-thirds of men on AS had a suspicious MR imaging. They found that a suspicious MR imaging increased the chance of finding clinically significant PCa on repeat biopsy, especially when the repeat biopsy incorporated a TB, and patients with a suspicious MR imaging who went on to RP were more likely to have Gleason upgrading, but not upstaging, than those with a nonsuspicious MR imaging. They also found that MR imaging at AS enrollment detected clinically significant cancer in one-third to one-half of men, but there was insufficient evidence for the use of MR imaging for monitoring during AS.

Radtke and colleagues[24] published a study of 149 patients on AS with low-risk PCa and eligible for AS by Prostate Cancer Research International Active Surveillance (PRIAS) criteria. Forty-five of them were initially diagnosed with PCa on 24-core transperineal SB with MR imaging–TRUS fusion TB. The rest (104) were initially diagnosed with PCa on standard 12-core SB. After 1 and 2 years, each patient underwent mpMRI with 24-core transperineal SB and MR imaging–TRUS fusion TB of suspicious lesions. The men diagnosed by each biopsy type initially had similar age and PSA, but despite this, the group diagnosed with PCa initially on 12-core SB had a 20% higher rate of reclassification at the interim biopsy, suggesting that the 12-core biopsy had underdiagnosed the degree of cancer present in that group.

Pepe and colleagues[25] reported 40 men with very-low-risk PCa enrolled on AS who had confirmatory biopsy with 30-core saturation biopsy. Each man also had mpMRI with TB for concerning lesions. In total, 25% of the patients had grade reclassification on that confirmatory saturation biopsy. mpMRI was 100% sensitive for the lesions that lead to grade reclassification; however, the TB accuracy was variable.

In a study by Almeida and colleagues,[26] 73 men eligible for AS by PRIAS criteria but who elected RP each underwent preoperative mpMRI. They found that PIRADS 4 to 5 scans had a sensitivity of 92% and 76% for upstaging and upgrading on RP pathology, respectively. On multivariable logistic regression, patients with PIRADS 5 scans had more than 16 times the odds of upstaging than patients with PIRADS 2 to 3 scans ($P = .05$).

Porpiglia and colleagues[27] reported a retrospective study of 120 patients eligible for AS by PRIAS criteria but all having RP. Each had preoperative mpMRI after biopsy. Having an MR imaging with a PIRADS ≥ 4 lesion had a sensitivity/specificity/PPV/NPV (%) of 73/61/62/73 for detecting significant cancer (defined as anything other than organ-confined Gleason 6 tumors, with the index tumor ≤ 1.3 mL and the total tumor volume ≤ 2.5 mL), which is associated with a false-negative rate of 27%.

Ouzzane and colleagues[28] reported a study of 281 men presenting for prostate biopsy because of abnormal PSA and/or DRE and eligible for AS based on their SB pathology. Each man had a pre-biopsy mpMRI with TB if the MR imaging was concerning. In total, 163 (58%) had suspicious lesions on MR imaging, and of those, 28 (10% of the total 281 patients) were made ineligible for AS based on the TB pathologies, which discovered unfavorable cancer by grade or volume. Most of those unfavorable TBs were anterior lesions. The investigators concluded that 10% of men eligible for AS by SB were disqualified by TB.

Kim and colleagues[29] conducted a study of 287 patients undergoing RP who were eligible for AS preoperatively. Each had a preoperative mpMRI. They found that patients with low apparent diffusion coefficient (ADC) value on MR imaging ($<0.830 \times 10^{-3}$ mm^2/s) had a significantly greater proportion of Gleason ≥ 7 cancer and non-organ-confined cancer.

Dianat and colleagues[30] published a study of 96 men on AS who had mpMRI within 1 year of AS enrollment. In total, 84 had lesions on MR imaging and 12 had no lesions on MR imaging (so they had MR imaging-invisible cancer). After 23 months of follow-up, MR imaging-invisibility was associated with a lower rate of clinically significant pathology on follow-up biopsy; however, $P > .05$.

MR imaging in prostate cancer active surveillance: monitoring for disease progression

Recabal and colleagues[36] reported 206 patients with Gleason score 3 + 3 PCa on AS undergoing surveillance mpMRI, SB, and MR imaging–TRUS fusion TB at ROIs. Overall, 66% of all patients had an ROI on MR imaging and 37% of men had grade reclassification. They found that a proprietary 5-point MR imaging score was predictive of grade reclassification. In total, 34% of the cohort had no ROI on MR imaging; however, 11% of those patients did have grade reclassification on SB. In patients with ROIs on MR imaging, TB did fail to identify some cancers that were detected by SB, but the rate that TB missed high-grade cancer was lower for increasing MR imaging score. This study shows that even for AS patients with ROIs on MR imaging, SB should not be omitted. It is unknown if cancer in the MR imaging ROIs would have been detected on SB in this study because the areas of the prostate sampled by TB were excluded on SB.

Ma and colleagues[12] reported a retrospective study of 103 men on AS with at least one PIRADS ≥ 3 lesion on mpMRI who underwent SB and TB. In total, 25 cases of Gleason score $\geq 3 + 4$ were discovered on biopsy, but only 3 of them were found by TB alone. Of all ROIs, only 5% had Gleason score $\geq 3 + 4$ cancer, and there were no differences in the rate of Gleason score $\geq 3 + 4$ cancer between PIRADS scores in those patients. These data show that SB remains an important component of AS monitoring, where scarring and prostatitis from prior biopsies may introduce false-positive results on MR imaging.

Felker and colleagues[35] reported a retrospective study of 49 men with Gleason score 3 + 3 cancer on AS who underwent mpMRI with TB at baseline and greater than 6 months after enrollment (mean 28 months). For predicting Gleason score $\geq 3 + 4$ on the second biopsy, the investigators found that including the second MR imaging findings in a model incorporating PSA density and baseline biopsy maximum cancer core length improved the performance of the model, with an area under the curve of 0.91.

Walton-Diaz and colleagues[34] published a retrospective study of 58 men choosing AS after meeting AS criteria on initial SB and confirmatory SB with MR imaging–TRUS fusion TB. They were followed with recurrent mpMRI and SB with TB. In total, 41 patients had stable MR images;

however, 8 (20%) of those patients had grade reclassification, of which 4 (10%) had grade reclassification in their TB. Conversely, 17 had MR imaging progression, and 9 (53%) of those had grade reclassification, of which 7 (41%) had grade reclassification in their TB. The PPV and NPV of MR imaging progression for detecting grade reclassification were 53% and 80%, respectively.

MR imaging in prostate cancer active surveillance: cost-effectiveness

The cost-effectiveness of MR imaging in AS is unclear. AS has been shown to be cost-effective versus definitive treatment for favorable-risk PCa for up to 10 years of follow-up,[43,44] so MR imaging at the time of cancer diagnosis may potentially be cost-effective if it can increase the utilization of AS, as has been shown in one economic modeling study.[45] MR imaging could also be cost-effective if it decreased the need for repeat biopsy, as was shown by one study suggesting a biopsy reduction rate as high as 68% in AS patients.[46] Further studies are certainly needed in this realm.

Combination of MR Imaging and Serum Markers

In a diagnostic biopsy setting of patients with and without a prior negative SB, Tosoian and colleagues[47] found that mpMRI and the PHI (a compound marker consisting of multiple PSA-isoforms) provided complementary information: in patients with negative MR images and aggressive cancer on SB, PHI was elevated (concerning). In patients with low (reassuring) PHI, patients with aggressive cancer were found to have suspicious lesions on MR imaging.

In a prior negative SB cohort undergoing MR imaging-guided transperineal SB with TB, Gnanapragasam and colleagues[48] found PHI to improve detection of any and clinically significant cancer. They found that using a PHI threshold of 35 led to an NPV of 97% for detecting clinically significant cancer when PHI was combined with MR imaging. PHI also improved prediction of significant cancer in men with negative MR images.

It is hoped that INNOVATE,[49] an ongoing trial in the United Kingdom, will further elucidate the advantages of combining mpMRI and biomarkers in the biopsy-naïve setting.

Future Directions

Although MR imaging has proven to be a big advancement for PCa diagnosis when compared with SB, it has limitations. In addition to the incorporation of various serum and urine biomarkers, molecular imaging has been proposed as one method of improving PCa diagnosis. One marker has shown particular promise: prostate-specific membrane antigen (PSMA), which is a membrane-bound protein highly expressed by PCa cells, for which several PET tracers currently exist.[50] Because PET has limited spatial resolution, it is often fused with computed tomographic (CT) images to facilitate anatomic localization of PET-avid sites.[51] However, intraprostatic lesion localization by CT is quite limited when compared with MR imaging, which has led to recent interest in PET-MR imaging fusion.[51] This promising technology is evolving and has the potential to improve lesion localization, characterization, and risk stratification.

SUMMARY

Diagnostic Performance of MR Imaging for the Detection of Prostate Cancer

The incidence of aggressive PCa is higher in a diagnostic setting than in an AS setting, where patients are selected for their favorable-risk disease. Accordingly, MR imaging–detected prostate lesions are less likely to represent aggressive PCa in the AS setting than in the diagnostic setting. The diagnostic performance of mpMRI for clinically significant PCa is widely variable across studies, but most found high sensitivity and low-moderate specificity. Conversely, for local staging, studies have found mpMRI to have low sensitivity and moderate-high specificity for the detection of locally advanced disease, with an apparent increase in sensitivity with increasing cancer risk-group.

MR Imaging in Prostate Cancer Screening

In the setting of elevated PSA, MR imaging may reduce overdiagnosis of PCa, with mixed results regarding increasing underdiagnosis. Incorporating MR imaging in PCa screening in men with low PSA might decrease PCa underdiagnosis but may do so at the cost of overdiagnosis. The cost-effectiveness of MR imaging in this setting is unknown.

MR Imaging in Prostate Cancer Active Surveillance

There is strong evidence for the use of MR imaging in men considering AS because it can identify clinically significant disease not found on SB. In men eligible for AS based on their SB, one-third to one-half will be made ineligible after MR imaging and TB. The evidence for monitoring patients on AS with MR imaging is less clear. Data do support not omitting SB in patients undergoing TB in that setting. Furthermore, in the AS setting, it is unclear if lesions with higher PIRADS scores are at increased risk of aggressive disease; however, PIRADS progression may represent an increased risk of grade reclassification. Last, if MR imaging leads to higher rates of AS versus curative treatment, then it will likely prove to be cost-effective, but definitive evidence for this is lacking.

Combination of MR Imaging and Serum Markers

The future of PCa diagnosis will likely involve using a combination of biomarkers and imaging. PHI is a promising serum biomarker that has been shown to provide complementary information to MR imaging and vice versa.

Future Directions

Advances in prostate imaging may improve the ability to diagnose and localize cancer. PET imaging (especially using PSMA) with MR imaging fusion provides one particularly attractive approach because it might allow for both molecular and anatomic cancer localization. Rigorous studies are needed.

REFERENCES

1. Loeb S, Bjurlin MA, Nicholson J, et al. Overdiagnosis and overtreatment of prostate cancer. Eur Urol 2014; 65(6):1046–55.
2. Moyer VA. U.S. preventive services task force. Screening for prostate cancer: U.S. Preventive Services Task Force recommendation statement. Ann Intern Med 2012;157(2):120–34.
3. Hugosson J, Carlsson S, Aus G, et al. Mortality results from the Göteborg randomised population-based prostate-cancer screening trial. Lancet Oncol 2010;11(8):725–32.
4. Schröder FH, Hugosson J, Roobol MJ, et al. Screening and prostate cancer mortality: results of the European Randomised Study of Screening for Prostate Cancer (ERSPC) at 13 years of follow-up. Lancet 2014;384(9959):2027–35.
5. Catalona WJ, Southwick PC, Slawin KM, et al. Comparison of percent free PSA, PSA density, and age-specific PSA cutoffs for prostate cancer detection and staging. Urology 2000;56(2):255–60.
6. Thompson IM, Pauler DK, Goodman PJ, et al. Prevalence of prostate cancer among men with a prostate-specific antigen level < or =4.0 ng per milliliter. N Engl J Med 2004;350(22):2239–46.
7. Godtman RA, Holmberg E, Khatami A, et al. Outcome following active surveillance of men with screen-detected prostate cancer. Results from the Göteborg randomised population-based prostate cancer screening trial. Eur Urol 2013;63(1):101–7.
8. Popiolek M, Rider JR, Andrén O, et al. Natural history of early, localized prostate cancer: a final report from three decades of follow-up. Eur Urol 2013; 63(3):428–35.
9. Catalona WJ, Partin AW, Sanda MG, et al. A multicenter study of [-2]pro-prostate specific antigen combined with prostate specific antigen and free prostate specific antigen for prostate cancer detection in the 2.0 to 10.0 ng/ml prostate specific antigen range. J Urol 2011;185(5):1650–5.
10. Tosoian JJ, Druskin SC, Andreas D, et al. Prostate health index density improves detection of clinically-significant prostate cancer. BJU Int 2017; 120(6):793–8.
11. Vedder MM, de Bekker-Grob EW, Lilja HG, et al. The added value of percentage of free to total prostate-specific antigen, PCA3, and a kallikrein panel to the ERSPC risk calculator for prostate cancer in pre-screened men. Eur Urol 2014;66(6):1109–15.
12. Ma TM, Tosoian JJ, Schaeffer EM, et al. The role of multiparametric magnetic resonance imaging/ultrasound fusion biopsy in active surveillance. Eur Urol 2017;71(2):174–80.
13. Ahmed HU, El-Shater Bosaily A, Brown LC, et al. Diagnostic accuracy of multi-parametric MRI and TRUS biopsy in prostate cancer (PROMIS): a paired validating confirmatory study. Lancet 2017; 389(10071):815–22.
14. Fütterer JJ, Briganti A, De Visschere P, et al. Can clinically significant prostate cancer be detected with multiparametric magnetic resonance imaging? A systematic review of the literature. Eur Urol 2015; 68(6):1045–53.
15. Grenabo Bergdahl A, Wilderäng U, Aus G, et al. Role of magnetic resonance imaging in prostate cancer screening: a pilot study within the Göteborg randomised screening trial. Eur Urol 2016;70(4): 566–73.
16. Thompson JE, Moses D, Shnier R, et al. Multiparametric magnetic resonance imaging guided diagnostic biopsy detects significant prostate cancer and could reduce unnecessary biopsies and over detection: a prospective study. J Urol 2014;192(1): 67–74.
17. Pokorny MR, de Rooij M, Duncan E, et al. Prospective study of diagnostic accuracy comparing prostate cancer detection by transrectal ultrasound-guided biopsy versus magnetic resonance (MR) imaging with subsequent MR-guided biopsy in men without previous prostate biopsies. Eur Urol 2014; 66(1):22–9.
18. Wysock JS, Mendhiratta N, Zattoni F, et al. Predictive value of negative 3T multiparametric prostate MRI on 12 core biopsy results. BJU Int 2016;118(4): 515–20.

19. Tosoian JJ, Carter HB, Lepor A, et al. Active surveillance for prostate cancer: current evidence and contemporary state of practice. Nat Rev Urol 2016; 13(4):205–15.

20. Mohler JL, Antonarakis ES, Armstrong AJ, et al. NCCN clinical practice guidelines in oncology-prostate cancer (2.2017). Available at: http://www.nccn.org/professionals/physician_gls/pdf/prostate.pdf. Accessed April 10, 2017.

21. Mottet N, Bellmunt J, Briers E, et al. EAU-ESTRO-SIOG guidelines on prostate cancer - 2016. Available at: https://uroweb.org/wp-content/uploads/EAU-Guidelines-Prostate-Cancer-2016.pdf. Accessed January 13, 2017.

22. Ward JF, Eggener SE. Active surveillance monitoring: the role of novel biomarkers and imaging. Asian J Androl 2015;17(6):882–4 [discussion:883].

23. Schoots IG, Petrides N, Giganti F, et al. Magnetic resonance imaging in active surveillance of prostate cancer: a systematic review. Eur Urol 2015;67(4): 627–36.

24. Radtke JP, Kuru TH, Bonekamp D, et al. Further reduction of disqualification rates by additional MRI-targeted biopsy with transperineal saturation biopsy compared with standard 12-core systematic biopsies for the selection of prostate cancer patients for active surveillance. Prostate Cancer Prostatic Dis 2016;19(3):283–91.

25. Pepe P, Garufi A, Priolo G, et al. Can MRI/TRUS fusion targeted biopsy replace saturation prostate biopsy in the re-evaluation of men in active surveillance? World J Urol 2016;34(9):1249–53.

26. Almeida GL, Petralia G, Ferro M, et al. Role of multiparametric magnetic resonance image and PIRADS score in patients with prostate cancer eligible for active surveillance according PRIAS criteria. Gynecol Obstet Invest 2016;96(4):459–69.

27. Porpiglia F, Cantiello F, De Luca S, et al. In-parallel comparative evaluation between multiparametric magnetic resonance imaging, prostate cancer antigen 3 and the prostate health index in predicting pathologically confirmed significant prostate cancer in men eligible for active surveillance. BJU Int 2016; 118(4):527–34.

28. Ouzzane A, Renard-Penna R, Marliere F, et al. Magnetic resonance imaging targeted biopsy improves selection of patients considered for active surveillance for clinically low risk prostate cancer based on systematic biopsies. The J Urol 2015;194(2): 350–6.

29. Kim TH, Jeong JY, Lee SW, et al. Diffusion-weighted magnetic resonance imaging for prediction of insignificant prostate cancer in potential candidates for active surveillance. Eur Radiol 2015;25(6):1786–92.

30. Dianat SS, Carter HB, Pienta KJ, et al. Magnetic resonance-invisible versus magnetic resonance-visible prostate cancer in active surveillance: a preliminary report on disease outcomes. Urology 2015;85(1):147–53.

31. Ahmed H, Emberton M. Focal therapy for prostate cancer. In: Wein A, Kavoussi L, Partin AW, et al, editors. Campbell-Walsh urology. 11th edition. Amsterdam: Elsevier; 2015. p. 2712.

32. Epstein JI, Feng Z, Trock BJ, et al. Upgrading and downgrading of prostate cancer from biopsy to radical prostatectomy: incidence and predictive factors using the modified Gleason grading system and factoring in tertiary grades. Eur Urol 2012;61(5): 1019–24.

33. Ouzzane A, Puech P, Lemaitre L, et al. Combined multiparametric MRI and targeted biopsies improve anterior prostate cancer detection, staging, and grading. Urology 2011;78(6):1356–62.

34. Walton-Diaz A, Shakir NA, George AK, et al. Use of serial multiparametric magnetic resonance imaging in the management of patients with prostate cancer on active surveillance. Urol Oncol 2015;33(5):202.e1–7.

35. Felker ER, Wu J, Natarajan S, et al. Serial magnetic resonance imaging in active surveillance of prostate cancer: incremental value. J Urol 2016;195(5): 1421–7.

36. Recabal P, Assel M, Sjoberg DD, et al. The efficacy of multiparametric magnetic resonance imaging and magnetic resonance imaging targeted biopsy in risk classification for patients with prostate cancer on active surveillance. J Urol 2016;196(2): 374–81.

37. Radtke JP, Schwab C, Wolf MB, et al. Multiparametric magnetic resonance imaging (MRI) and MRI-transrectal ultrasound fusion biopsy for index tumor detection: correlation with radical prostatectomy specimen. Eur Urol 2016;70(5): 846–53.

38. de Rooij M, Hamoen EHJ, Witjes JA, et al. Accuracy of magnetic resonance imaging for local staging of prostate cancer: a diagnostic meta-analysis. Eur Urol 2016;70(2):233–45.

39. Somford DM, Hamoen EH, Fütterer JJ, et al. The predictive value of endorectal 3 Tesla multiparametric magnetic resonance imaging for extraprostatic extension in patients with low, intermediate and high risk prostate cancer. J Urol 2013;190(5): 1728–34.

40. Gupta RT, Faridi KF, Singh AA, et al. Comparing 3-T multiparametric MRI and the Partin tables to predict organ-confined prostate cancer after radical prostatectomy. Urol Oncol 2014;32(8):1292–9.

41. Carroll PR, Parsons JK, Andriole G, et al. NCCN clinical practice guidelines in oncology prostate cancer early detection, version 2.2016. Available at: https://www.nccn.org/professionals/physician_gls/pdf/prostate_detection.pdf. Published 2016. Accessed November 16, 2016.

42. National Collaborating Centre for Cancer (UK). Prostate cancer: diagnosis and treatment. Cardiff (UK): National Collaborating Centre for Cancer (UK); 2014 Jan. (NICE Clinical Guidelines, No. 175.). Available at: https://www.ncbi.nlm.nih.gov/books/NBK247469/pdf/Bookshelf_NBK247469.pdf. Accessed March 15, 2017.

43. Keegan KA, Dall'Era MA, Durbin-Johnson B, et al. Active surveillance for prostate cancer compared with immediate treatment: an economic analysis. Cancer 2012;118(14):3512–8.

44. Laviana AA, Ilg AM, Veruttipong D, et al. Utilizing time-driven activity-based costing to understand the short- and long-term costs of treating localized, low-risk prostate cancer. Cancer 2016;122(3): 447–55.

45. Gordon LG, James R, Tuffaha HW, et al. Cost-effectiveness analysis of multiparametric MRI with increased active surveillance for low-risk prostate cancer in Australia. J Magn Reson Imaging 2016; 198(Suppl 3):540.

46. Siddiqui MM, Truong H, Rais-Bahrami S, et al. Clinical implications of a multiparametric magnetic resonance imaging based nomogram applied to prostate cancer active surveillance. The J Urol 2015;193(6):1943–9.

47. Tosoian JJ, Druskin SC, Andreas D, et al. Use of the prostate health index for detection of prostate cancer: results from a large academic practice. Prostate Cancer Prostatic Dis 2017;20(2): 228–33.

48. Gnanapragasam VJ, Burling K, George A, et al. The prostate health index adds predictive value to multi-parametric MRI in detecting significant prostate cancers in a repeat biopsy population. Sci Rep 2016; 6(1):35364.

49. Johnston E, Pye H, Bonet-Carne E, et al. INNOVATE: a prospective cohort study combining serum and urinary biomarkers with novel diffusion-weighted magnetic resonance imaging for the prediction and characterization of prostate cancer. BMC Cancer 2016;16(1):816.

50. Maurer T, Eiber M, Schwaiger M, et al. Current use of PSMA-PET in prostate cancer management. Nat Rev Urol 2016;13(4):226–35.

51. Lindenberg L, Ahlman M, Turkbey B, et al. Advancement of MR and PET/MR in prostate cancer. Semin Nucl Med 2016;46(6):536–43.

Prostate MR Imaging for Posttreatment Evaluation and Recurrence

Sonia Gaur, BS, Baris Turkbey, MD*

KEYWORDS

- Prostate cancer • Recurrence • mpMRI • Radical prostatectomy • Radiation therapy
- Focal therapy

KEY POINTS

- Multiparametric MR imaging (mpMRI) can help in evaluation of posttreatment changes after diagnosis and treatment of prostate cancer as well as for diagnosis of locally recurrent disease.
- After radical prostatectomy, radiation therapy, or focal therapy, there are certain expected changes in the remaining tissue.
- Many of the mpMRI patterns of recurrent disease are similar to those of primary prostate cancer. In diagnosis of recurrence, however, normal posttreatment changes and possible inflammation must remain considerations in the interpretation of imaging findings.

INTRODUCTION

Prostate cancer (PCa) is the most common solid organ malignancy and second most common cause of cancer-related deaths among men in the United States. Last year, approximately 190,000 men were newly diagnosed with PCa and 26,000 men died of this disease.[1] Increasingly, timely diagnosis of high-grade disease is achieved with use of prostate multiparametric MR imaging (mpMRI), giving patients with localized disease (stages I–III) early options for definitive treatment. Treatment commonly includes radical prostatectomy (RP) or radiation therapy (RT), which can include external-beam RT (EBRT) or brachytherapy. Generally, RP is preferred for younger men with localized tumors and RT is preferred for elder patients or patients who are not ideal surgery candidates.[2] More recently, patients with a certain pattern of disease visualized on mpMRI may also be offered prostate-sparing focal therapy

treatment options that utilize laser technology, microwave ablation, cryotherapy, or high-intensity focused ultrasound (HIFU).[3,4] Unfortunately, despite advances in diagnosis and management of PCa, the disease recurs after definitive treatment in up to 40% of patients.[5] Therefore, detection and treatment of recurrent disease has become a relevant focus across multiple disciplines. From an imaging perspective, prostate mpMRI not only can provide insight into primary PCa but also can achieve good anatomic spatial resolution and provide functional data for visualization of recurrent disease.[6]

After treatment, patients are followed closely for biochemical recurrence (BCR), defined based on serum prostate-specific antigen (PSA) criteria specific for each treatment option.[7–9] PSA nadir achieved after each treatment option differs, because in RT and in focal therapy, PSA-producing prostate parenchyma is not completely eradicated.[9] After RP, PSA nadir of undetectable

Disclosure Statement: Authors have nothing to disclose.
Molecular Imaging Program, National Cancer Institute, National Institutes of Health, 10 Center Drive, Building 10, Room B3B85, Bethesda, MD 20814, USA
* Corresponding author.
E-mail address: turkbeyi@mail.nih.gov

Radiol Clin N Am 56 (2018) 263–275
https://doi.org/10.1016/j.rcl.2017.10.008
0033-8389/18/Published by Elsevier Inc.

levels is expected, whereas after RT or focal therapy, a PSA nadir greater than zero is achieved within weeks or months after completion of therapy. Accordingly, in RP patients, recurrence is suspected with an increase in PSA above the threshold greater than or equal to 0.2 ng/mL with a second confirmatory level, whereas in RT patients, an increase in PSA 2.0 ng/mL above the established posttreatment nadir is suspicious.[10] PSA patterns are monitored after focal therapy as well, although consensus about kinetics and a threshold value is still being investigated.[9] In patients who receive definitive therapy, BCR indicates locally recurrent disease in up to two-thirds of patients, and this must be extensively evaluated for appropriate subsequent management.[11–13] Distinction of PSA-producing benign etiologies from local recurrence and distant metastasis is vital. Prostate mpMRI can greatly assist this by aiding visualization of local structures posttreatment, with some considerations.[14–16] This is clinically important because localized recurrence that can be visualized on mpMRI can be offered local salvage treatment, which is drastically different from systemic options offered to patients with distant metastatic disease.

Evaluation and imaging of recurrent disease with mpMRI require certain considerations based on treatment received. Prostate mpMRI's strength lies in combining anatomic data (T1-weighted [T1W] and T2-weighted [T2W] MR imaging) with functional data (diffusion-weighted imaging [DWI] and dynamic contrast-enhanced imaging [DCE]) to provide maximum information about the location and character of possible disease. Established guidelines for characterizing and reporting suspicious areas on prostate mpMRI, such as Prostate Imaging—Reporting and Data System, Version 2, are designed only for characterization of primary cancer.[17] Although baseline pulse sequences (**Box 1**) used are the same for posttreatment evaluation, treatment greatly changes anatomy visualized, can change signal intensity on certain sequences, and can introduce artifact that compromises sequence utility. For example, after RP, a drastically different anatomy is visualized on imaging and image artifact may be introduced with use of surgical clips during the procedure. In contrast, after RT, although the general anatomic structures remain the same, the prostate shrinks greatly in size and has different signal pattern on T2W imaging. The purpose of this article is to discuss general guidelines for identifying normal posttreatment changes and possible recurrence on mpMRI as well as pitfalls of mpMRI interpretation after the various treatments for PCa.

MULTIPARAMETRIC MR IMAGING AFTER RADICAL PROSTATECTOMY

RP is a common active treatment chosen for PCa patients with localized disease, with approximately 40% of patients undergoing definitive therapy choosing this option.[18] RP includes total removal of the prostate and seminal vesicles, along with pelvic lymph node dissection to varying extents for evaluation of local metastasis.[19] Subsequent pathology analysis evaluates surgical margins and lymph nodes for staging. Risk for future BCR is a consideration at this point, because certain characteristics of the original PCa can increase risk of recurrence, such as seminal vesical invasion, positive surgical margins, extraprostatic extension, perineural invasion, lymphovascular invasion, and increased tumor volume.[18] After successful surgery, PSA should drop to undetectable levels within 2 weeks to 3 weeks and patients should be followed with serial serum PSA measurements for early detection of possible BCR. According to the American Urological Association guidelines, BCR after RP is defined as a serum PSA measurement greater than or equal to 0.2 ng/mL, followed by a second confirmatory serum PSA measurement of greater than or equal to 0.2 ng/mL.[7] Post-RP, approximately 35% of patients experience BCR within 10 years, and there are certain parameters that make this recurrence more likely to be found as localized disease.[20–24] These include PSA increase more than 3 years post-RP, PSA doubling time greater than 11 months, original Gleason score less than or equal to 7, and stage less than or equal to pT3a pN0, pTx with negative surgical margins. In contrast, systemic disease can be predicted if PSA increases in less than 1 year post-RP, PSA doubling time is in 4 months to 6 months, original

---

Box 1
Pulse sequences used for posttreatment evaluation with multiparametric MR imaging

mpMRI protocol in recurrent PCa work-up

Triplane T2W MR imaging

Diffusion-weighted MR imaging

  ADC map

  High *b*-value DW MR imaging (>1400) (acquired or calculated)

DCE MR imaging

Pelvic T1W MR imaging

Gleason score was 8 to 10, and stage pT3b, pTxpN1.[10] Imaging can aid with distinguishing between local and distant metastatic disease, and, if local disease seems likely, mpMRI specifically can play an important subsequent role in evaluation.

After surgery, the male pelvic anatomy is greatly changed, and this is an important consideration when evaluating the area with imaging. Use of mpMRI is ideal for evaluation of the postsurgical bed, because its functional components allow the important differentiation between recurrent cancer, residual prostate tissue, inflammatory tissue, and fibrosis. Presurgical anatomy is relatively consistent between patients—going superior to inferiorly, the bladder neck lies above the prostate base, seminal vesicles appear between the prostate base and bladder neck, and then the prostate is clearly visualized base to apex. Postsurgical anatomy on mpMRI is drastically different due to the open prostatectomy fossa left behind from where the prostate is removed. Imaging should show the bladder neck descended into the prostatectomy fossa with a more conical shape, the vesicourethral anastomosis (VUA) inferior to the bladder neck, and the retrovesical bed posterior to these structures on the sagittal view. Fat stranding may be present around the bladder base on anatomic imaging. In addition to changed anatomy, there are certain expected post-RP signal patterns and artifacts to consider. The VUA should be visualized as a ring of postoperative fibrosis, exhibiting low signal intensity on all sequences of mpMRI. In certain situations, such as if there was extensive hemorrhage at the time of surgery or if there is inflammatory tissue postoperatively, some VUA hyperintense tissue may be seen on T2W imaging. These circumstances are discussed more extensively with other recurrent PCa mimics later. Patterns of fibrosis may differ between patients, based on surgical approach used.[25] If metallic clips were used in the surgery, these can be seen as hyperintense structures on T2W imaging. In up to 20% of cases, seminal vesicles may be left behind in the body, and these can be seen in their presurgical locations with their characteristic tubular structure on T1W or T2W anatomic imaging.[26] They appear as intermediate to high intensity on T2W imaging, may show restricted diffusion on DWI, and often show early enhancement on DCE[27,28] (Fig. 1). On postoperative imaging of the wider pelvic field of view, it is possible to see lymphoceles in patients who undergo pelvic lymph node dissection. These form due to the accumulation of lymph from damage to the lymphatic system in the resection.[29] These are visualized at the locations of former lymph nodes as hyperintense thin-walled cystlike

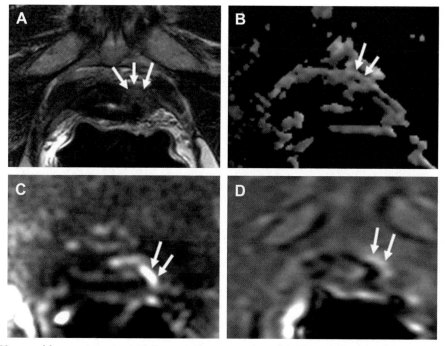

Fig. 1. A 68-year-old man, status post-RP 5 years prior, presenting with PSA = 0.47 ng/mL for mpMRI evaluation. Axial T2W MR imaging (*A*), ADC map (*B*), b-2000 DW MR imaging (*C*), and DCE MR imaging (*D*) recurrent lesion (*arrows*). The area suspicious for recurrence appears at the VUA, relatively hyperintense on T2W, corresponding with a hypointense area on the ADC map, hyperintense area on b-2000, and early hyperenhancement on DCE MR imaging.

structures on T2Ww imaging and exhibit no enhancement on DCE.

The individual mpMRI sequences vary in utility for post-RP imaging, especially for detection of recurrence. T2W imaging is always used in evaluation postsurgery for anatomy orientation and evaluation of signal patterns. Generally, DWI utility is highly dependent on whether or not surgical clips were used in the surgery. If clips were used, their metallic property introduces susceptibility artifacts to the DWI images, greatly reducing the value of DWI in evaluation.[30] If a patient does not have clips in the postsurgical bed, however, DWI can be useful for distinguishing tumor from mimicking etiologies, such as inflammation or residual benign tissue. Overall, DCE is much more reliable than DWI and has been proved as the most useful sequence for detecting recurrence. If looking at a normal postoperative DCE MR imaging sequence, early enhancement should not be seen in the arterial phase, but there should be some general low-level enhancement of the surgical bed during the venous phase. Changes in early enhancement on DCE MR imaging are very sensitive for being locally recurrent disease.[31]

Locally recurrent PCa in the post-RP patient may occur anywhere in or around the surgical bed but most commonly occurs at the VUA.[19] Recurrence tends to appear nodular and relatively hyperintense in comparison to pelvic muscle signal intensity on T2W imaging.[32] On DCE, these areas readily enhance during the arterial phase with quick washout during the venous phase.[33] This DCE enhancement appears as a focal nodular enhancement that contrasts sharply with the general background low-level venous enhancement at the VUA and has been proved important in the MR imaging evaluation. In 1 study evaluating 46 post-RP BCR patients, Casciani and colleagues[34] found that addition of DCE to T2W for evaluation increased sensitivity from 48% to 88% and increased specificity from 52% to 100%. Cirillo and colleagues[31] reported similar findings with their cohort of 72 post-RP BCR patients, with a sensitivity of 84.1% (compared with 61.4%) and specificity of 89.3% (compared with 82.1%) when DCE was combined with T2W compared with T2W only. Finally, if DWI has not been compromised by use of surgical clips, recurrent disease appears hypointense on the apparent diffusion coefficient (ADC) map and hyperintense on high *b*-value imaging.[35] Therefore, overall signal patterns are similar to those of in situ primary PCa. Recurrent disease, however, is more difficult to identify due to the changed anatomy and missing background of normal prostatic tissue. Additionally, unlike in imaging evaluation for primary PCa, DCE serves as the most important sequence in detection.

There are some common mimics and pitfalls that the radiologist should keep in mind when identifying areas suspicious for post-RP recurrent disease. First, there is always a possibility of residual glandular tissue postsurgery, and this is PSA-producing and may mimic recurrent disease on imaging. Residual glandular tissue may take on a nodular appearance on T2W, resembling PCa. The functional data, however, for this area on MR should help differentiate this benign etiology—it should not have any signal abnormality on DWI and should not enhance early in the arterial phase on DCE.[28] PSA kinetics should also help; PSA doubling time for residual benign tissue should be much longer than for recurrent disease.[15] Second, after surgery, it is possible that granulation tissue or hemorrhage is present near the VUA due to the procedure and subsequent natural inflammation. Granulation tissue appears hyperintense on T2W imaging, similar to recurrent tumor, and hyperenhances on an early DCE phase due to hypervascularity. Extensive hemorrhage also hyperenhances early on DCE. These mimics can be best separated from recurrent disease on DWI, on which they should appear benign with no notable signal abnormalities. Third, the appearance of fibrosis after RP is variable for each patient and may be confused with recurrence. Fibrotic tissue is highly cellular and thus may have restricted diffusion similar to recurrent tumor on DWI sequences.[36] It is also possible that on T2 alone, it may be difficult to distinguish local recurrence from mimicking fibrosis if it occurs in a nodular formation. On T2W and DCE imaging, however, fibrotic tissue should appear as more hypointense than recurrent tumor with a delayed thin layer of enhancement during the venous phase.[19,37]

Various studies have been performed testing the utility of mpMRI in detection of recurrence after prostatectomy. In 84 consecutive post-RP BCR-risk patients, Panebianco and colleagues[38] found that MR imaging had higher diagnostic accuracy (sensitivity 92% and specificity 75%) than the alternative PET/CT modality (sensitivity 62% and specificity 50%) in detection of local recurrence. The same group later verified this with other studies, reporting that mpMRI is the most promising technique for post-RP local recurrence detection.[39] Of all the mpMRI sequences, DCE MR imaging is repeatedly reported as adding exceptional value to detection. In 1 analysis of 80 post-RP patients, different mpMRI combinations were tested for detection value. The combinations of T2W + DCE and T2W + DWI + DCE had significantly higher detection rates (76.5%–82.4%) than

T2W alone or T2W + DWI (detection rates 25%–29.4%).[40] This incremental value of DCE is verified in a separate study conducted by Wassberg and colleagues,[41] which showed that detection increases along with inter-reader agreement (58% from 39% agreement) with use of DCE MR imaging. In a different study with 262 high-risk post-RP patients conducted by Panebianco and colleagues,[28] T2W + DCE gave high sensitivity, specificity, and accuracy (98%, 94%, and 93%, respectively). In addition, they found that when DWI is able to be used, it can produce comparable detection in combination with T2W (93% sensitivity, 89% specificity, and 88% accuracy). There is no true consensus, however, on the value of DWI, with other studies reporting T2W + DWI sensitivity as low as 46% to 49%.[30]

In summary, post-RP, there are many considerations when performing local imaging with mpMRI, including changed anatomy, new signal patterns, and abnormalities indicative of recurrent disease. DCE MR imaging provides significantly more value in detection of recurrent disease compared with primary tumors, and optimal imaging may be achieved with use of all 3 sequences. Caution should be used, with radiologists remaining vigilant for disease that is difficult to identify against a reduced prostate background while also keeping common mimics and pitfalls in mind.

MULTIPARAMETRIC MR IMAGING AFTER RADIATION THERAPY

The second most common definitive treatment chosen for stages I to III PCa is RT, given to up to 40% of patients over 65 years old and up to 25% of patients under 65 years old.[42] RT can be offered as EBRT or brachytherapy. EBRT is generally used for earlier-stage disease and may be offered in forms, such as intensity-modulated RT or stereotactic body RT. In this approach, all radiation is delivered externally and focused through beams to the prostate. In contrast, brachytherapy uses radioactive pellets that are implanted into the prostate. The seeds internally give off radiation to treat the prostate, and this is best used for low-grade disease and in smaller prostates. For higher-grade disease, brachytherapy may be combined with EBRT for improved cancer treatment.[43] All RT may be combined with hormonal therapy in an effort to shrink the prostate for maximal treatment efficacy.[11] The method of radiation delivery and the incorporation of hormones in treatment are important considerations for posttreatment imaging.

After RT, PSA nadir is not achieved as quickly because it is post-RP, and the decrement is more variable. Generally, patients take approximately 18 months to reach PSA nadir but may even take up to 3 years.[44–46] Establishment of PSA nadir may be further complicated by an observed PSA bounce that can occur at 9 months to 21 months that lasts for several months and is eventually followed by PSA decrease to nadir.[46–49] Once nadir is established, the patient should be followed with serial serum PSA immunoassays. The American Society for Therapeutic Radiology and Oncology (ASTRO) defines post-RP BCR using the Phoenix criteria, defined as 2 successive measurements showing a rise in serum PSA of at least 2 ng/mL above the nadir.[8] In patients with high-risk disease, up to approximately 30% can have BCR post-RT, and risk factors include higher initial clinical tumor stage, higher pretreatment Gleason score, and a shorter time interval from the end of radiotherapy until the detection of BCR.[50,51] After BCR is first detected, median times to distant metastasis and PCa-specific mortality are 5 years and 10 years, respectively.[52] Unfortunately, when attempting to determine if BCR initially represents localized or metastatic disease, RT has less established risk factors compared with RP. Generally, it has been shown that faster PSA kinetics are associated with more adverse disease; higher initial clinical tumor stage has a worse BCR prognosis; and, if PSA doubles in less than 8 months, especially in the first year after treatment, this can be a predictor for metastatic disease.[13] A majority of post-RT recurrences have been shown to be local, with top site of recurrence the prostate; therefore, evaluation with prostate mpMRI is essential in the follow-up of BCR.[52,53]

If localized disease is present in an RT patient, it most commonly occurs at the site of original tumor. Therefore, a baseline mpMRI study showing the primary tumor site can be helpful for subsequent posttreatment evaluation.[32] Expected posttreatment changes of the prostate on imaging are different based on the mode of radiation delivery used.

Multiparametric MR Imaging After External-Beam Radiation Therapy

EBRT causes overall changes in signal intensity and structure of the prostate. The irradiated prostate appears smaller as a result of gland atrophy and differentiation of the zones is made difficult by effacement of the prostatic tissue.[54] The entire prostate appears hypointense on T2W imaging, further complicating differentiation between zones as well as distinction between benign versus tumor tissue.[55] DWI and DCE appearance of the prostate is impacted as well; postradiation gland fibrosis is less cellular and has diminished vascularity compared with pretreatment prostate tissue. Changes on DWI and DCE, however, are not as drastic as on T2W, and the functional sequences are best for detecting locally recurrent disease.

On anatomic T2 imaging, structures surrounding the prostate appear different as well compared with their pretreatment appearance. Seminal vesicles appear shrunken from effects of radiation and all the muscles appear relatively hyperintense compared with pretreatment.[55,56] Bone marrow visualized around the pelvis are hypointense on T2W imaging as a result of fatty replacement of the bone marrow from the effect of radiation.

Identification of post-EBRT local recurrence is made difficult by the glandular changes that occur from treatment. On T2W imaging, recurrence appears as a nodular structure that often exhibits a capsular bulge. The nodular structure is relatively hypointense compared with normal prostatic tissue and may appear as a bulge due to the rapid growth of tumor relative to the atrophic gland.[35] Recurrence most commonly appears at the original site of the primary tumor, with only 4% to 9% of local recurrent disease appearing elsewhere.[57,58] Unfortunately, due to the changed background signal within the prostate, T2W imaging has marked limitations and is not most important for posttreatment evaluation or recurrence detection. In 1 study with 64 patients with post-EBRT recurrence suspicion, Westphalen and colleagues[59] found an area under the curve (AUC) of only 67% in correct detection of recurrent disease

on T2 alone. This was verified by another study, conducted by Sala and colleagues,[60] analyzing a cohort of 45 patients with BCR post-EBRT. They found that sensitivity for T2W alone ranged from 36% to 75%, and specificity ranged from 65% to 81%. Because T2W seems limited as an independent sequence, the functional sequences of mpMRI play a more dominant role in detection of post-RT recurrence. On DWI, signal characteristics of post-RT recurrence are similar to characteristics of primary PCa, with a focal hypointensity on the ADC map and hyperintensity on high b-value imaging corresponding with a nodular area visualized on T2W imaging. Studies analyzing the utility of DWI combined with T2W compared with T2W alone show great promise for the utility of DWI in post-RT imaging. In 1 study of a cohort of 36 patients with post-RT BCR, T2W + DWI achieved significantly higher AUC compared with T2W alone, at 88% versus 61%.[61] In another study analyzing 16 post-EBRT patients, Hara and colleagues[62] found that patient-based sensitivity and specificity for DWI were 100%, with region-based accuracy of 89%. DCE has been proved important in post-EBRT evaluation as well. Although the vascularity of the overall irradiated prostate decreases with gland atrophy, recurrent tumors retain their highly vascular network.[63,64] Recurrence shows early hyperenhancement on DCE MR imaging relative to the treated prostate, and this is especially powerful if it can be correlated with abnormality on T2 or DWI[65] (Fig. 2). In 1 study of 33 post-EBRT patients conducted by Haider and

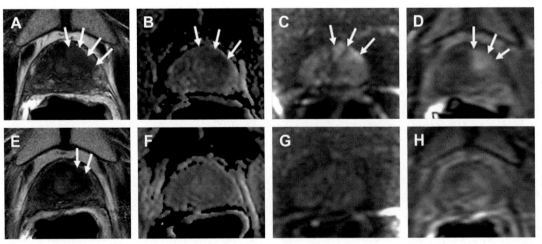

Fig. 2. A 55-year-old man, status post–EBRT, presenting with pretreatment PSA = 7.96 ng/mL. Axial T2W (A), ADC map (B), b-2000 DW MR imaging (C), and DCE MR imaging (D) show the original tumor in the left midanterior transition zone (arrows). On 1 year posttreatment follow-up, patient presented with PSA = 0.76 ng/mL. Posttreatment axial T2W MR imaging (E), ADC map (F), b-2000 DW MR imaging (G), and DCE MR imaging (H) show the prostate decreased in size and overall gland intensity changes. The tumor (arrows) is smaller and appears less concerning with indistinct DWI signal intensity and no focal enhancement on DCE MR imaging.

colleagues,[66] significantly higher sensitivity (72% vs 38%), positive predictive value (49% vs 24%), and negative predictive value (95% vs 88%) were found for DCE compared with T2W imaging. Finally, Kim and colleagues[67] tested utility of both functional sequences and found that DWI and DCE are both important for detection of recurrent disease. In their cohort of 24 patients, DWI + DCE was able to achieve significantly higher AUC (86%) than T2W, DWI, or DCE alone (*P*<.05).

Multiparametric MR Imaging After Brachytherapy

Posttreatment changes to the prostate gland are similar in brachytherapy to EBRT, however, with the addition of visualization of the radioactive seeds used. Brachytherapy seeds are radioactive material contained in small nonradioactive metallic capsules. These metallic capsules introduce magnetic resonance (MR) susceptibility artifacts, which can distort DWI the most and make interpretation difficult. On T2W imaging, the brachytherapy seeds appear as small hypointense ellipsoid structures scattered throughout the prostate gland. The gland itself is hypointense compared with pretreatment imaging, and, as seen in post-EBRT imaging, zonal and tissue differentiation are made difficult by the signal change. As a patient completes a brachytherapy course, the prostate gland becomes progressively more atrophic and the seeds gradually migrate peripherally within the gland as it shrinks in size.

Fortunately, recurrence is less of a concern after brachytherapy than it is after EBRT, due to a majority of the patients having very-low-risk primary disease. If BCR is detected and local recurrence is present, the recurrence appears as a hypointense nodule on T2W imaging that shows rapid hyperenhancement on DCE MR imaging. If DWI is not too limited, recurrent tumor appears hypointense on the ADC map and hyperintense on high *b*-value imaging. Just as with EBRT, T2W interpretation should be performed with caution due to the changed glandular background. The general signal properties remain the same between EBRT and brachytherapy; however, fewer studies have been performed to support the use of mpMRI postbrachytherapy, likely because BCR rates are so low. It is suggested that DCE is more important postbrachytherapy than it is post-EBRT due to the seed artifact on DWI.[37] Similar to EBRT, however, the most common site of recurrence postbrachytherapy is at the location of the original tumor.

Thus far, the traditional low-dose rate (LDR) brachytherapy has been described, but a new form of brachytherapy is offered in temporary high-dose rate (HDR) form. The advantage of HDR is that the source dwell time and position can be modulated, allowing more exact dosimetry.[68] Postbrachytherapy imaging differs with HDR, because the seeds are removed, so the quality does not suffer from susceptibility artifacts. Because HDR is so new and BCR postbrachytherapy occurs less frequently, data validating the use of mpMRI post-HDR are limited. In a study of 16 HDR patients conducted by Tamada and colleagues,[69] DWI shows high sensitivity for detection of recurrence and remains noncompromised with the removal of seeds, and DCE shows early hyperenhancement in recurrent disease. T2W sensitivity is limited due to the limitation of gland background (**Fig. 3**).

Many of the pitfalls encountered when performing post-RT imaging overlap with usual pitfalls encountered in mpMRI evaluation for primary tumor detection.[70] False-positive results seen on the mpMRI sequences often correspond with prostatitis, hemorrhage, dysplasia, or benign prostatic hyperplasia, even in the irradiated prostate.[71] Specific to post-RT imaging, however, a focal hypointensity on T2 may actually be treated tumor. Mimics like this are most unclear if there is no pretreatment imaging available. Finally, it is important to make note of whether a patient received hormonal therapy in conjunction with RT. Hormonal therapy can cause additional changes to the gland, which can make interpretation even more difficult. Post–androgen deprivation, the prostate shrinks in size, overall ADC values significantly increase, and gland vascularity decreases.[72,73]

In summary, post-RT, there are various factors to consider in local imaging evaluation. If a patient is post-EBRT, overall gland changes must be accounted for. Similar changes must be accounted for in postbrachytherapy patients, with the addition of imaging artifact from the brachytherapy seeds used. Generally, the functional sequences of mpMRI remain best for detecting local disease post-RT.

MULTIPARAMETRIC MR IMAGING AFTER FOCAL THERAPY

Focal therapy is a newly emerging treatment option for patients with localized PCa that falls within a certain criteria that allows the index tumor to be directly targeted. Focal therapy relies on use of various energies for local destruction of cancer cells in the gland, such as microwave, focal laser ablation (FLA), cryotherapy, and HIFU. Regardless of which energy is used, there are numerous posttreatment changes seen on follow-up MR imaging that are important to

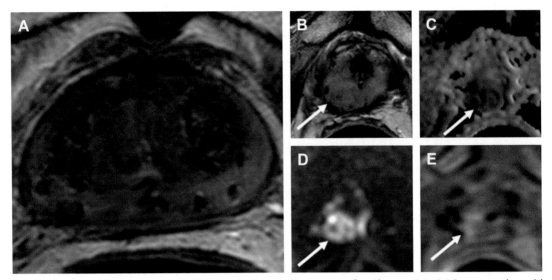

Fig. 3. A 77-year-old man, status post-LDR brachytherapy 8 years ago for Gleason 4 + 4 PCa, presenting with PSA = 11.97 ng/mL. He underwent endorectal coil 3T MR imaging after treatment, and then 8 years later for recurrence suspicion. Axial T2W image shows normal posttreatment changes of the gland, with brachytherapy seeds visible as hypointense structures and the background of the gland hypointense with zonal differentiation made difficult (*A*). Axial T2W (*B*), ADC map (*C*), *b*-2000 DW MR imaging (*D*), and DCE MR imaging (*E*) at distal apex of the prostate shows the recurrent lesion (*arrows*).

consider for success of treatment as well as for evaluation of possible recurrence. After a patient receives focal therapy, a good treatment response is defined as a negative control biopsy, absence of a persistent lesion on posttreatment imaging, and a decrease in PSA of at least 50%.[9] Focal therapy is still greatly in its investigative stages and seems to demonstrate reasonable efficacy. PSA, however, is not very reliable in postfocal therapy follow-up because there is preservation of a large amount of prostate tissue postablation and thus no agreement on a definition for BCR.[4] The consensus is that postablation PSA surveillance should be judged based on PSA kinetics. Many institutions use the Phoenix or ASTRO (increase in 3 successive PSA measurements) criteria for monitoring BCR after focal therapy, but these were both designed for surveillance of whole-gland disease.[74–78] Therefore, an integrated approach, incorporating mpMRI for imaging surveillance, has been recommended for postfocal therapy follow-up.[9]

In postfocal therapy follow-up, it is important to establish posttreatment changes very soon after the energy is applied to the prostate and to pay attention to the PSA nadir that is established after treatment. In 2014, attempt at standardization of postfocal therapy follow-up was made using the Delphi consensus method, by Muller and colleagues.[79] Right after treatment, it is prudent to establish a baseline with regular follow-up: a postablation control biopsy that includes targeting of the

treated area should be performed, and follow-up should be done with mpMRI for a minimum of 5 years (**Fig. 4**). mpMRI should include the standard sequences T1W, T2W, DWI (ADC map and high *b*-value >1000), and DCE, optimized at 3T with endorectal coil. It is also suggested by some that an mpMRI be obtained within 2 days to 7 days after treatment to capture early posttreatment findings.[80] Generally, the appearance that focal therapy has on mpMRI can make it difficult to assess for recurrence, because the changes that the therapy induces in the prostatic architecture overlap greatly with tumor appearance.[32]

Posttreatment appearance of the prostate varies somewhat based on energy used in the therapy. Cryotherapy alternates freeze-thaw cycles, producing coagulative necrosis within the prostate gland. The visualized area affected by the cycles is often larger than the actual area of cells killed, and imaging can underestimate true effect of the cryotherapy. The treatment area shows drastically changed architecture and hypointensity on T2.[81] HIFU, which uses focused ultrasound for heating, shows similar heterogenous hypointensity on T2 but may also show DCE perfusion at the periphery of the treatment area.[81,82] Finally, FLA shows the heterogenous T2 hypointensity along with restricted diffusion on DWI.[6] Generally, all treatments eventually result in atrophy of the treated area, causing decreased T2 signal, lower signal on DWI, and lower perfusion on DCE[35] (**Fig. 5**).

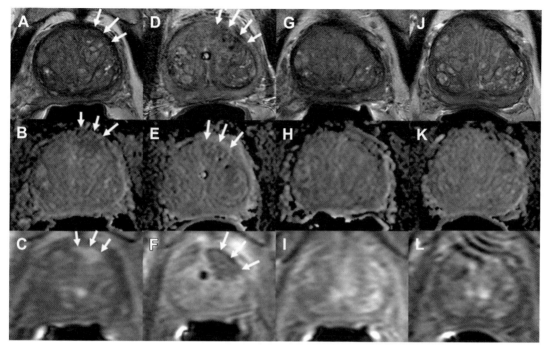

Fig. 4. A 74-year-old man, initially presenting with PSA = 7.33 ng/mL. Axial T2W (A), ADC map (B), and DCE MR imaging (C) show the site of original tumor in the left mid anterior transition zone (arrows), found positive for Gleason 3 + 4 PCa on targeted biopsy. The patient was offered FLA, and 1 day posttreatment axial T2W (D) shows a hypointensity within the treated area (arrows) with some focal changes in prostatic architecture, ADC map (E) shows corresponding restricted diffusion in the treated area (arrows), and DCE MR imaging (F) shows low perfusion of this region (arrows). On follow-up 1 year later, patient presented with PSA = 2.59 ng/mL and axial T2W (G), ADC map (H), and DCE MR imaging (I) show shrinkage of the original tumor area with less distinct findings on all sequences. Targeted biopsy of the treated area was negative for disease. At 2-year posttreatment follow-up, patient presented with PSA = 5.58 ng/mL with axial T2W (J), ADC map (K), and DCE MR imaging (L) showing overall slightly changed architecture in the left midanterior transition zone compared with baseline but no signal findings indicative of disease. A 2-year follow-up targeted biopsy of the treated area was negative for disease.

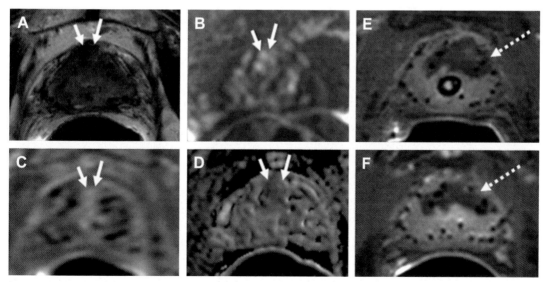

Fig. 5. A 62-year-old man, status post–LDR brachytherapy presenting with PSA = 1.98 ng/mL. Axial T2W (A), b2000 DW MR imaging (B), DCE MR imaging (C), and ADC map (D) show recurrent lesion in the midline anterior transition zone (arrows). This area was subsequently biopsied and came back positive for PCa. After diagnosis of postbrachytherapy focal recurrence, patient was offered FLA. The 1-day postablation DWI image is shown (E), with the treatment area (dotted arrows) shrinking in size 1 year postablation, as shown in (F). Postablation, biopsy of the area was benign, and PSA = 0.21 ng/mL.

Most focal therapy methods do not have long follow-up times reported, but there are some data about recurrent disease in current studies. Postcryotherapy, 20% to 40% of treated patients have can have BCR, reported up to 10 years from treatment.[83,84] For post-HIFU follow-up, a 160-patient study conducted by Mearini and colleagues[85] found that BCR-free rate in 72 months was 70% for low-risk disease and 41% for intermediate-risk disease. Finally, in a phase II study of FLA in 27 patients, Eggener and colleagues[86] found cancer in 10 patients at 12-month follow-up, with 27% tumors found in the ablation zone and 73% found outside the ablation zone. Appearance of recurrence itself after all treatments takes on signal properties similar to primary disease. Recurrence may be most difficult to differentiate from normal posttreatment on T2, however, making the functional sequences more important for identification.[35]

SUMMARY

Prostate mpMRI offers promising potential for visualization of posttreatment changes and for evaluation of local recurrent disease in the context of BCR. Because the mpMRI evaluation is so important in detection of localized recurrence, it is vital that radiologists be communicative with the multidisciplinary team. The referring urologist, radiation oncologist, or medical oncologist should be aware that the radiologist will be acquiring and interpreting a dedicated MR imaging for posttreatment follow-up and recurrence detection. Therefore, referring physicians should provide all the information that they can about a patient, including entire PCa history, PSA measurements, past treatments, and any past imaging (Box 2). Referring physicians should also advise their patients that for optimal imaging, they will receive a full mpMRI with endorectal coil, acquired at 3T with contrast injection.

Box 2
What the referring physician needs to know for local imaging evaluation after treatment of prostate cancer

- This is a dedicated high-resolution MR imaging for posttreatment follow-up
- Essential to provide
  - Complete PCa history
  - PSA measurements
  - All past treatments
  - Any past imaging

Radiologists can make an important difference in the care of a posttreatment PCa patient. They should be comfortable not only with interpretation of mpMRI for detection of primary PCa but also with the evaluation of posttreatment local imaging. Diagnosis and timely treatment of recurrent PCa are vital because care of primary cancer improves and course of disease is followed more closely. In cases of a rising PSA, it is important for any radiologist reading prostate images to be familiar with treatment types, with posttreatment anatomy, with appearance of recurrent disease, and with common pitfalls.

REFERENCES

1. Siegel RL, Miller KD, Jemal A. Cancer statistics, 2016. CA Cancer J Clin 2016;66(1):7–30.
2. Lu-Yao GL, Yao SL. Population-based study of long-term survival in patients with clinically localised prostate cancer. Lancet 1997;349(9056):906–10.
3. Trewartha D, Carter K. Advances in prostate cancer treatment. Nat Rev Drug Discov 2013;12(11):823–4.
4. Bozzini G, Colin P, Nevoux P, et al. Focal therapy of prostate cancer: energies and procedures. Urol Oncol 2013;31(2):155–67.
5. Babaian RJ, Troncoso P, Bhadkamkar VA, et al. Analysis of clinicopathologic factors predicting outcome after radical prostatectomy. Cancer 2001; 91(8):1414–22.
6. Mertan FV, Greer MD, Borofsky S, et al. Multiparametric magnetic resonance imaging of recurrent prostate cancer. Top Magn Reson Imaging 2016; 25(3):139–47.
7. Stephenson AJ, Kattan MW, Eastham JA, et al. Defining biochemical recurrence of prostate cancer after radical prostatectomy: a proposal for a standardized definition. J Clin Oncol 2006;24(24): 3973–8.
8. Roach M 3rd, Hanks G, Thames H Jr, et al. Defining biochemical failure following radiotherapy with or without hormonal therapy in men with clinically localized prostate cancer: recommendations of the RTOG-ASTRO Phoenix consensus conference. Int J Radiat Oncol Biol Phys 2006;65(4):965–74.
9. Barret E, Harvey-Bryan KA, Sanchez-Salas R, et al. How to diagnose and treat focal therapy failure and recurrence? Curr Opin Urol 2014;24(3):241–6.
10. Heidenreich A, Bastian PJ, Bellmunt J, et al. EAU guidelines on prostate cancer. Part II: treatment of advanced, relapsing, and castration-resistant prostate cancer. Eur Urol 2014;65(2):467–79.
11. Bolla M, Van Tienhoven G, Warde P, et al. External irradiation with or without long-term androgen suppression for prostate cancer with high metastatic risk: 10-year results of an EORTC randomised study. Lancet Oncol 2010;11(11):1066–73.

12. Siegel R, Ward E, Brawley O, et al. Cancer statistics, 2011: the impact of eliminating socioeconomic and racial disparities on premature cancer deaths. CA Cancer J Clin 2011;61(4):212–36.

13. Zagars GK, Pollack A. Kinetics of serum prostate-specific antigen after external beam radiation for clinically localized prostate cancer. Radiother Oncol 1997;44(3):213–21.

14. Panebianco V, Barchetti F, Sciarra A, et al. Multiparametric magnetic resonance imaging vs. standard care in men being evaluated for prostate cancer: a randomized study. Urol Oncol 2015;33(1):17.e1-e7.

15. Notley M, Yu J, Fulcher AS, et al. Pictorial review. Diagnosis of recurrent prostate cancer and its mimics at multiparametric prostate MRI. Br J Radiol 2015;88(1054):20150362.

16. Abd-Alazeez M, Ramachandran N, Dikaios N, et al. Multiparametric MRI for detection of radiorecurrent prostate cancer: added value of apparent diffusion coefficient maps and dynamic contrast-enhanced images. Prostate Cancer Prostatic Dis 2015;18(2): 128–36.

17. Weinreb JC, Barentsz JO, Choyke PL, et al. PI-RADS prostate imaging - reporting and data system: 2015, version 2. Eur Urol 2016;69(1):16–40.

18. Adamis S, Varkarakis IM. Defining prostate cancer risk after radical prostatectomy. Eur J Surg Oncol 2014;40(5):496–504.

19. Lopes Dias J, Lucas R, Magalhaes Pina J, et al. Post-treated prostate cancer: normal findings and signs of local relapse on multiparametric magnetic resonance imaging. Abdom Imaging 2015;40(7): 2814–38.

20. Freedland SJ, Humphreys EB, Mangold LA, et al. Risk of prostate cancer-specific mortality following biochemical recurrence after radical prostatectomy. JAMA 2005;294(4):433–9.

21. Han M, Partin AW, Pound CR, et al. Long-term biochemical disease-free and cancer-specific survival following anatomic radical retropubic prostatectomy. The 15-year Johns Hopkins experience. Urol Clin North Am 2001;28(3):555–65.

22. Roehl KA, Han M, Ramos CG, et al. Cancer progression and survival rates following anatomical radical retropubic prostatectomy in 3,478 consecutive patients: long-term results. J Urol 2004;172(3): 910–4.

23. Hull GW, Rabbani F, Abbas F, et al. Cancer control with radical prostatectomy alone in 1,000 consecutive patients. J Urol 2002;167(2 Pt 1):528–34.

24. Amling CL, Blute ML, Bergstralh EJ, et al. Long-term hazard of progression after radical prostatectomy for clinically localized prostate cancer: continued risk of biochemical failure after 5 years. J Urol 2000;164(1):101–5.

25. Allen SD, Thompson A, Sohaib SA. The normal post-surgical anatomy of the male pelvis following radical prostatectomy as assessed by magnetic resonance imaging. Eur Radiol 2008;18(6):1281–91.

26. Sella T, Schwartz LH, Hricak H. Retained seminal vesicles after radical prostatectomy: frequency, MRI characteristics, and clinical relevance. AJR Am J Roentgenol 2006;186(2):539–46.

27. Vargas HA, Wassberg C, Akin O, et al. MR imaging of treated prostate cancer. Radiology 2012;262(1): 26–42.

28. Panebianco V, Barchetti F, Sciarra A, et al. Prostate cancer recurrence after radical prostatectomy: the role of 3-T diffusion imaging in multi-parametric magnetic resonance imaging. Eur Radiol 2013; 23(6):1745–52.

29. Keskin MS, Argun OB, Obek C, et al. The incidence and sequela of lymphocele formation after robot-assisted extended pelvic lymph node dissection. BJU Int 2016;118(1):127–31.

30. Cha D, Kim CK, Park SY, et al. Evaluation of suspected soft tissue lesion in the prostate bed after radical prostatectomy using 3T multiparametric magnetic resonance imaging. Magn Reson Imaging 2015;33(4):407–12.

31. Cirillo S, Petracchini M, Scotti L, et al. Endorectal magnetic resonance imaging at 1.5 Tesla to assess local recurrence following radical prostatectomy using T2-weighted and contrast-enhanced imaging. Eur Radiol 2009;19(3):761–9.

32. Grant K, Lindenberg ML, Shebel H, et al. Functional and molecular imaging of localized and recurrent prostate cancer. Eur J Nucl Med Mol Imaging 2013;40(Suppl 1):S48–59.

33. Sella T, Schwartz LH, Swindle PW, et al. Suspected local recurrence after radical prostatectomy: endorectal coil MR imaging. Radiology 2004;231(2):379–85.

34. Casciani E, Polettini E, Carmenini E, et al. Endorectal and dynamic contrast-enhanced MRI for detection of local recurrence after radical prostatectomy. AJR Am J Roentgenol 2008;190(5): 1187–92.

35. McCammack KC, Raman SS, Margolis DJ. Imaging of local recurrence in prostate cancer. Future Oncol 2016;12(21):2401–15.

36. De Visschere PJ, De Meerleer GO, Futterer JJ, et al. Role of MRI in follow-up after focal therapy for prostate carcinoma. AJR Am J Roentgenol 2010;194(6): 1427–33.

37. Rouviere O, Vitry T, Lyonnet D. Imaging of prostate cancer local recurrences: why and how? Eur Radiol 2010;20(5):1254–66.

38. Panebianco V, Sciarra A, Lisi D, et al. Prostate cancer: 1HMRS-DCEMR at 3T versus [(18)F]choline PET/CT in the detection of local prostate cancer recurrence in men with biochemical progression after radical retropubic prostatectomy (RRP). Eur J Radiol 2012;81(4):700–8.

39. Alfarone A, Panebianco V, Schillaci O, et al. Comparative analysis of multiparametric magnetic resonance and PET-CT in the management of local recurrence after radical prostatectomy for prostate cancer. Crit Rev Oncol Hematol 2012; 84(1):109–21.

40. Kitajima K, Hartman RP, Froemming AT, et al. Detection of local recurrence of prostate cancer after radical prostatectomy using endorectal coil MRI at 3 T: addition of DWI and dynamic contrast enhancement to T2-Weighted MRI. AJR Am J Roentgenol 2015;205(4):807–16.

41. Wassberg C, Akin O, Vargas HA, et al. The incremental value of contrast-enhanced MRI in the detection of biopsy-proven local recurrence of prostate cancer after radical prostatectomy: effect of reader experience. AJR Am J Roentgenol 2012;199(2): 360–6.

42. Siegel R, DeSantis C, Virgo K, et al. Cancer treatment and survivorship statistics, 2012. CA Cancer J Clin 2012;62(4):220–41.

43. Moon DH, Efstathiou JA, Chen RC. What is the best way to radiate the prostate in 2016? Urol Oncol 2017;35(2):59–68.

44. Kuban DA, Thames HD, Levy LB, et al. Long-term multi-institutional analysis of stage T1-T2 prostate cancer treated with radiotherapy in the PSA era. Int J Radiat Oncol Biol Phys 2003;57(4):915–28.

45. Shipley WU, Thames HD, Sandler HM, et al. Radiation therapy for clinically localized prostate cancer: a multi-institutional pooled analysis. JAMA 1999; 281(17):1598–604.

46. Pickles T, British Columbia Cancer Agency Prostate Cohort Outcomes Initiative. Prostate-specific antigen (PSA) bounce and other fluctuations: which biochemical relapse definition is least prone to PSA false calls? An analysis of 2030 men treated for prostate cancer with external beam or brachytherapy with or without adjuvant androgen deprivation therapy. Int J Radiat Oncol Biol Phys 2006; 64(5):1355–9.

47. Kim DN, Straka C, Cho LC, et al. Early and multiple PSA bounces can occur following high-dose prostate stereotactic body radiation therapy: subset analysis of a phase 1/2 trial. Pract Radiat Oncol 2017;7(1):e43–9.

48. Horwitz EM, Levy LB, Thames HD, et al. Biochemical and clinical significance of the posttreatment prostate-specific antigen bounce for prostate cancer patients treated with external beam radiation therapy alone: a multiinstitutional pooled analysis. Cancer 2006;107(7):1496–502.

49. Caloglu M, Ciezki JP, Reddy CA, et al. PSA bounce and biochemical failure after brachytherapy for prostate cancer: a study of 820 patients with a minimum of 3 years of follow-up. Int J Radiat Oncol Biol Phys 2011;80(3):735–41.

50. Rosenbaum E, Partin A, Eisenberger MA. Biochemical relapse after primary treatment for prostate cancer: studies on natural history and therapeutic considerations. J Natl Compr Canc Netw 2004; 2(3):249–56.

51. Spratt DE, Pei X, Yamada J, et al. Long-term survival and toxicity in patients treated with high-dose intensity modulated radiation therapy for localized prostate cancer. Int J Radiat Oncol Biol Phys 2013; 85(3):686–92.

52. Zumsteg ZS, Spratt DE, Romesser PB, et al. The natural history and predictors of outcome following biochemical relapse in the dose escalation era for prostate cancer patients undergoing definitive external beam radiotherapy. Eur Urol 2015;67(6): 1009–16.

53. Zumsteg ZS, Spratt DE, Romesser PB, et al. Anatomical patterns of recurrence following biochemical relapse in the dose escalation era of external beam radiotherapy for prostate cancer. J Urol 2015;194(6):1624–30.

54. Sugimura K, Carrington BM, Quivey JM, et al. Postirradiation changes in the pelvis: assessment with MR imaging. Radiology 1990;175(3):805–13.

55. Chan TW, Kressel HY. Prostate and seminal vesicles after irradiation: MR appearance. J Magn Reson Imaging 1991;1(5):503–11.

56. Coakley FV, Teh HS, Qayyum A, et al. Endorectal MR imaging and MR spectroscopic imaging for locally recurrent prostate cancer after external beam radiation therapy: preliminary experience. Radiology 2004;233(2):441–8.

57. Arrayeh E, Westphalen AC, Kurhanewicz J, et al. Does local recurrence of prostate cancer after radiation therapy occur at the site of primary tumor? Results of a longitudinal MRI and MRSI study. Int J Radiat Oncol Biol Phys 2012;82(5):e787–93.

58. Jalloh M, Leapman MS, Cowan JE, et al. Patterns of local failure following radiation therapy for prostate cancer. J Urol 2015;194(4):977–82.

59. Westphalen AC, Kurhanewicz J, Cunha RM, et al. T2-Weighted endorectal magnetic resonance imaging of prostate cancer after external beam radiation therapy. Int Braz J Urol 2009;35(2):171–80 [discussion: 181–2].

60. Sala E, Eberhardt SC, Akin O, et al. Endorectal MR imaging before salvage prostatectomy: tumor localization and staging. Radiology 2006;238(1):176–83.

61. Kim CK, Park BK, Lee HM. Prediction of locally recurrent prostate cancer after radiation therapy: incremental value of 3T diffusion-weighted MRI. J Magn Reson Imaging 2009;29(2):391–7.

62. Hara T, Inoue Y, Satoh T, et al. Diffusion-weighted imaging of local recurrent prostate cancer after radiation therapy: comparison with 22-core three-dimensional prostate mapping biopsy. Magn Reson Imaging 2012;30(8):1091–8.

63. Rouviere O, Valette O, Grivolat S, et al. Recurrent prostate cancer after external beam radiotherapy: value of contrast-enhanced dynamic MRI in localizing intraprostatic tumor–correlation with biopsy findings. Urology 2004;63(5):922–7.

64. Franiel T, Ludemann L, Taupitz M, et al. MRI before and after external beam intensity-modulated radiotherapy of patients with prostate cancer: the feasibility of monitoring of radiation-induced tissue changes using a dynamic contrast-enhanced inversion-prepared dual-contrast gradient echo sequence. Radiother Oncol 2009;93(2):241–5.

65. Barchetti F, Panebianco V. Multiparametric MRI for recurrent prostate cancer post radical prostatectomy and postradiation therapy. Biomed Res Int 2014;2014:316272.

66. Haider MA, Chung P, Sweet J, et al. Dynamic contrast-enhanced magnetic resonance imaging for localization of recurrent prostate cancer after external beam radiotherapy. Int J Radiat Oncol Biol Phys 2008;70(2):425–30.

67. Kim CK, Park BK, Park W, et al. Prostate MR imaging at 3T using a phased-arrayed coil in predicting locally recurrent prostate cancer after radiation therapy: preliminary experience. Abdom Imaging 2010; 35(2):246–52.

68. Skowronek J. Low-dose-rate or high-dose-rate brachytherapy in treatment of prostate cancer - between options. J Contemp Brachytherapy 2013; 5(1):33–41.

69. Tamada T, Sone T, Jo Y, et al. Locally recurrent prostate cancer after high-dose-rate brachytherapy: the value of diffusion-weighted imaging, dynamic contrast-enhanced MRI, and T2-weighted imaging in localizing tumors. AJR Am J Roentgenol 2011; 197(2):408–14.

70. Hamstra DA, Rehemtulla A, Ross BD. Diffusion magnetic resonance imaging: a biomarker for treatment response in oncology. J Clin Oncol 2007;25(26): 4104–9.

71. Venkatesan AM, Stafford RJ, Duran C, et al. Prostate magnetic resonance imaging for brachytherapists: anatomy and technique. Brachytherapy 2017; 16(4):679–87.

72. Hotker AM, Mazaheri Y, Zheng J, et al. Prostate cancer: assessing the effects of androgen-deprivation therapy using quantitative diffusion-weighted and dynamic contrast-enhanced MRI. Eur Radiol 2015; 25(9):2665–72.

73. Kim AY, Kim CK, Park SY, et al. Diffusion-weighted imaging to evaluate for changes from androgen deprivation therapy in prostate cancer. AJR Am J Roentgenol 2014;203(6):W645–50.

74. Ellis DS, Manny TB Jr, Rewcastle JC. Focal cryosurgery followed by penile rehabilitation as primary treatment for localized prostate cancer: initial results. Urology 2007;70(6 Suppl):9–15.

75. Lindner U, Weersink RA, Haider MA, et al. Image guided photothermal focal therapy for localized prostate cancer: phase I trial. J Urol 2009;182(4): 1371–7.

76. Truesdale MD, Cheetham PJ, Hruby GW, et al. An evaluation of patient selection criteria on predicting progression-free survival after primary focal unilateral nerve-sparing cryoablation for prostate cancer: recommendations for follow up. Cancer J 2010; 16(5):544–9.

77. Ward JF, Jones JS. Focal cryotherapy for localized prostate cancer: a report from the national Cryo On-Line Database (COLD) Registry. BJU Int 2012; 109(11):1648–54.

78. Ahmed HU, Hindley RG, Dickinson L, et al. Focal therapy for localised unifocal and multifocal prostate cancer: a prospective development study. Lancet Oncol 2012;13(6):622–32.

79. Muller BG, van den Bos W, Brausi M, et al. Follow-up modalities in focal therapy for prostate cancer: results from a Delphi consensus project. World J Urol 2015;33(10):1503–9.

80. Ahmed HU, Moore C, Lecornet E, et al. Focal therapy in prostate cancer: determinants of success and failure. J Endourol 2010;24(5):819–25.

81. Martino P, Scattoni V, Galosi AB, et al. Role of imaging and biopsy to assess local recurrence after definitive treatment for prostate carcinoma (surgery, radiotherapy, cryotherapy, HIFU). World J Urol 2011; 29(5):595–605.

82. Kirkham AP, Emberton M, Hoh IM, et al. MR imaging of prostate after treatment with high-intensity focused ultrasound. Radiology 2008; 246(3):833–44.

83. Levy DA, Ross AE, ElShafei A, et al. Definition of biochemical success following primary whole gland prostate cryoablation. J Urol 2014;192(5):1380–4.

84. Long JP, Bahn D, Lee F, et al. Five-year retrospective, multi-institutional pooled analysis of cancer-related outcomes after cryosurgical ablation of the prostate. Urology 2001;57(3):518–23.

85. Mearini L, D'Urso L, Collura D, et al. High-intensity focused ultrasound for the treatment of prostate cancer: a prospective trial with long-term follow-up. Scand J Urol 2015;49(4):267–74.

86. Eggener SE, Yousuf A, Watson S, et al. Phase II evaluation of magnetic resonance imaging guided focal laser ablation of prostate cancer. J Urol 2016;196(6): 1670–5.

Multiparametric MR imaging of the Prostate
Pitfalls in Interpretation

Stephen Thomas, MD*, Aytekin Oto, MD, MBA

KEYWORDS

• MR imaging • Prostate MR imaging • Multiparametric • Prostate cancer • Pitfalls in interpretation

KEY POINTS

• Normal anatomic structures such as the normal central zone, anterior fibromuscular stroma, capsular insertions, surgical capsule, and periprostatic venous plexus may be misinterpreted as prostate cancer.
• Benign lesions such as focal prostate atrophy, prostatitis, transition zone nodules, benign prostatic hyperplasia nodules in the peripheral zone, and prostate calcifications may confound the diagnosis of prostate cancer.
• Prostate hemorrhage can persist for several weeks to months after biopsy and may mimic prostate cancer.
• It is crucial for radiologists to be aware of these pitfalls for accurate interpretation of multiparametric prostate MR imaging.

INTRODUCTION

Prostate cancer is the most common diagnosed cancer in males and is the second cause of cancer related death in men.[1] Screening for prostate cancer includes serum prostate-specific antigen (PSA) and digital rectal examination. Diagnosis of prostate cancer is done with transrectal ultrasound (TRUS)-guided prostate biopsy, and the TNM (tumor, node, and metastasis) stage is obtained from these variables. Multiparametric MR imaging (mpMRI) has shown significant clinical utility, not only in the diagnosis and staging of prostate cancer, but also in the workup of high-risk patients with elevated PSA with multiple negative prostate biopsies.[2] It is used to guide focused biopsies of high-risk targets, either as fusion targeted (ultrasound + MR imaging) or magnetic resonance-guided biopsy. In patients with biopsy-proven low-grade disease, mpMRI is used to complement or replace TRUS biopsy in active surveillance.

mpMRI examination of the prostate is best performed on a high field magnetic resonance unit with or without an endorectal coil and after administration of an antispasmodic agent to reduce bowel motion-related artifacts. The standard set of pulse sequences for mpMRI for the application of PI-RADS v2 includes multiplanar T2W, diffusion-weighted imaging (DWI), and dynamic contrast-enhanced MR imaging (DCE-MR imaging). Magnetic resonance spectroscopy is not formally included in PI-RADS v2 protocols or image assessment.[3]

Evaluation of mpMRI of the prostate gland has several pitfalls, with both normal anatomic structures and abnormal benign entities having similar imaging characteristics features as prostate cancer. When present, these lesions and pseudo-lesions can present diagnostic challenges. Knowledge of the magnetic resonance features of these mimics and their characteristic locations where

Department of Radiology, University of Chicago, 5841 South Maryland Avenue, MC 2026, Chicago, IL 60637, USA
* Corresponding author.
E-mail address: sthomas@hotmail.com

Radiol Clin N Am 56 (2018) 277–287
https://doi.org/10.1016/j.rcl.2017.10.009

they occur within the prostate can help differentiate these entities from prostate carcinoma.

NORMAL CENTRAL ZONE

The contemporary prostate zonal anatomy is based on the classical work done by McNeal,[4] who proposed different prostate zones. The seminal vesicles are located superiorly to the prostate and drain into the mid prostatic urethra via the ejaculatory ducts in the region of the verumontanum. The central zone is distinct from the transition zone. It surrounds the ejaculatory ducts and is located posterior to the transition zone and the urethra proximal to the verumontanum and extends to the prostate base adjacent to the seminal vesicles.[5]

The central zone forms a homogenous low T2W structure that is symmetric on either side of ejaculatory ducts, and low uniform ADC mimicking magnetic resonance features of prostate cancer (Fig. 1). On DCE-MR imaging, however, the central zone shows a type 1 (progressive) or type 2 (plateau) enhancement.[6] The central zone is symmetric on axial and coronal T2W sequences. When the transition zone is hypertrophic, it extends superiorly from the verumontanum and compresses and displaces the central zone superiorly and laterally to the base, just inferior to the seminal vesicles.[7] If the hypertrophy is asymmetric, this can cause asymmetric displacement of the central zone, which may be mistaken for prostate cancer. Its enhancement on DCE-MR imaging can be helpful in its differentiation from cancer, especially when there is asymmetry of the central zone.

Central zone cancers account for 0.5% to 2.5% of all prostate cancers. They tend to have a higher Gleason grade, are likely to invade the seminal vesicles, and have extracapsular extension (Fig. 2). They are also prone to biochemical recurrence after prostatectomy.[8] Therefore, their differentiation from normal central zone is critical.

ANTERIOR FIBROMUSCULAR STROMA

The anterior fibromuscular stroma (AFMS) forms the anterior surface of the prostate located anterior to the transition zone. It is composed of connective tissue, smooth muscle, and some skeletal muscle. There is a smooth transition from the capsule to the AMFS, with the AFMS increased in thickness medially. In most cases (89%), the AFMS forms the only anterior covering of the prostate. Laterally, the AFMS fuses with the lateral pelvic fascia and covers the outermost regions of the lateral and anterior surfaces of the prostate in most cases (85%).[9]

AFMS typically has low signal on T2-weighted and high b value DW images and ADC maps (Fig. 3). Therefore, can either obscure or mimic PCa.[10] On DCE-MR imaging, the AFMS shows a type 1 (progressive) enhancement curve. AFMS is the most delayed enhancing component of the prostate because of its fibrous and muscular histology.

In an analysis of radical prostatectomy specimens, pure anterior cancers account for 20% of all cancers, and in cases of multifocal cancer pure anterior cancers are involved at least 50% of the time. Anterior cancers tend to have higher rates of extracapsular extension.[11] Anterior cancers are hyperintense on high b-value DWI, and usually have a type 3 enhancement pattern that can help with differentiation (Fig. 4).[10]

CAPSULAR AND FASCIA INSERTION AT MIDLINE OF THE PERIPHERAL ZONE

Posterior prostatic fascia and seminal vesicles fascia (Denonvillier fascia) are composed of

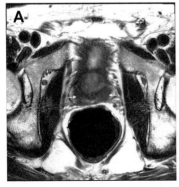 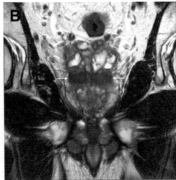 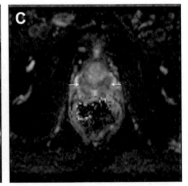

Fig. 1. 64-year-old man with elevated PSA. (A, B) Axial and coronal T2W images show the normal central zone near the base of the prostate as symmetric low-intensity structures (arrows). (C) ADC maps of the area show the same area as areas of low ADC (arrows).

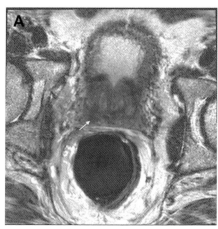
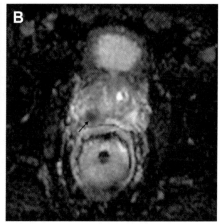

Fig. 2. 67-year-old man with biopsy-proven prostate cancer. (*A*) Axial T2W image shows small focal asymmetric mass in the right central zone (*arrow*). (*B*) ADC maps show focal restricted diffusion in the mass (*arrow*).

collagenous fibers and occasional muscle fibers that fuse with the capsule at midline near the base of the prostate at the insertion of the seminal vesicles.[9,12] This causes a smooth thickening of the prostatic capsule at the junction of the 2 lobes (**Fig. 5**).

This area is imaged as low T2 signal intensity focus and might show some diffusion restriction mimicking prostate cancer. Differentiating this focus from prostate cancer is based on its central location, smooth concave contour, and a type 1 or type 2 enhancement curve.[13]

PERIPHERAL ZONE-TRANSITION ZONE PSEUDOCAPSULE (SURGICAL CAPSULE)

In the boundary between the transition zone and peripheral zone is a concentric band of fibromuscular and compressed glandular tissue. This band is referred to as the surgical capsule as it provides a landmark for enucleation or ablation

of transitional zone benign prostate hyperplastic nodules.[14] This band of tissue can hypertrophy with age and with enlargement of the transition zone.[15]

The surgical capsule is hypointense on T2W and ADC maps because of the compressed fibromuscular tissue and does not enhance (**Fig. 6**). Its symmetric crescentic band-like shape and location should help identify this anatomic landmark.

PERIPROSTATIC VENOUS PLEXUS

The arterial supply to the prostate is via the inferior vesicle and middle rectal arteries. Venous drainage is via the prostatic venous plexus that lies mostly along the gland's lateral aspect. This communicates with dorsal venous plexus (santorini) and hemorrhoidal venous plexus posteriorly to drain in to the internal iliac vein.[16]

The periprostatic venous plexus is imaged as tubular structures outside the prostatic capsule

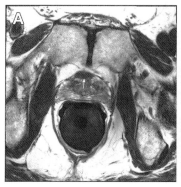
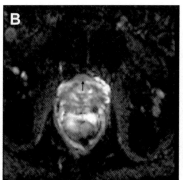
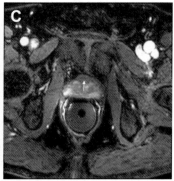

Fig. 3. 70-year-old man with prostate cancer. (*A*) Axial T2W image area of band like symmetric hypointensity anterior to the gland (*arrow*). (*B*) ADC map of the area does not show diffusion restriction (*arrow*). (*C*) DCE-MR imaging shows late enhancement, which is characteristic for AFMS (*arrow*).

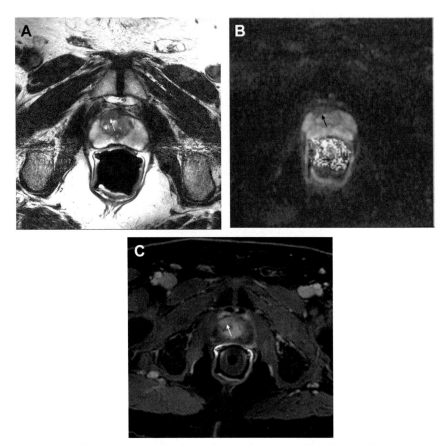

Fig. 4. 68-year-old man with negative biopsies in the face of increasing PSA. (*A*)Axial T2 image shows focal thickening and asymmetry in the region of the right AFMS (*arrow*); note normal AFMS on the left. (*B*) ADC map of the area shows a focal area of restricted diffusion on the right (*arrow*). (*C*) DCE-MR imaging shows early asymmetric early enhancement of the area (*arrow*). Prostatectomy confirmed Gleason 4 + 3 central zone cancer.

and becomes less prominent as a function of increasing age.[17] Prominent veins are hypointense on T2W and ADC. They may be mistaken for intraprostatic lesions, particularly in areas where the prostatic pseudocapsule is sparse. At the apex, there is sparseness of the pseudocapsule with intermixing of the periprostatic supporting tissue and glandular tissue sparse.[18] Because the veins

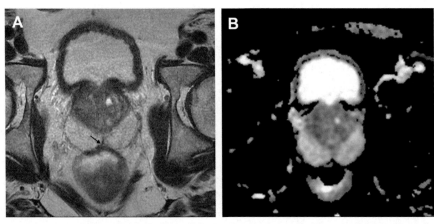

Fig. 5. 61-year-old man with elevated PSA. (*A*) Axial T2W image shows focal area of thickening of the prostate capsule at the junction of the 2 lobes (*arrow*). (*B*) ADC map of the area shows no focal restricted diffusion. Prostatectomy did not reveal cancer in that zone.

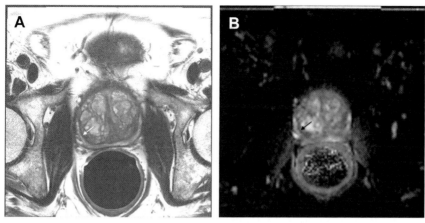

Fig. 6. 68-year-old man undergoing active surveillance for Gleason score 6 prostate cancer. (*A*) Axial T2W image shows thickening of the surgical capsule as a dark band (*arrow*). (*B*) ADC maps of the area shows band like area of low ADC (*arrow*). This is a normal variant and needs to be differentiated from prostate cancer.

directly drain the prostate gland, they enhance avidly on DCE-MR imaging (Fig. 7). Tracing their linear morphology on multiple slices and planes will allow the reader to identify them.

FOCAL PROSTATE ATROPHY

Focal prostate atrophy (FPA) is a common histologic diagnosis found in 73% of biopsy specimens with proliferative inflammatory atrophy (PIA) being

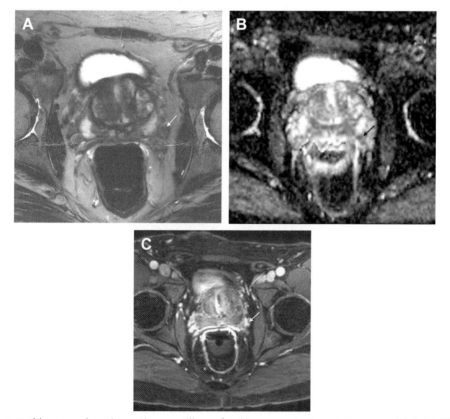

Fig. 7. 68-year-old man undergoing active surveillance for Gleason score 6 prostate cancer. (*A*) Axial T2W image shows low intensity tubular structures outside the prostate (*arrow*). (*B*) ADC maps of the area show mild hypointensity in the periprostatic area (*arrow*). (*C*) DCE-MR imaging shows brisk enhancement of venous plexus (*arrow*).

the most common type.[19,20] It has not been proven to have an association with prostate cancer. Finding PIA in negative biopsies correlates with a decreased frequency of detecting prostate cancer in men with persistent suspicion of prostate cancer.[21] FPA can mimic prostate cancer on histology and MR imaging and may lead to overdiagnosis.[20] There is a positive and significant association between the extent of atrophy and the total or free serum PSA elevation, possibly due to damaged epithelial cells in atrophic acini.[22]

Focal atrophy has volume loss and appears hypointense on T2W, with moderate diffusion restriction and moderate enhancement on DCE-MR imaging (Fig. 8). The degree of diffusion restriction and tissue enhancement is usually less marked than with prostate cancer.[23]

POSTBIOPSY HEMORRHAGE

Postbiopsy hemorrhage occurs along the needle track and tends to be larger than what would be expected from the needle. Postbiopsy hemorrhage is imaged as focal, diffuse, or striated high signal on T1W (Fig. 9) and can cause decreased T2 signal intensity that can mimic or obscure an area of tumor.[24] The intrinsic high T1 signal may limit qualitative interpretation of DCE-MR images. Subtraction images are critical for accurate interpretation of DCE-MR imaging in these cases.

Postbiopsy hemorrhage can be detected up to 4 months after biopsy. This is possibly because of the production of citrate by the gland, which has an anticoagulant effect.[24] Hemorrhage is seen in about 49% of patients at 21 days.[24] A delay of 6 to 8 weeks after biopsy has been suggested to decrease the confounding imaging findings of hemorrhage.[25]

Identifying prostate cancer in areas of hemorrhage can be difficult. Prostate cancer tends to have lower homogenous T2 signal and ADC values compared with hemorrhagic and nonhemorrhagic benign peripheral zone (PZ).[26] Using subtraction images may improve performance of DCE-MR imaging. Prostate cancer has decreased levels of citrate, leading to less hemorrhage in areas of cancer than surrounding benign PZ, producing a hemorrhage exclusion sign. Areas in the PZ where hemorrhage is excluded in conjunction with a corresponding area of homogeneous low-signal intensity at T2-weighted imaging are highly accurate for cancer identification.[27]

PROSTATITIS/INFLAMMATION

Acute prostatitis is usually caused by an acute bacterial infection of the prostate gland. It is estimated to comprise up to 10% of all prostatitis diagnoses, and its incidence peaks in persons 20 to 40 years of age and in persons older than 70 years.[28] Most cases of acute bacterial prostatitis are caused by ascending urethral infection or intraprostatic reflux caused by multiple risk factors.[29] Acute bacterial prostatitis is most frequently caused by *Escherichia coli*, followed by *Pseudomonas aeruginosa*.[29]

Chronic bacterial prostatitis may result from undertreated acute prostatitis and is thought to be caused by infection moving from the distal urethra to the prostate and has a lifetime prevalence of 1.8% to 8.2%.[30]

Prostatitis can be focal or diffuse, involving both the PZ and the transition zone (TZ). On MR imaging, the affected areas are low on T2W and ADC with mild-to-moderate diffusion restriction caused by the increased inflammatory cellular infiltrate

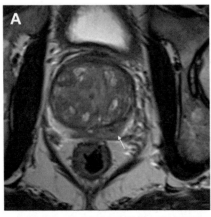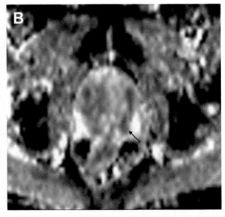

Fig. 8. 67-year-old with elevated PSA. (A) Axial T2W image shows a mass with low signal in the left PZ (*arrow*). (B) ADC map shows of the area shows low ADC (*arrow*). The area was biopsied under MR imaging guidance, and histology confirmed proliferative inflammatory atrophy.

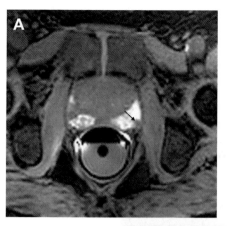
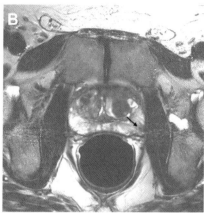
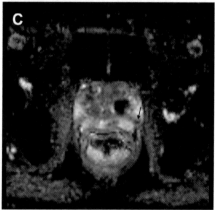

Fig. 9. 67-year-old with biopsy-proven Gleason score 4 + 3 prostate cancer for staging. (*A*) Axial precontrast T1 shows diffuse striated T1 hyperintensity in the PZ. Note focal area of sparing in the left PZ (hemorrhage exclusion sign, *arrow*). (*B*) Axial T2W image shows scattered low signal in the PZ with more focal area of signal abnormality corresponding to the area of sparing on T1W image (*arrow*). (*C*) ADC maps show low signal in the PZ with a focal area of restricted diffusion corresponding to the area of cancer proven by prostatectomy (*arrow*).

(Fig. 10). The diffusion restriction in chronic prostatitis is lower than in prostate cancer.[31] On DCE-MR imaging, areas of prostatitis can have early enhancement and washout similar to prostate cancer but have a band-like or wedge-shaped morphology.[7,32]

Granulomatous prostatitis is a benign inflammatory condition histologically characterized by epithelioid granulomas with or without other inflammatory cells.[33] It is caused by urinary tract infection, systemic infection, fungal infection, or intravesical administration of Bacillus Calmette–Guerin (BCG) for bladder cancer.[33] Although uncommon, its diagnosis in increasing due to increased transurethral resection of the prostate (TURP), needle biopsy procedures, and extensive use of intravesical BCG instillation for the treatment of nonmuscle-invasive bladder cancer (NMIBC).[33,34]

Clinically, granulomatous prostatitis can present with a firm palpable nodule or a hard and fixed nodule on digital rectal examination with elevated PSA. It can coexist with areas of prostate cancer, and diagnosis is based on needle biopsy and pathologic analysis.[33] On MR imaging, granulomatous prostatitis has low signal on T2W, and low ADC, making it difficult to discriminate from PCa.[35,36] Foci of granulomatous prostatitis can be mischaracterized on mpMRI as a moderate to highly suspicious lesion for prostate cancer leading to false-negative MR imaging findings on targeted biopsies.[36]

TRANSITION ZONE NODULES

Benign prostatic hyperplasia (BPH) refers to the stromal and glandular epithelial hyperplasia that occurs in the TZ of the prostate.[37] Some of the BPH nodules can have low T2 and ADC signal and demonstrate early enhancement with wash-out on DCE-MR images mimicking PCa.[38] Because 24% of prostate cancers are found in the in the TZ, it is important to differentiate between benign BPH nodules and TZ cancers.[39] TZ cancers tend to be larger, have high preoperative PSA, and lower Gleason scores compared with PZ cancers.[40] T2W can be used evaluate the morphology of the lesion in the TZ. The

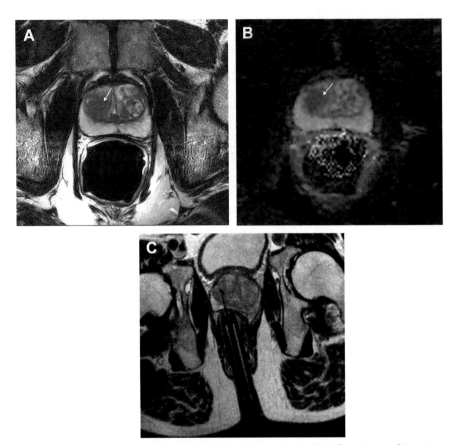

Fig. 10. 54-year-old man with elevated PSA. (*A*) Axial T2W image shows ill-defined area of hypointensity in the right TZ (*arrow*). (*B*) ADC maps of the area show low signal (*arrow*). (*C*) Transrectal MR imaging-guided biopsy of the area showed acute on chronic prostatitis on histology.

morphology and texture of the TZ nodules are important in distinguishing between BPH nodules and TZ cancers. Benign BPH nodules have a well-defined margin, rounded. TZ cancers tend to have irregular margins and lenticular shaped, larger and possibly show invasion (**Fig. 11**).[7,41] Typically, TZ cancers tend to have lower ADC values compared with BPH.

It is important to understand the imaging features of BPH nodules and TZ cancers, as

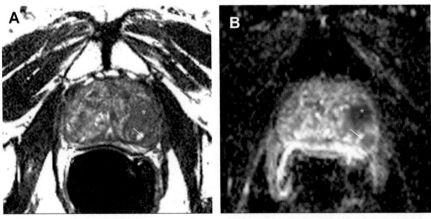

Fig. 11. 85-year-old man with elevated PSA and biopsy-proven Gleason 3 + 4 prostate cancer. (*A*) Axial T2W image shows ill-defined area of hypointensity in the left TZ (*asterisk*) and adjacent focal nodule with well-defined margins and low T2 signal (*arrow*). (*B*) ADC map of the area shows increased restricted diffusion in the biopsy-proven cancer (*asterisk*) compared with the benign prostatic hyperplasia nodule (*arrow*).

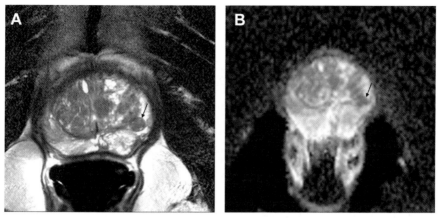

Fig. 12. 54-year-old man with elevated PSA. (*A*) Axial T2W image shows a well-defined nodule in the left PZ (*arrow*). (*B*) ADC map of the region shows restricted diffusion of the BPH nodule (*arrow*).

anterior predominant tumors are often undersampled on conventional TRUS biopsy, and MR imaging is usually performed in these patients with initial negative biopsy in the face of increasing PSA caused by large anterior cancers.[42]

BENIGN PROSTATIC HYPERPLASIA NODULES IN THE PERIPHERAL ZONE

Benign prostatic nodules can occasionally originate in the PZ of the prostate and are histologically similar to TZ nodules.[43,44] Histologic tissue

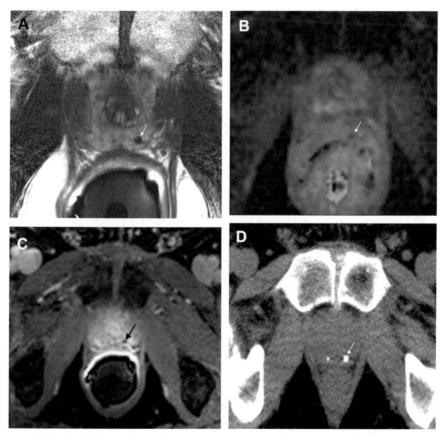

Fig. 13. 72-year-old man with biopsy-proven Gleason 3 + 4 prostate cancer. (*A*) Axial T2W image shows a focal area devoid of signal in the PZ (*arrow*). (*B*) ADC map shows focal hypointensity in the same area (*arrow*). (*C*) DCE-MR imaging of the area shows no enhancement corresponding in the focus of signal abnormality (*arrow*). (*D*) Computed tomography scan confirms the presence of a focal calcification (*arrow*) at that location.

analysis suggests some of these nodules originate from the PZ and are not the extension or herniation of TZ nodules.[45] They tend to be purely glandular in etiology. They are usually well circumscribed, ovoid, or round, and do not extend to the capsule.[43] They have low T2 and ADC signal with avid early enhancement and wash-out similar to PZ cancers (**Fig. 12**). Their well-defined borders and round shape are the 2 important imaging findings in their differentiation from PZ cancer.

PROSTATIC CALCIFICATIONS

Prostatic calcifications are relatively common radiologic findings and increase with age over 40. They can be associated with disease processes such as BPH, infection, and metabolic abnormalities.[46] Corpora amylacea are presumably precursors to calcified stones. Analysis of the proteins in prostatic corpora amylacea and calculi found that the predominant proteins comprising these concretions are proteins involved in acute inflammation, and in particular proteins contained in neutrophil granules.[47] Prostate calcifications are typically hypointense on T2W and ADC and do not enhance (**Fig. 13**). Complete lack of enhancement on MR imaging is important in their differentiation from prostate cancer. Correlation with computed tomography can be useful in confirming focal calcification. Corpora amylacea can occur within foci of prostatic adenocarcinoma; however, incidence is low and more associated with low Gleason grade cancers.[48]

SUMMARY

mpMRI is widely embraced for the diagnosis, staging, and surveillance of prostate cancer. However, normal anatomic structures and many benign entities have overlapping imaging features with prostate cancer. Although some of these entities require biopsy and histopathologic diagnosis, some have characteristic imaging features that are suggestive of their diagnosis. Knowledge of these pitfalls is important in establishing a correct diagnosis and avoiding unnecessary biopsies, as these entities are encountered routinely in clinical practice.

REFERENCES

1. Group USCSW. United States cancer statistics: 1999–2013 incidence and mortality Web-based report. 2013. Available at: http://www.cdc.gov/uscs. Accessed May 1, 2017.
2. Murphy G, Haider M, Ghai S, et al. The expanding role of MRI in prostate cancer. AJR Am J Roentgenol 2013;201(6):1229–38.
3. American College of Radiology. MR prostate imaging reporting and data system version 2.0. Washington, DC: American College of Radiology; 2015. Available at: http://www.acr.org/Quality-Safety/Resources/PIRADS/. Accessed May 1, 2017.
4. McNeal JE. Regional morphology and pathology of the prostate. Am J Clin Pathol 1968;49(3):347–57.
5. Vargas HA, Akin O, Franiel T, et al. Normal central zone of the prostate and central zone involvement by prostate cancer: clinical and MR imaging implications. Radiology 2012;262(3):894–902.
6. Hansford BG, Karademir I, Peng Y, et al. Dynamic contrast-enhanced MR imaging features of the normal central zone of the prostate. Acad Radiol 2014;21(5):569–77.
7. Rosenkrantz AB, Taneja SS. Radiologist, be aware: ten pitfalls that confound the interpretation of multiparametric prostate MRI. AJR Am J Roentgenol 2014;202(1):109–20.
8. Cohen RJ, Shannon BA, Phillips M, et al. Central zone carcinoma of the prostate gland: a distinct tumor type with poor prognostic features. J Urol 2008;179(5):1762–7 [discussion: 1767].
9. Kiyoshima K, Yokomizo A, Yoshida T, et al. Anatomical features of periprostatic tissue and its surroundings: a histological analysis of 79 radical retropubic prostatectomy specimens. Jpn J Clin Oncol 2004;34(8):463–8.
10. Ward E, Baad M, Peng Y, et al. Multi-parametric MR imaging of the anterior fibromuscular stroma and its differentiation from prostate cancer. Abdom Radiol (NY) 2017;42(3):926–34.
11. Koppie TM, Bianco FJ Jr, Kuroiwa K, et al. The clinical features of anterior prostate cancers. BJU Int 2006;98(6):1167–71.
12. Walz J, Epstein JI, Ganzer R, et al. A critical analysis of the current knowledge of surgical anatomy of the prostate related to optimisation of cancer control and preservation of continence and erection in candidates for radical prostatectomy: an update. Eur Urol 2016;70(2):301–11.
13. Yu J, Fulcher AS, Turner MA, et al. Prostate cancer and its mimics at multiparametric prostate MRI. Br J Radiol 2014;87(1037):20130659.
14. Kahokehr AA, Gilling PJ. Which laser works best for benign prostatic hyperplasia? Curr Urol Rep 2013; 14(6):614–9.
15. Semple JE. Surgical capsule of the benign enlargement of the prostate. Its development and action. Br Med J 1963;1(5346):1640–3.
16. Cristini C, Di Pierro GB, Leonardo C, et al. Safe digital isolation of the santorini plexus during radical retropubic prostatectomy. BMC Urol 2013;13:13.
17. Allen KS, Kressel HY, Arger PH, et al. Age-related changes of the prostate: evaluation by MR imaging. AJR Am J Roentgenol 1989;152(1):77–81.
18. Ayala AG, Ro JY, Babaian R, et al. The prostatic capsule: does it exist? Its importance in the staging

and treatment of prostatic carcinoma. Am J Surg Pathol 1989;13(1):21–7.

19. Benedetti I, Bettin A, Reyes N. Inflammation and focal atrophy in prostate needle biopsy cores and association to prostatic adenocarcinoma. Ann Diagn Pathol 2016;24:55–61.

20. Freitas DM, Andriole GL Jr, Castro-Santamaria R, et al. Extent of baseline prostate atrophy is associated with lower incidence of low- and high-grade prostate cancer on repeat biopsy. Urology 2017;103:161–6.

21. Servian P, Celma A, Planas J, et al. Clinical significance of proliferative inflammatory atrophy in negative prostatic biopsies. Prostate 2016;76(16):1501–6.

22. Billis A, Meirelles LR, Magna LA, et al. Extent of prostatic atrophy in needle biopsies and serum PSA levels: is there an association? Urology 2007;69(5):927–30.

23. Kitzing YX, Prando A, Varol C, et al. Benign conditions that mimic prostate carcinoma: MR imaging features with histopathologic correlation. Radiographics 2016;36(1):162–75.

24. White S, Hricak H, Forstner R, et al. Prostate cancer: effect of postbiopsy hemorrhage on interpretation of MR images. Radiology 1995;195(2):385–90.

25. Qayyum A, Coakley FV, Lu Y, et al. Organ-confined prostate cancer: effect of prior transrectal biopsy on endorectal MRI and MR spectroscopic imaging. AJR Am J Roentgenol 2004;183(4):1079–83.

26. Rosenkrantz AB, Kopec M, Kong X, et al. Prostate cancer vs. post-biopsy hemorrhage: diagnosis with T2- and diffusion-weighted imaging. J Magn Reson Imaging 2010;31(6):1387–94.

27. Barrett T, Vargas HA, Akin O, et al. Value of the hemorrhage exclusion sign on T1-weighted prostate MR images for the detection of prostate cancer. Radiology 2012;263(3):751–7.

28. Roberts RO, Lieber MM, Rhodes T, et al. Prevalence of a physician-assigned diagnosis of prostatitis: the Olmsted County Study of Urinary Symptoms and Health Status Among Men. Urology 1998;51(4):578–84.

29. Coker TJ, Dierfeldt DM. Acute bacterial prostatitis: diagnosis and management. Am Fam Physician 2016;93(2):114–20.

30. Holt JD, Garrett WA, McCurry TK, et al. Common questions about chronic prostatitis. Am Fam Physician 2016;93(4):290–6.

31. Gurses B, Tasdelen N, Yencilek F, et al. Diagnostic utility of DTI in prostate cancer. Eur J Radiol 2011;79(2):172–6.

32. Sciarra A, Panebianco V, Ciccariello M, et al. Magnetic resonance spectroscopic imaging (1H-MRSI) and dynamic contrast-enhanced magnetic resonance (DCE-MRI): pattern changes from inflammation to prostate cancer. Cancer Invest 2010;28(4):424–32.

33. Shukla P, Gulwani HV, Kaur S. Granulomatous prostatitis: clinical and histomorphologic survey of the disease in a tertiary care hospital. Prostate Int 2017;5(1):29–34.

34. Stillwell TJ, Engen DE, Farrow GM. The clinical spectrum of granulomatous prostatitis: a report of 200 cases. J Urol 1987;138(2):320–3.

35. Bour L, Schull A, Delongchamps NB, et al. Multiparametric MRI features of granulomatous prostatitis and tubercular prostate abscess. Diagn Interv Imaging 2013;94(1):84–90.

36. Rais-Bahrami S, Nix JW, Turkbey B, et al. Clinical and multiparametric MRI signatures of granulomatous prostatitis. Abdom Radiol (NY) 2017;42(7):1956–62.

37. Aaron L, Franco OE, Hayward SW. Review of prostate anatomy and embryology and the etiology of benign prostatic hyperplasia. Urol Clin North Am 2016;43(3):279–88.

38. Oto A, Kayhan A, Jiang Y, et al. Prostate cancer: differentiation of central gland cancer from benign prostatic hyperplasia by using diffusion-weighted and dynamic contrast-enhanced MR imaging. Radiology 2010;257(3):715–23.

39. McNeal JE, Redwine EA, Freiha FS, et al. Zonal distribution of prostatic adenocarcinoma. Correlation with histologic pattern and direction of spread. Am J Surg Pathol 1988;12(12):897–906.

40. King CR, Ferrari M, Brooks JD. Prognostic significance of prostate cancer originating from the transition zone. Urol Oncol 2009;27(6):592–7.

41. Hoeks CM, Hambrock T, Yakar D, et al. Transition zone prostate cancer: detection and localization with 3-T multiparametric MR imaging. Radiology 2013;266(1):207–17.

42. Lawrentschuk N, Haider MA, Daljeet N, et al. 'Prostatic evasive anterior tumours': the role of magnetic resonance imaging. BJU Int 2010;105(9):1231–6.

43. Oyen RH, Van de Voorde WM, Van Poppel HP, et al. Benign hyperplastic nodules that originate in the peripheral zone of the prostate gland. Radiology 1993;189(3):707–11.

44. Liu X, Tang J, Yang JC, et al. An autopsy specimen study of benign hyperplastic nodules in the peripheral zone of the prostate. Zhonghua Nan Ke Xue 2008;14(4):307–10 [in Chinese].

45. Tang J, Yang JC, Zhang Y, et al. Does benign prostatic hyperplasia originate from the peripheral zone of the prostate? A preliminary study. BJU Int 2007;100(5):1091–6.

46. Klimas R, Bennett B, Gardner WA Jr. Prostatic calculi: a review. Prostate 1985;7(1):91–6.

47. Sfanos KS, Wilson BA, De Marzo AM, et al. Acute inflammatory proteins constitute the organic matrix of prostatic corpora amylacea and calculi in men with prostate cancer. Proc Natl Acad Sci U S A 2009;106(9):3443–8.

48. Christian JD, Lamm TC, Morrow JF, et al. Corpora amylacea in adenocarcinoma of the prostate: incidence and histology within needle core biopsies. Mod Pathol 2005;18(1):36–9.

MR Imaging–Targeted Prostate Biopsies

Saradwata Sarkar, PhD[a], Sadhna Verma, MD, FSAR[b],*

KEYWORDS

- Prostate cancer • Prostate biopsy • In-gantry MR imaging–targeted biopsy
- Cognitive MR imaging–ultrasound fusion targeted biopsy
- Software-guided MR imaging–ultrasound fusion targeted biopsy

KEY POINTS

- Conventional ultrasound imaging has limited tissue contrast for localizing prostate cancer during prostate biopsies. Multiparametric MR imaging offers improved localization of prostatic tumors allowing tumor-targeted biopsies.
- In-gantry MR imaging–targeted biopsies provide improved targeting and accuracy validation compared with other biopsy approaches. The in-gantry approach requires increased procedure times and costs.
- MR imaging–ultrasound fusion biopsies are a practical, cost-effective approach to performing MR imaging–targeted biopsies outside the MR imaging scanner in an office setting.
- Cognitive MR imaging–ultrasound fusion targeted biopsies are cost-effective but require considerable operator expertise. Software MR imaging–ultrasound fusion targeted biopsies are less operator-dependent and allow accurate targeting with relatively lower costs compared with in-gantry biopsies.
- MR imaging–targeted biopsies result in higher detection rates of clinically significant cancer and lower detection rates of clinically insignificant cancer compared with conventional ultrasound-guided biopsies.

INTRODUCTION

Prostate cancer (PCa) is the most frequently diagnosed cancer in American men and the second leading cause of cancer-related death.[1] Currently, the only definitive way to confirm the presence of PCa is through pathologic analysis of tissue samples obtained from prostate biopsy. Conventionally, prostate biopsies involve the systematic extraction of 12 or more tissue samples from different parts of the prostate under transrectal ultrasound image guidance (TRUS-B). This procedure is often referred to as "blind" systematic biopsy because ultrasound imaging offers limited tissue contrast differentiating malignant prostate cancer from other benign abnormalities of the prostate. As such, conventional systematic ultrasound-guided prostate biopsies have been shown to cause underdetection of clinically significant PCa (usually, but not always, defined as tumors with total Gleason score ≥7) and overdetection of clinically insignificant PCa.[2–4]

Multiparametric MR imaging (mpMRI) provides improved visualization and localization of clinically significant prostate cancer compared with ultrasound imaging.[5] The term multiparametric MR imaging refers to an MR imaging examination protocol with multiple scan sequences that image both the anatomic as well as the functional aspects of prostate tumors. A typical mpMRI

Disclosures: No disclosures.
[a] Research and Development, Eigen, 13366 Grass Valley Avenue, Grass Valley, CA 95945, USA; [b] Department of Radiology, University of Cincinnati, College of Medicine, 234 Goodman Street, Cincinnati, OH 45267-0762, USA
* Corresponding author.
E-mail address: vermasm@ucmail.uc.edu

radiologic.theclinics.com

acquisition protocol for the prostate may include T2-weighted imaging (T2WI) to assess defects in zonal anatomy, diffusion weighted imaging (DWI) with apparent diffusion coefficient (ADC) maps to assess impeded water mobility, and dynamic contrast-enhanced (DCE) MR imaging to assess hyper-vascularity and angiogenesis.[6,7]

In 2015, the Prostate Imaging–Reporting and Data System (PI-RADS) steering committee published the PI-RADS v2 acquisition and reporting guidelines recognizing the importance of mpMRI for prostate cancer diagnosis.[8] With improved standardization and advancements in biopsy targeting technologies, MR imaging is playing an increasingly vital role in PCa detection and diagnosis. Following prebiopsy mpMRI, a potentially cancerous tumor can be localized and then targeted for biopsy in MR gantry or indirectly using image fusion techniques. In this article, we focus on the technical and clinical aspects of various techniques that use MR imaging for direct or indirect targeting of prostatic lesions during prostate biopsies.

MR IMAGING–TARGETED PROSTATE BIOPSY TECHNIQUES

Lesions identified on mpMRI as suspicious for harboring PCa can be targeted for biopsy either directly within the MR imaging scanner, referred to as in-gantry MR imaging–targeted prostate biopsy (IG-TB), or indirectly outside the MR imaging scanner by fusing the MR images with a secondary imaging modality, such as ultrasound (FUS-TB). The use of MR imaging as a preprocedure planning modality and ultrasound for real-time intraprocedure imaging necessitates the incorporation of multimodality image fusion techniques into the biopsy process. Multimodality image fusion allows the "transfer" of lesions from MR imaging to ultrasound images, thereby enabling the operator to target the mpMRI-identified lesions outside the gantry. If during biopsy the MR imaging–ultrasound image fusion is performed cognitively or visually by the operator, it is referred to as cognitive MR imaging–ultrasound fusion targeted prostate biopsy (COG-TB). If the image fusion is performed algorithmically using the assistance of image fusion software, it is referred to as software-guided fusion targeted prostate biopsy (SW-TB). The following sections discuss the aforementioned techniques in further detail.

In-Gantry MR Imaging–Targeted Biopsy

This biopsy technique is performed while the patient is in the MR gantry and allows direct visualization of the path of biopsy guide needle to confirm its position in the MR target before tissue samples are obtained. These biopsies can be performed on open low-field systems or closed 1.5-T and 3.0-T systems.[9–20] The most commonly used in-gantry approach is the transrectal biopsy. However, in-gantry MR imaging–targeted biopsy also can be performed using a transperineal[21] or transgluteal approach.

A commonly used device for transrectal biopsies is the DynaTRIM system (Invivo, Gainesville, FL), compatible with all MR vendors. It features a holding mechanism for a disposable needle sleeve that is inserted into the rectum for targeting lesions. The biopsy system is mounted on a base plate that is fitted on the MR table (Fig. 1). During the procedure, the needle sleeve can be viewed on MR images over its entire length, which allows for a visual inspection of the needle path in the MR images before needle insertion (Fig. 2). This system includes an interventional planning software (DynaLOC; Invivo) to assist in appropriate needle guide placement and biopsy.

In a cohort of 265 patients with prior negative TRUS-B, Hoeks and colleagues[22] used IG-TB for a cancer detection rate of 41%, 87% of which were clinically significant. In a systematic review by Overduin and colleagues,[23] including 10 studies, IG-TB detected PCa in the range of 8% to 59% (median: 42%) and 81% to 93% of detected cancers were clinically significant. The advantages of IG-TB are accurate targeting of the lesion, precise documentation of the biopsy sample site, obtaining fewer cores for each patient, and increased detection of clinically relevant tumors. However, IG-TB has a wide range of reported durations for biopsy, largely dependent on the number of samples extracted as well as the experience of the operator.[12,15] The potential for longer procedure time is the biggest challenge of in-gantry MR biopsies, as it adds to patient discomfort and increased cost expenses.[22–24]

MR Imaging–Ultrasound Fusion Targeted Biopsy

MR imaging–ultrasound fusion targeted prostate biopsies offer a viable, cost-effective alternative to IG-TB that combines the best of both worlds of MR imaging and ultrasound. In other words, fusion imaging combines the real-time imaging and cost-effectiveness of ultrasound with the lesion detection and localization capabilities of mpMRI for prostate cancer diagnosis.

The general workflow of an MR imaging–ultrasound fusion biopsy procedure consists of 3 major steps, as shown in Fig. 3. A patient first gets a multiparametric MR imaging examination

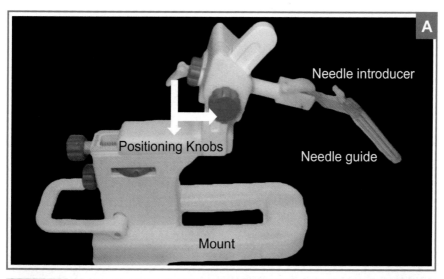

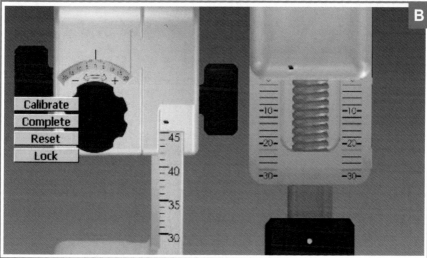

Fig. 1. (A) Photograph shows an MR-compatible prostate biopsy device with a needle guide attached. After the patient is placed prone on the MR table, the biopsy device mount is fitted on the MR table and this guide is inserted into the patient's rectum. Multiplanar localization sequences are performed to identify the ROIs, typically using a T2-weighted fast spin echo sequence. The gadolinium-filled needle guide is then directed toward the lesion by means of the biopsy device and guidance sequences are performed between needle guide adjustments. (B) Photograph shows the display at an independent workstation running an automated software that provides automated adjustment parameters for the needle. The guidance sequences used are usually T2W fast spin echo or single-shot fast spin echo (SSFSE) obtained either in the sagittal or oblique axial planes that contain the needle. (*Courtesy of* Dr A. Oto, Chicago, IL.)

that images both the anatomic and functional aspects of the prostate (see **Fig. 3**A). The radiologist analyzes the mpMR images (typically using a planning software) and assesses regions within the prostate that may harbor clinically significant PCa. The clinically suspicious regions of interest (ROIs) are marked on the MR imaging (see **Fig. 3**B). On biopsy day, the MR images with the marked ROIs are aligned with the intraprocedure ultrasound images either cognitively (COG-TB) or with the assistance of a fusion biopsy software (SW-TB) for targeted biopsy of the MR imaging–identified regions (see **Fig. 3**C). In the following sections we discuss both the cognitive and software-driven techniques of fusion-guided biopsies.

Cognitive MR imaging–ultrasound fusion targeted biopsy
Cognitive MR imaging–ultrasound fusion prostate biopsy refers to the technique in which the

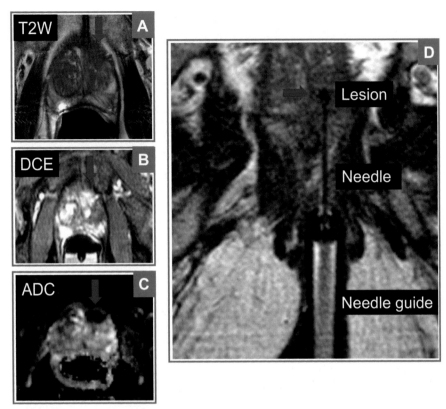

Fig. 2. Prostate mpMRI demonstrating an anterior transition zone lesion (*red arrows*) in a 57-year-old man with elevated PSA of 6.5 ng/mL and 1 set of negative transrectal prostate biopsy. Axial T2WI shows a homogeneous hypointense lesion in the left midgland anterior transition zone (*A*) with focal enhancement on dynamic contrast images (*B*) and with restricted diffusion on ADC map derived from DWI (*C*) highly suspicious for malignancy. Image obtained with the needle guide in the appropriate position for biopsy shows the insertion of an 18-gauge MR-compatible biopsy needle (*D*). Pathology yielded Gleason score 9 (4 + 5) prostate adenocarcinoma. This region was not included in the systematic TRUS biopsy zones. (*Courtesy of* Dr A. Oto, Chicago, IL.)

operator targets MR imaging–identified lesions by visually or cognitively aligning the preprocedure MR images with intraprocedure ultrasound images. This method avoids the capital investment and training time involved in becoming operationally effective with an in-gantry or fusion software device. In a cognitive-fusion setting, the operator studies the prostatic lesion location on the mpMR images and then manually determines the anatomic location of the virtual MR imaging lesion on real-time ultrasound prostate images. During the visual registration, the operator pays close attention to the zonal topography of the prostate and uses the presence of any internal landmarks, such as cysts, calcifications, or benign prostatic hyperplasia nodules for guidance.[25] Although theoretically possible, the cognitive registration process is challenging because the patient orientation during the MR imaging examination (supine) is different from that during an ultrasound biopsy (lateral decubitus or lithotomy), which changes the planes of acquisition of the MR imaging and ultrasound images.

A multicenter prospective study of 95 patients by Puech and colleagues[26] demonstrated a 10% increase in overall PCa detection and a 15% increase in clinically significant PCa detection when comparing MR imaging–targeted cognitive and software fusion biopsies versus systematic biopsies. The study showed no statistical difference between cancer detection rates using cognitive versus software fusion biopsies. In a study of 125 men with 172 identified MR imaging–suspicious lesions, Wysock and colleagues[27] compared software fusion biopsies with expert cognitive-fusion biopsies. On a per-target analysis, software fusion biopsies detected more clinically significant PCa than cognitive fusion (20.3% vs 15.1%, $P = .0523$). Although COG-TB can be quite effective in the hands of the expert user, its operator dependence makes it less adoptable in the wider community. A randomized blinded controlled trial

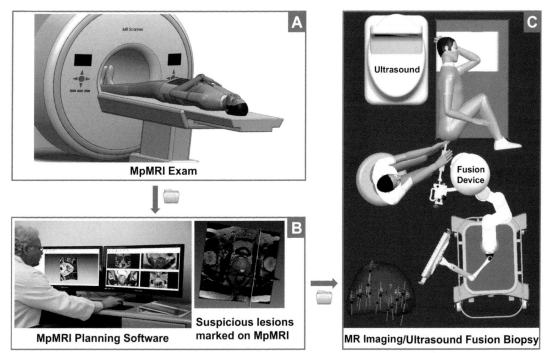

Fig. 3. Figure demonstrating the typical workflow in an MR imaging–ultrasound targeted fusion prostate biopsy. Patient gets an mpMRI examination (typically T2WI, DWI/ADC, DCE) before the biopsy (*A*). The radiologist annotates suspicious regions on the patient's acquired mpMR images using a planning software (*B*). At the time of biopsy, the annotated preoperative MR imaging and intraoperative ultrasound images are registered either cognitively or using a fusion biopsy device, which helps map the suspicious areas from MR imaging to ultrasound. The fusion process allows targeting of MR imaging–identified suspicious areas for biopsy using real-time ultrasound (*C*).

of 130 biopsy-naïve men undergoing prostate biopsy showed no improvement in cancer detection rate when COG-TB was added to routine TRUS-B. One of the major limitations of the study was the relative inexperience of the radiologists with prostate MR imaging and the differing experience levels of the urologists with cognitive fusion, which may well be reflective of typical community practices.[28]

Software-guided MR imaging–ultrasound fusion targeted biopsy

Commercially available MR imaging–ultrasound fusion devices attempt to address the operator dependency and poor reproducibility of cognitive MR imaging–ultrasound fusion biopsies through a software-based algorithmic approach. Currently, several MR imaging–ultrasound fusion platforms have multinational regulatory clearance for targeted prostate biopsies and are being increasingly used worldwide. Examples of some fusion biopsy devices (and their manufacturers) are Aplio Smart Fusion (Toshiba, Ōtawara, Japan),[29] Artemis (Eigen, Grass Valley, CA, USA),[30] BioJet (D&K Technologies GmbH, Barum, Germany),[31] BiopSee (MedCom, Darmstadt, Germany),[32]

Hitachi Real-time Virtual Sonography or HI RVS (Hitachi, Tokyo, Japan),[33] iSR'obot Mona Lisa (Biobot Surgical, Singapore, Singapore),[34] Logiq 9 (GE Healthcare, Little Chalfont, UK),[35] MIM Symphony Bx (MIM Software Inc, Cleveland, OH, USA),[36] Navigo (UC-Care, Yokneam, Israel),[37] UroNav (In Vivo/Philips, Gainesville, FL, USA),[38] Urostation (Koelis, La Tronche, France),[39] and Virtual Navigator (Esaote, Genoa, Italy).[40]

Despite a number of conceptual differences between the individual devices in terms of (1) the mode of ultrasound image acquisition, (2) the fusion technique used for overlaying MR imaging with ultrasound images, (3) the tracking mechanism used during probe navigation, and (4) the needle insertion route, the workflow of all devices have several common elements that are summarized in **Fig. 4** and **Table 1**. In the following sections, we discuss the workflow of a typical MR imaging–ultrasound fusion biopsy procedure in further detail while highlighting the similarities and differences of individual fusion biopsy devices.

Multiparametric MR imaging analysis and planning Following mpMRI acquisition (see **Fig. 3**A), the radiologist analyzes the images using

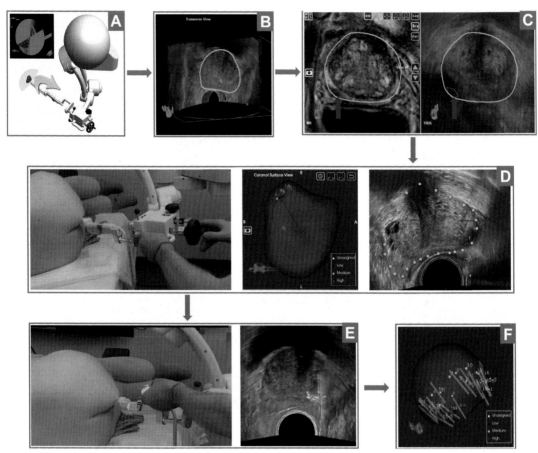

Fig. 4. Figure depicting a software-guided MR imaging–ultrasound fusion targeted biopsy workflow on procedure day. (*A*) Three-dimensional ultrasound image of the prostate is obtained via rotation, translation, or free hand sweep of a 2D ultrasound probe. (*B*) The prostate boundaries are semiautomatically outlined (*green*) on the grayscale ultrasound images. (*C*) The segmented MR imaging and ultrasound images are rigidly or elastically fused thereby mapping the lesion (*red arrow*) from the MR imaging (*left*) onto the ultrasound images (*right*). (*D*) Left: Real-time probe movement on the prostate is tracked (picture depicts tracking via position sensing mechanical arms on which the probe is mounted). Middle: Real-time location of the needle (*orange cylinder*) with respect to the lesion (*red*) and prostate (*brown*) is displayed on a graphical interface. Right: Live tracking accuracy feedback is provided to the operator (*green bubbles* around real-time prostate) as the probe is manipulated around the prostate. The depth of penetration required by the biopsy needle (*red bow-tie*) is displayed. (*E*) Left: The biopsy needle is inserted through a needle guide (picture depicts transrectal needle route). Right: The needle track is captured on live ultrasound (*red overlay on white needle path*). (*F*) All sampled biopsy core locations (*white tracks*) are mapped by the system onto a 3D prostate volume (*brown*) and may be used for future intervention.

dedicated image visualization, analysis, and biopsy planning software (see **Fig. 3**B). Individual fusion platforms use their own proprietary planning software, for example, DynaCAD (Invivo),[41] ProFuse (Eigen),[42] and UroFusion (Biobot Surgical).[34] The planning software provides the ability to query-retrieve and send mpMRI Digital Imaging and Communications in Medicine data to and from a Picture Archiving and Communication System (PACS). In a typical workflow, the radiologist outlines or segments the boundary of the prostate on anatomic T2WI that offers the best visualization of the prostate zonal anatomy. This is followed by

delineation of lesions on coregistered anatomic and functional mpMRI image sequences, such as T2WI, DWI/ADC, and DCE. As per the PI-RADS v2 guidelines, DWI/ADC images and T2W images play a dominant role in the identification of peripheral zone and transition zone lesions, respectively.[8] Computer-aided detection software may also be used by the radiologist at this stage to identify lesions via extrapolated high b-value DWI or perfusion analysis.[43] The output of this step is a 3-dimensional (3D) MR image (typically T2WI) with the prostate gland contoured and the lesions suspicious of harboring PCa outlined on the 3D

Table 1
Workflow steps and technique of an MR imaging–ultrasound fusion biopsy procedure stratified by fusion biopsy device

Workflow Step/Technique	Biopsy Device
Ultrasound image acquisition	
Base-to-apex sweep of 2-dimensional (2D) ultrasound probe	UroNav, Virtual Navigator
Cranio-caudal translation of 2D ultrasound probe	BiopSee, iSR'obot Mona Lisa, MIM Symphony Bx
Biplanar transrectal ultrasound acquisition	HI RVS, NaviGo
End-fire transrectal ultrasound acquisition	Aplio Smart Fusion, Logiq 9
Rotation along probe axis of 2D ultrasound probe	Artemis, BioJet
Image stitching of panoramic 3D ultrasound images	Urostation
MR imaging–ultrasound fusion	
Rigid	Aplio Smart Fusion, BiopSee, HI RVS, Logiq 9, MIM Symphony Bx, NaviGo, Virtual Navigator
Elastic	Artemis, BioJet, iSR'obot Mona Lisa, UroNav, Urostation
Tracking and navigation	
Electromagnetic	Aplio Smart Fusion, HI RVS, Logiq 9, NaviGo, UroNav, Virtual Navigator
Mechanical articulated arm with positional encoders	Artemis
Mechanical with position-encoded stepper	BioJet, BiopSee, MIM Symphony Bx
Software-controlled robotic arm	iSR'obot Mona Lisa
3D ultrasound-ultrasound fusion	Urostation
Biopsy targeting route	
Transrectal	Aplio Smart Fusion, Logiq 9, NaviGo, Virtual Navigator
Transperineal	iSR'obot Mona Lisa, MIM Symphony Bx
Transrectal or transperineal	Artemis, BioJet, BiopSee, HI RVS, UroNav, Urostation
Biopsy core recording	
Archive sampled locations	All devices

image. These marked images are transferred to the fusion biopsy device via PACS, network, or cloud.

Subsequent steps in the fusion biopsy are summarized in **Fig. 4** and described in further detail below.

MR-transrectal ultrasound biopsy workflow

Ultrasound image acquisition and segmentation At the time of biopsy, the MR images with marked ROIs are downloaded onto the fusion device and the fusion device is connected to an ultrasound machine. The first task at the start of a fusion biopsy procedure is to acquire and reconstruct a 3D ultrasound reference image

(see **Fig.** 4A). Accurate 3D ultrasound volume reconstruction is critical to the integrity of the procedure because this is used later in the workflow to fuse with the 3D MR image. As conventional endocavity ultrasound probes used during prostate biopsies generate 2D images only, the software algorithmically reconstructs a set of 2D ultrasound images into a composite 3D volume. Based on the device used, the 2D ultrasound image set may be acquired using a freehand base-to-apex sweep (eg, UroNav), a motorized cranio-caudal translation (eg, iSR'obot Mona Lisa, MIM Symphony Bx) or a mechanically stabilized rotation of the probe along its long axis (eg, Artemis). The Urostation system differs from the other devices in that it uses a 3D ultrasound probe to acquire multiple images that span the dimensions of the prostate. These images are then stitched together into a panorama 3D ultrasound volume by the software. Some devices use mechanical stabilization during acquisition, whereas some others use freehand probe manipulation. During freehand acquisitions, care must be taken to ensure an even and smooth sweep for accurate 3D reconstruction.[44]

Post-acquisition and 3D reconstruction, the operator semiautomatically segments or contours the outer boundary of the prostate in the software. This step helps in partitioning the acquired 3D ultrasound volume into prostatic and nonprostatic tissue. The output of this step is a 3D ultrasound image with the prostate boundary outlined on the image (see **Fig. 4**B).

MR imaging–ultrasound image fusion The segmented MR imaging and ultrasound volumes serve as the input for the multimodality image fusion step that is performed in this step. Lesions identified on preprocedure mpMRIs are mapped onto the intraprocedure ultrasound images using image fusion or image registration techniques. This critical step allows the operator to "see" the MR imaging–identified lesions on the ultrasound image (see **Fig. 4**C).

The fusion technique used by the biopsy device may be broadly classified as rigid or elastic based on the transformation model used to register the 3D MR imaging and ultrasound image volumes. Rigid registration uses a shape-preserving transformation model that helps account for global orientation (rotation and translation) differences between the MR imaging and ultrasound prostate volumes. Examples of devices that use this transformation include HI RVS and Virtual Navigator.[40] Nonrigid or elastic registration techniques account for local geometric differences between the 2 images and may be necessary to account for deformations that occur between volumes due to differences in patient orientation, bladder/rectal filling, and pressure of the endorectal coil or TRUS probe. Examples of devices that use this technique include Artemis[45] and Urostation.[40]

Tracking and navigation Tracking refers to the ability of the fusion device to provide real-time or near real-time 3D localization of the TRUS probe with respect to the prostate. This localization provides the operator the ability to navigate to specific areas of the prostate, such as MR imaging–identified lesions (see **Fig. 4**D).

Devices that track based on electromagnetic technology (eg, UroNav, HI RVS) need a special sensor that attaches to the ultrasound probe. A low intensity (~0.1 T) electromagnetic field generator is placed in the vicinity of the patient. As the ultrasound probe moves within this electromagnetic field, the attached sensor relays the 3D position of the probe to the device software.[46] Other devices (eg, Artemis, BioJet, BiopSee) use positional encoders attached to a mechanical arm or stepper mechanism. Movement of the probe triggers differences in encoder readings that are relayed to the device software and displayed on a graphical interface.[24] Although these platforms use a combination of hardware and software for prospective tracking and navigation, the Urostation platform uses an entirely software-driven approach based on retrospective 3D-3D elastic registration between interval ultrasound images.[47]

Regardless of the fusion device used, attention must be paid to ensure that tracking is accurate during the procedure. Unlike in-gantry procedures, near real-time needle track visualization on MR images is not available during fusion biopsies. Accurate targeting of MR imaging–identified lesions depends not only on the quality of the fusion but also on accurate tracking of probe movement with respect to the prostate during the procedure.

Biopsy route Tissue extraction during biopsy may be done with a transrectal approach (ie, the biopsy needle is routed through the rectum, see **Fig. 4**E) or using a transperineal approach (ie, the biopsy needle goes through the skin at the perineum). Based on the fusion device used, the operator may have the option of using the transrectal (eg, Virtual Navigator) or transperineal (eg, iSR'obot Mona Lisa) targeting method. Some devices offer both transrectal and transperineal approaches (eg, Artemis, BioJet, UroNav, Urostation). A vast majority of biopsies are performed with the transrectal approach under local anesthesia. Needle insertion via the perineum using the transperineal approach avoids the rectal mucosa and reduces the likelihood of serious bacterial infections post biopsy. In a systematic review of 85 studies cataloging complications occurring after prostate biopsies, Borghesi and colleagues[48] found that transperineal approaches were associated with reduced rates of serious infections.

Biopsy core recording All fusion biopsy devices offer the ability to record the ROI-biopsied locations on the 3D model (see **Fig. 4**F). This is a significant advantage for future intervention in terms of focal therapy or for disease tracking in active surveillance patients.

Summary of studies involving software fusion targeted biopsies Studies involving SW-TB have largely shown an increased detection of clinically significant PCa and decreased detection of clinically insignificant PCa. In a systematic review of 15 studies, Valerio and colleagues[49] compared the detection rate of clinically significant PCa between SW-TB and TRUS-B. The investigators found that SW-TB detected more clinically significant PCa (median: 33.3% vs 23.6%) using far fewer biopsy cores (median: 9.2 vs 37.1) compared with TRUS-B. SW-TB detected approximately 9% clinically significant PCa that would have been missed using TRUS-B alone. In a large cohort study of 1003 men undergoing targeted and random systematic biopsies, Siddiqui and colleagues[38] found that targeted biopsy detected 30% more high-risk cancer ($P<.001$) and 17% fewer low-risk cancer ($P<.001$) than systematic biopsies.

SW-TB addresses the issues associated with increased costs of IG-TB and the operator dependence of COG-TB and may be the most practical approach for performing MR imaging–targeted biopsies at this time. However, the time and financial investment required in acquiring, maintaining and training on fusion biopsy devices is still significant and a barrier to widespread adoption.[50]

DISCUSSION

Conventional ultrasound-guided prostate biopsies have been known to cause overdetection of clinically insignificant cancer leading to possible overtreatment and underdetection of clinically significant cancer that may potentially prove lethal. MR imaging–targeted biopsies address these limitations. Regardless of the MR imaging–targeted approach used, evidence supports increased detection of clinically significant PCa and decreased clinically insignificant PCa detection through incorporation of MR imaging targeting. In a meta-analysis of 43 studies, Wegelin and colleagues[51] evaluated if MR imaging–targeted biopsies increase detection rate of PCa compared with TRUS-B. They also evaluated which of 3 MR imaging–targeted techniques (in-gantry, cognitive-fusion, and software fusion) had a higher cancer detection rate. They found that although MR imaging–targeted biopsies and TRUS biopsies had a similar overall cancer detection rate, the detection of clinically significant PCa was higher with MR imaging–targeted biopsies than TRUS biopsies (relative sensitivity ratio 1.16) and the detection of clinically insignificant PCa was lower (relative sensitivity ratio 0.47). The investigators found a statistically significant advantage ($P = .02$) in overall PCa detection using in-gantry targeted biopsies compared with cognitive-fusion biopsies, but no statistically significant difference among the 3 MR imaging–targeted techniques in terms of clinically significant PCa detection.

If MR imaging–targeted prostate biopsies can improve detection rate of clinically significant PCa and lower the detection rate of indolent tumors, it may lead to improved survival and considerable cost savings through improved risk stratification and avoidance of unnecessary treatment side effects. In a 2014 study, de Rooij and colleagues[52] developed a decision analytical model to evaluate diagnostic accuracy, survival, quality of life, and costs associated with IG-TB and TRUS-B in men with elevated prostate-specific antigen (PSA) levels. They found that although the MR imaging–guided approach had higher upfront costs, the ultimate cost was quite similar to TRUS-B when adjusted for the improvement in quality of life due to the reduction of overdiagnosis and overtreatment. Another recent study by Venderink and colleagues[53] found cost-effectiveness of FUS-TB to be more than TRUS-B, which the investigators attributed to improved accuracy of diagnosis using FUS-TB.

MR imaging–targeted biopsies have been used for prostate cancer detection in all cohorts of men: men with no known cancer (whether biopsy naïve or prior negative) or in men with known diagnosis of cancer (prior positive). In men with no previous biopsy, MR imaging–targeted biopsies increase detection rate of clinically significant cancer while reducing detection of indolent disease.[54] In men with a previous negative biopsy, the combination of MR imaging–targeted and systematic biopsies has been shown to detect more clinically significant PCa than using systematic biopsies alone.[54] A consensus statement by the American Urological Association and the Society of Abdominal Radiology Prostate Cancer Disease-Focused Panel supports the use of MR imaging and targeted biopsies for prior negative patients to facilitate detection of clinically significant PCa.[55] Among men on active surveillance with low-risk disease, MR imaging–targeted repeat biopsies improve risk stratification via disease reclassification and may also reduce the number of repeat biopsies.[56]

Despite advancements in MR imaging technology and standardization of interpretation, several challenges remain for widespread implementation of MR imaging–targeted prostate biopsies. A successful program requires multidisciplinary coordination and feedback among radiologists, urologists, and pathologists. Accurate prostate MR imaging interpretation and analysis performed by experienced radiologists is key to the success of MR imaging–targeted prostate biopsies. The upfront capital investment associated with acquiring and maintaining MR imaging scanning equipment and/or a fusion biopsy device remains a significant barrier for widespread adoption. Improvements in MR imaging, reporting, and advancement of fusion biopsy technologies is expected to continue to address several of these challenges. It is conceivable that in the future, obtaining a prebiopsy MR imaging and then using MR imaging for direct or indirect targeting may become standard of care for patients suspected of having PCa.

REFERENCES

1. Siegel RL, Miller KD, Jemal A. Cancer statistics, 2015. CA Cancer J Clin 2015;65(1):5–29.
2. Singh H, Canto EI, Shariat SF, et al. Predictors of prostate cancer after initial negative systematic 12 core biopsy. J Urol 2004;171(5):1850–4.
3. Taira AV, Merrick GS, Galbreath RW, et al. Performance of transperineal template-guided mapping biopsy in detecting prostate cancer in the initial and repeat biopsy setting. Prostate Cancer Prostatic Dis 2010;13(1):71–7.
4. Zaytoun OM, Moussa AS, Gao T, et al. Office based transrectal saturation biopsy improves prostate cancer detection compared to extended biopsy in the repeat biopsy population. J Urol 2011;186(3):850–4.
5. Barentsz JO, Richenberg J, Clements R, et al. ESUR prostate MR guidelines 2012. Eur Radiol 2012;22(4):746–57.
6. Verma S, Rajesh A. A clinically relevant approach to imaging prostate cancer: review. AJR Am J Roentgenol 2011;196(3_supplement):S1–10.
7. Sarkar S, Das S. A review of imaging methods for prostate cancer detection. Biomed Eng Comput Biol 2016;7(Suppl 1):1–15.
8. Weinreb JC, Barentsz JO, Choyke PL, et al. PI-RADS prostate imaging—reporting and data system: 2015, version 2. Eur Urol 2016;69(1):16–40.
9. Anastasiadis AG, Lichy MP, Nagele U, et al. MRI-guided biopsy of the prostate increases diagnostic performance in men with elevated or increasing PSA levels after previous negative TRUS biopsies. Eur Urol 2006;50(4):738–48 [discussion: 748–9].
10. Beyersdorff D, Winkel A, Hamm B, et al. MR imaging-guided prostate biopsy with a closed MR unit at 1.5 T: initial results. Radiology 2005;234(2):576–81.
11. D'Amico AV, Tempany CM, Cormack R, et al. Transperineal magnetic resonance image guided prostate biopsy. J Urol 2000;164(2):385–7.
12. Engelhard K, Hollenbach HP, Kiefer B, et al. Prostate biopsy in the supine position in a standard 1.5-T scanner under real time MR-imaging control using a MR-compatible endorectal biopsy device. Eur Radiol 2006;16(6):1237–43.
13. Franiel T, Stephan C, Erbersdobler A, et al. Areas suspicious for prostate cancer: MR-guided biopsy in patients with at least one transrectal US-guided biopsy with a negative finding–multiparametric MR imaging for detection and biopsy planning. Radiology 2011;259(1):162–72.
14. Hambrock T, Futterer JJ, Huisman HJ, et al. Thirty-two-channel coil 3T magnetic resonance-guided biopsies of prostate tumor suspicious regions identified on multimodality 3T magnetic resonance imaging: technique and feasibility. Invest Radiol 2008;43(10):686–94.
15. Hambrock T, Somford DM, Hoeks C, et al. Magnetic resonance imaging guided prostate biopsy in men with repeat negative biopsies and increased prostate specific antigen. J Urol 2010;183(2):520–7.
16. Hata N, Jinzaki M, Kacher D, et al. MR imaging-guided prostate biopsy with surgical navigation software: device validation and feasibility. Radiology 2001;220(1):263–8.
17. Susil RC, Menard C, Krieger A, et al. Transrectal prostate biopsy and fiducial marker placement in a standard 1.5T magnetic resonance imaging scanner. J Urol 2006;175(1):113–20.
18. Yakar D, Hambrock T, Hoeks C, et al. Magnetic resonance-guided biopsy of the prostate: feasibility, technique, and clinical applications. Top Magn Reson Imaging 2008;19(6):291–5.
19. Zangos S, Eichler K, Engelmann K, et al. MR-guided transgluteal biopsies with an open low-field system in patients with clinically suspected prostate cancer: technique and preliminary results. Eur Radiol 2005;15(1):174–82.
20. Yacoub JH, Verma S, Moulton JS, et al. Imaging-guided prostate biopsy: conventional and emerging techniques. Radiographics 2012;32(3):819–37.
21. Penzkofer T, Tuncali K, Fedorov A, et al. Transperineal in-bore 3-T MR imaging-guided prostate biopsy: a prospective clinical observational study. Radiology 2015;274(1):170–80.
22. Hoeks CM, Schouten MG, Bomers JG, et al. Three-Tesla magnetic resonance-guided prostate biopsy in men with increased prostate-specific antigen and repeated, negative, random, systematic, transrectal ultrasound biopsies: detection of clinically significant prostate cancers. Eur Urol 2012;62(5):902–9.
23. Overduin CG, Futterer JJ, Barentsz JO. MRI-guided biopsy for prostate cancer detection: a systematic review of current clinical results. Curr Urol Rep 2013;14(3):209–13.
24. Marks L, Young S, Natarajan S. MRI-ultrasound fusion for guidance of targeted prostate biopsy. Curr Opin Urol 2013;23(1):43–50.
25. Puech P, Ouzzane A, Gaillard V, et al. Multiparametric MRI-targeted TRUS prostate biopsies using visual registration. Biomed Res Int 2014;2014:819360.

26. Puech P, Rouviere O, Renard-Penna R, et al. Prostate cancer diagnosis: multiparametric MR-targeted biopsy with cognitive and transrectal US-MR fusion guidance versus systematic biopsy–prospective multicenter study. Radiology 2013;268(2):461–9.

27. Wysock JS, Rosenkrantz AB, Huang WC, et al. A prospective, blinded comparison of magnetic resonance (MR) imaging-ultrasound fusion and visual estimation in the performance of MR-targeted prostate biopsy: the PROFUS trial. Eur Urol 2014; 66(2):343–51.

28. Tonttila PP, Lantto J, Paakko E, et al. Prebiopsy multiparametric magnetic resonance imaging for prostate cancer diagnosis in biopsy-naive men with suspected prostate cancer based on elevated prostate-specific antigen values: results from a randomized prospective blinded controlled trial. Eur Urol 2016;69(3):419–25.

29. Jelidi A, Ohana M, Labani A, et al. Prostate cancer diagnosis: efficacy of a simple electromagnetic MRI-TRUS fusion method to target biopsies. Eur J Radiol 2017;86:127–34.

30. Sonn GA, Natarajan S, Margolis DJ, et al. Targeted biopsy in the detection of prostate cancer using an office based magnetic resonance ultrasound fusion device. J Urol 2013;189(1):86–91.

31. Shoji S, Hiraiwa S, Ogawa T, et al. Accuracy of real-time magnetic resonance imaging-transrectal ultrasound fusion image-guided transperineal target biopsy with needle tracking with a mechanical position-encoded stepper in detecting significant prostate cancer in biopsy-naive men. Int J Urol 2017;24(4):288–94.

32. Hansen N, Patruno G, Wadhwa K, et al. Magnetic resonance and ultrasound image fusion supported transperineal prostate biopsy using the Ginsburg protocol: technique, learning points, and biopsy results. Eur Urol 2016;70(2):332–40.

33. Miyagawa T, Ishikawa S, Kimura T, et al. Real-time virtual sonography for navigation during targeted prostate biopsy using magnetic resonance imaging data. Int J Urol 2010;17(10):855–60.

34. Kroenig M, Schaal K, Benndorf M, et al. Diagnostic accuracy of robot-guided, software based transperineal MRI/TRUS fusion biopsy of the prostate in a high risk population of previously biopsy negative men. Biomed Res Int 2016;2016:2384894.

35. Junker D, Schafer G, Heidegger I, et al. Multiparametric magnetic resonance imaging/transrectal ultrasound fusion targeted biopsy of the prostate: preliminary results of a prospective single-centre study. Urol Int 2015;94(3):313–8.

36. Akhter W, Khan M, Karim O, et al. PE59: early experience with the MIM symphony software registration for MRI-targeted transperineal prostate biopsies. Eur Urol Suppl 2014;13(3):38.

37. Gayet M, van der Aa A, Schmitz P, et al. 3D Navigo versus TRUS-guided prostate biopsy in prostate cancer detection. World J Urol 2016;34(9):1255–60.

38. Siddiqui MM, Rais-Bahrami S, Turkbey B, et al. Comparison of MR/ultrasound fusion-guided biopsy with ultrasound-guided biopsy for the diagnosis of prostate cancer. JAMA 2015;313(4):390–7.

39. Mozer P, Roupret M, Le Cossec C, et al. First round of targeted biopsies using magnetic resonance imaging/ultrasonography fusion compared with conventional transrectal ultrasonography-guided biopsies for the diagnosis of localised prostate cancer. BJU Int 2015;115(1):50–7.

40. Delongchamps NB, Peyromaure M, Schull A, et al. Prebiopsy magnetic resonance imaging and prostate cancer detection: comparison of random and targeted biopsies. J Urol 2013;189(2):493–9.

41. Liddell H, Jyoti R, Haxhimolla HZ. mp-MRI prostate characterised PIRADS 3 lesions are associated with a low risk of clinically significant prostate cancer—a retrospective review of 92 biopsied PIRADS 3 lesions. Curr Urol 2015;8(2):96–100.

42. Verma S, Sarkar S, Young J, et al. Evaluation of the impact of computed high b-value diffusion-weighted imaging on prostate cancer detection. Abdom Radiol (NY) 2016;41(5):934–45.

43. Rosenkrantz AB, Parikh N, Kierans AS, et al. Prostate cancer detection using computed very high b-value diffusion-weighted imaging: how high should we go? Acad Radiol 2016;23(6):704–11.

44. Tay KJ, Gupta RT, Rastinehad AR, et al. Navigating MRI-TRUS fusion biopsy: optimizing the process and avoiding technical pitfalls. Expert Rev Anticancer Ther 2016;16(3):303–11.

45. Westhoff N, Siegel FP, Hausmann D, et al. Precision of MRI/ultrasound-fusion biopsy in prostate cancer diagnosis: an ex vivo comparison of alternative biopsy techniques on prostate phantoms. World J Urol 2017;35(7):1015–22.

46. Kongnyuy M, George AK, Rastinehad AR, et al. Magnetic resonance imaging-ultrasound fusion-guided prostate biopsy: review of technology, techniques, and outcomes. Curr Urol Rep 2016;17(4):32.

47. Ukimura O, Desai MM, Palmer S, et al. 3-dimensional elastic registration system of prostate biopsy location by real-time 3-dimensional transrectal ultrasound guidance with magnetic resonance/transrectal ultrasound image fusion. J Urol 2012;187(3):1080–6.

48. Borghesi M, Ahmed H, Nam R, et al. Complications after systematic, random, and image-guided prostate biopsy. Eur Urol 2017;71(3):353–65.

49. Valerio M, Donaldson I, Emberton M, et al. Detection of clinically significant prostate cancer using magnetic resonance imaging-ultrasound fusion targeted biopsy: a systematic review. Eur Urol 2015; 68(1):8–19.

50. Tyson MD, Arora SS, Scarpato KR, et al. Magnetic resonance-ultrasound fusion prostate biopsy in the diagnosis of prostate cancer. Urol Oncol 2016; 34(7):326–32.

51. Wegelin O, van Melick HH, Hooft L, et al. Comparing three different techniques for magnetic resonance imaging-targeted prostate biopsies: a systematic review of in-bore versus magnetic resonance imaging-transrectal ultrasound fusion versus cognitive registration. Is there a preferred technique? Eur Urol 2017;71(4):517–31.

52. de Rooij M, Crienen S, Witjes JA, et al. Cost-effectiveness of magnetic resonance (MR) imaging and MR-guided targeted biopsy versus systematic transrectal ultrasound-guided biopsy in diagnosing prostate cancer: a modelling study from a health care perspective. Eur Urol 2014; 66(3):430–6.

53. Venderink W, Govers TM, de Rooij M, et al. Cost-effectiveness comparison of imaging-guided prostate biopsy techniques: systematic transrectal ultrasound, direct in-bore MRI, and image fusion. AJR Am J Roentgenol 2017;208(5):1058–63.

54. Bjurlin MA, Rosenkrantz AB, Taneja SS. Role of MRI prebiopsy in men at risk for prostate cancer: taking off the blindfold. Curr Opin Urol 2017;27(3):246–53.

55. Rosenkrantz AB, Verma S, Choyke P, et al. Prostate magnetic resonance imaging and magnetic resonance imaging targeted biopsy in patients with a prior negative biopsy: a consensus statement by AUA and SAR. J Urol 2016;196(6):1613–8.

56. Bjurlin MA, Mendhiratta N, Wysock JS, et al. Multi-parametric MRI and targeted prostate biopsy: improvements in cancer detection, localization, and risk assessment. Cent European J Urol 2016;69(1): 9–18.

MR Imaging–Guided Focal Treatment of Prostate Cancer: An Update

Sherif G. Nour, MD, FRCR[a,b,c],*

KEYWORDS

- MR imaging • Focal treatment • Prostate cancer • Update

KEY POINTS

- Focal treatment of prostate cancer has evolved from a concept to a practice in the recent few years and is projected to fill an existing need, bridging the gap between conservative and radical traditional treatment options.
- With its low morbidity and rapid recovery time compared with whole-gland treatment alternatives, focal therapy is poised to gain more acceptance among patients and health care providers.
- As our experience with focal treatment matures and evidence continues to accrue, the landscape of this practice might look quite different in the future.

INTRODUCTION

Minimally invasive targeted therapy has steadily developed into an integral part of cancer treatment paradigms over the last 2 decades. The urologic oncology community has witnessed the materialization of percutaneous ablative technology into a well-established alternative to nephron-sparing surgeries in selected patients with small renal malignancies. The same concept of organ-sparing treatment has been appealing to clinicians and researchers interested in prostate cancer care over many years, since Onik and colleagues[1] published a small series of focal nerve-sparing cryosurgery for the treatment of primary prostate cancer as a new approach to preserving potency. The growing concern that patients with low- and intermediate-risk prostate cancer are being offered either no treatment (ie, active surveillance) or overly aggressive radical treatment options has kept the momentum to explore a middle ground, minimally invasive treatment option for this patient population.

The implementation of the concept of focal treatment has, however, been restricted by the lack of technology to accurately visualize and sample focal prostate cancer. The advent of multi-parametric prostate MR imaging (mpMRI) and the integration of interventional MR imaging technology in prostate cancer care have been the major catalysts behind the recently revived interest in focal treatment because of the significantly improved ability to visualize, sample, and treat localized disease within the prostate gland.

[a] Division of Abdominal Imaging, Interventional MRI Program, Department of Radiology and Imaging Sciences, Emory University Hospitals and School of Medicine, Room BG-42, 1364 Clifton Road Northeast, Atlanta, GA 30322, USA; [b] Division of Interventional Radiology, Interventional MRI Program, Department of Radiology and Imaging Sciences, Emory University Hospitals and School of Medicine, Room BG-42, 1364 Clifton Road Northeast, Atlanta, GA 30322, USA; [c] Division of Image-Guided Medicine, Interventional MRI Program, Department of Radiology and Imaging Sciences, Emory University Hospitals and School of Medicine, Room BG-42, 1364 Clifton Road Northeast, Atlanta, GA 30322, USA
* Divisions of Abdominal Imaging, Interventional Radiology and Image-Guided Medicine, Interventional MRI Program, Department of Radiology and Imaging Sciences, Emory University Hospitals and School of Medicine, 1364 Clifton Road Northeast, Atlanta, GA 30322.
E-mail address: sherif.nour@emoryhealthcare.org

Radiol Clin N Am 56 (2018) 301–318
https://doi.org/10.1016/j.rcl.2017.10.011
0033-8389/18/© 2017 Elsevier Inc. All rights reserved.

THE CASE FOR FOCAL PROSTATE TREATMENT

The lack of benefit from radical therapy in patients with low-risk prostate cancer has been proven by level 1 evidence derived from multiple randomized controlled clinical trials[2–4] in recent years. Wilt and colleagues[5] just published their experience with nearly 20 years of follow-up among men with localized prostate cancer and reported that surgery was not associated with significantly lower all-cause or prostate-cancer mortality than observation. In a large earlier study of the incidence of initial local therapy among men with low-risk prostate cancer in the United States, Miller and colleagues[6] evaluated 24,405 patients with low-risk prostate cancer and found that 55% of them were treated with radical prostatectomy or radiation therapy. This population could potentially benefit from more conservative treatment approaches that might limit overtreatment while improving the quality of care.

Active surveillance, on the other hand, may be an attractive option for patients with low-risk prostate cancer but may not represent an effective management strategy for those with intermediate-risk disease.[7,8] In addition, active surveillance is limited by the current lack of validated criteria to select candidates for initial enrollment and by the lack of solid grounds to trigger active intervention. As a result, various active surveillance protocols are being implemented, with current protocols ranging from recommending an annual biopsy after diagnosis[9,10] to a more conservative approach whereby biopsies are repeated every 2 to 3 years.[11,12] This uncertainty in treatment direction may add a considerable deal to the underlying patient anxiety associated with the presence of known untreated cancer.[13]

Patients with recurrent prostate cancer following radical treatment pose another dimension of challenge to existing treatment modalities. The reported 5-year biochemical relapse-free survival rates are 30% to 40% after salvage radical prostatectomy, 10% to 77% after salvage radiotherapy, and 20% to 87% after salvage brachytherapy.[14]

Introducing a minimally invasive treatment option for localized low- and intermediate-risk de novo disease and possibly for locally recurrent cancer does, therefore, seem to fit an important existing need in prostate cancer care. This option is particularly relevant given the magnitude of the prostate cancer problem that affects 1 in every 7 American men and represents the second most common cancer in this population, being surpassed only by skin cancer. The American Cancer Society estimates the number of new prostate cancer cases in 2017 at 161,360 with 26,730 estimated deaths from this disease during the same year, qualifying prostate cancer as the second deadliest cancer in American men after lung cancer.[15]

THE CASE AGAINST FOCAL PROSTATE TREATMENT

One of the primary arguments against the concept of focal prostate cancer treatment is the often multifocal nature of this disease.[16] In a study examining the histologic details in 486 men treated with radical retropubic prostatectomy, Wise and colleagues[17] found that only 17% of all cases had a single focus of prostate cancer, with multifocal disease representing the prevalent histologic pattern. Adopting a focal treatment approach is, therefore, likely to leave behind untreated cancer.

The possible progression of conservatively managed low-risk prostate cancer, resulting in the development of metastases and death, has been used to advocate the need for definitive treatment particularly among patients with an estimated life expectancy exceeding 15 years.[18] With reported cancer-specific mortality rates of 6% to 30% over 15 years[19,20] and 46% beyond 15 years of follow-up[18] of conservatively managed low-risk prostate cancer, a focal treatment strategy may be associated with suboptimally treated malignancy and potential subsequent disease dissemination.

CHALLENGING THE CASE AGAINST FOCAL PROSTATE TREATMENT

Prostate cancer has been shown on autopsy specimens to exist in almost a third of men aged 50 years or older and in 46% of men in the 70 to 81-year-old age group, who happened to die of unrelated causes.[21,22] This high prevalence of undetected and nonfatal cancerous foci mismatches the much lower lifetime risk of developing clinically detected prostate cancer, which is estimated to be around 18%.[19,23,24] These findings have led to an increasing recognition of the concept of index tumor in prostate cancer. Multifocal prostate cancer is often composed of a histologically dominant focal tumor along with a smaller burden of nondominant tumors that rarely contain higher-grade disease than the primary lesion. These secondary tumors in multifocal prostate cancer have been shown to lack significance as predictors of biochemical failure after radical prostatectomy.[25] The theory of focal prostate cancer treatment, therefore, revolves around a targeted eradication of the dominant primary lesion while sparing the rest of the gland. Achieving this goal is hypothesized to control the denominator for disease progression while trading the reduced morbidity and improved functional outcomes for possible residual insignificant secondary tumors.[16,17,26–28]

The reports of low-risk prostate cancer progressing to metastatic disease and leading to cancer-specific mortality[18–20] should be interpreted in view of the limited ability to reliably map and accurately sample intraprostatic disease at the time of these reports. The information obtained from prostate-specific antigen (PSA) levels, digital rectal examinations, and systematic biopsies may not identify significant prostate cancer if it exists in a small volume or in a unifocal pattern.[26] The technique of systematic transrectal ultrasound (TRUS) biopsy of the prostate does not rely on visualizing a target for biopsy but rather uses methodical sampling of representative parts of the prostate gland. It is conceivable to expect that some foci of significant cancer may be missed because of the essentially random nature of this technique, which is notoriously known for missing anterior and apical prostate lesions, particularly in larger-volume glands. Previous work examining repeat TRUS biopsies performed during active surveillance in men with low-risk prostate cancer showed that approximately a third of this population are initially undergraded.[29,30] It is noteworthy to observe the proximity of this figure to the previously reported mortality rates in conservatively managed low-risk prostate cancer.[18–20] The author, therefore, thinks that the likelihood of a true low-risk prostate cancer to progress into metastatic disease is very slim and that a higher-risk cancer is usually present but undetected in those patients who experience disease progression while receiving conservative management for their presumed low-risk cancer.

CANDIDATE SELECTION FOR FOCAL PROSTATE TREATMENT

Patients with small-volume, low- or intermediate-risk cancer (Table 1) confined to one or limited parts of the gland without extracapsular extension, lymphadenopathy, or distant metastases are generally considered appropriate candidates for focal treatment. Reliable identification and risk stratification of cancerous foci are, therefore, central to a successful decision to proceed with focal therapy.

This decision cannot be made based on information obtained from clinical and laboratory assessment, supplemented solely by a traditional systematic 12-core ultrasound (US)-guided biopsy. The inability of these methods to pinpoint the dominant focal cancer and to reliably exclude additional significant disease has led to ablative treatments being offered on a whole-gland basis since the 1960s.[31] This approach to prostate ablation is synonymous with an aggressive whole-gland treatment, has been associated with many complications, and represents an entirely different concept from the proposed focal ablative treatment.

A method for extensive template-guided transperineal pathologic mapping of the prostate (3-dimensional pathologic mapping) has been proposed[32] to improve the reliability of patient selection for focal cryoablation. This method uses a transperineal brachytherapy grid to obtain a median number of 46 (SD ± 19) core biopsies of the prostate and has been reported to improve the reliability of identifying true unilateral disease. Bilateral cancer was demonstrated using this method in 55% of patients previously deemed to have unilateral cancer on TRUS biopsy, who would otherwise be erroneously considered suitable candidates for the treatment of one side of the gland.[33] This invasive sampling process is performed under general anesthesia or deep

Table 1						
Common 3-group prostate cancer risk stratification system						
	Gleason Grade		**PSA**			**Clinical Stage**
Low risk	GS ≤6	And	PSA ≤10	And		T1–T2a
Intermediate risk	GS = 7	Or	PSA >10 to ≤20	Or		T2b
High risk	GS ≥8	Or	PSA >20	Or		≥T2c

The system was first proposed by D'Amico and colleagues[80] in 1998 and endorsed by the American Urologic Association[81] and the European Association of Urology.[82]

Abbreviation: GS, Gleason score.

Data from D'Amico AV, Whittington R, Malkowicz SB, et al. Biochemical outcome after radical prostatectomy, external beam radiation therapy, or interstitial radiation therapy for clinically localized prostate cancer. JAMA 1998;280(11):969–74.

sedation, provides evidence that pertains to unilateral versus bilateral disease involvement, and may be used to support candidate selection for hemi-ablation of the side of the prostate harboring a significant tumor.

In order to contemplate a true focal and minimally invasive treatment of prostate cancer, the focus of a significant tumor should be unequivocally identified and the presence of additional high-risk foci should be ruled out. Historically, imaging played a limited role in prostate cancer care and was primarily used to evaluate patients for gross local invasion and metastatic disease. The advent of mpMRI in the recent years has placed a strong emphasis on imaging for prostate cancer detection and risk stratification through its ability to not only identify minor extracapsular disease but to also map disease burden within the confines of the intact capsule. The reported negative predictive value (NPV) of mpMRI in ruling out clinically significant prostate cancer varies based on the reference standard used. When systematic TRUS biopsy is used as the reference test,[16,23–26] the NPV is 88% to 100%; when transperineal template mapping biopsy is used as the reference test,[23,27–29] the NPV is 79% to 89%. Much lower NPVs have been, however, reported for detecting small clinically significant cancers when prostatectomy specimens are used as the reference test, as discussed next in the "Multi-parametric MR imaging and prostate cancer risk stratification" section.

MULTI-PARAMETRIC MR IMAGING AND PROSTATE CANCER RISK STRATIFICATION

The interpretation of mpMRI findings in patients with suspected confined prostate cancer revolves around identifying intraglandular cancer suspicious foci and assigning them specific levels of suspicion. There have been several attempts by investigators to create a scoring system that can reproducibly translate the imaging findings into a numerical score to reflect the likelihood of cancer in a certain focus. The latest group effort in this regard is exemplified by the collaborative work of the American College of Radiology, the European Society of Urogenital Radiology, and the AdMeTech Foundation resulting in the publication of the Prostate Imaging-Reporting and Data System Version 2 (PI-RADS v2) in late 2015.[34] These collaborative efforts continue to modify and refine the scoring system based on feedback[35,36] from users around the world, and the PI-RADS v3 is currently in the works at the time of this writing.

The specifics of mpMRI features related to each cancer suspicion level are beyond the scope of

this article and may be reviewed elsewhere.[34,37] A more relevant discussion to the topic of definite risk stratification and candidate appropriateness for focal therapy is whether the science has reached a sufficient maturity level that allows a completely noninvasive vetting before assigning certain patients to focal therapy. Most readers would rightfully argue that direct tissue sampling is currently an essential component of establishing the diagnosis and treatment direction of prostate cancer. The debate about the extent of this tissue sampling remains, however, quite unsettled. Although some practices implement a sampling approach that targets only highly suspicious lesions (category 4 and 5 lesions, PI-RADS v2) during MR imaging–guided biopsies, others still follow a more conservative strategy of comprehensive sampling of all MR imaging–visible lesions regardless of their suspicion level. Some experts may even pursue a standard 12-core TRUS biopsy to supplement the result of a targeted MR imaging biopsy before offering focal treatment of prostate cancer. The current version of the PI-RADS system (PI-RADS v2, 2015) does not include recommendations for specific management of MR imaging findings. It states that biopsy may or may not be appropriate for PI-RADS assessment categories 2 or 3 (ie, low and intermediate suspicion for cancer).[23]

Studies correlating PI-RADS scoring categories with pathologic findings demonstrated an overall good correlation between the presence of lesions scoring 4 or greater and the presence of clinically significant cancer, with a reported accuracy of greater than 80% for experienced readers.[36,38] However, clinically significant cancer has been repeatedly reported at sites of low or no suspicion on mpMRI. Using MR imaging/TRUS fusion prostate biopsies, cancer detection rates for PI-RADS (v1) category 2 and 3 lesions were reported at 16% (with 60% rate of significant tumors) and 26% (with 66% rate of significant tumors), respectively.[38] Similarly, Filson and colleagues[39] found on a recent large prospective study that the combination of targeted MR imaging/TRUS fusion and nontargeted systematic biopsies detected more clinically significant prostate cancer than either modality alone. They also reported that systematic biopsies revealed clinically significant prostate cancer in 16% of men with no suspicious MR imaging target. Seo and colleagues[36] just reported a limited utility of the new PI-RADS system (PI-RADS v2, 2015) in the detection of small clinically significant cancers, using pathologic analysis of radical prostatectomy specimens as the reference standard. With a cutoff score of 4 or greater, they described low NPVs of 38.8% and 50.0% by 2 readers. A total of 81.3% and 66.7% of the clinically significant cancers missed by 2 experienced readers had tumor volumes less than 1 cm³. Similar findings were also reported by Vargas and colleagues[40] who found a limited value of PI-RADS v2 in the assessment of prostate cancer foci 0.5 cm³ or less, even for detecting clinically significant cancer of Gleason score 4 + 3 or greater.

Acknowledging the current limitations in imaging technology, the author thinks that limited sampling of PI-RADS assessment categories 4 and 5 constitutes an insufficient workup before embarking in focal treatment of prostate cancer and may result in overall poor outcomes related to this treatment concept. More comprehensive sampling may include in-bore MR imaging–guided biopsies or MR imaging/TRUS fusion biopsies targeting foci at all levels of cancer suspicion or standard 12-core systematic TRUS biopsies to supplement the targeted sampling of high suspicion foci intended for focal treatment. In addition, patients with clearly unifocal disease on MR imaging should be subjected to additional contralateral sampling before their final approval for focal therapy. Focal treatment candidates presenting with limited low- or intermediate-risk cancer diagnosed solely on a 12-core systematic TRUS biopsy should be carefully evaluated to ensure that the treatment target on mpMRI correlates with the site of positive cores on TRUS biopsy. Because the exact sources of standard TRUS biopsy cores cannot be accurately documented, additional direct sampling of the planned treatment area with in-bore MR imaging–guided or MR imaging/TRUS fusion biopsy is often required.

FOCAL TREATMENT OPTIONS FOR PROSTATE CANCER

Once the candidacy for focal treatment has been established, the choice of ablative therapy may include cryoablation, high-intensity focused/directional US, laser, or irreversible electroporation (IRE). With the currently limited long-term outcome data and the lack of evidence-based superiority of one modality versus another, focal ablative treatments presently offered at various institutions are essentially related to device and skill availability rather than to established practice guidelines. Similar to prior experience with ablative treatments in other body organs, the efficacy of prostate focal ablative therapy will likely prove to be primarily related to proper candidate selection, sound ablative technique, reliable monitoring of energy deployment, and adequate posttreatment follow-up rather than to the choice of ablative modality itself.

Cryoablation

Cryoablation is probably one of the earliest ablative techniques applied to the prostate gland and its initial use in the 1960s was associated with many complications.[31] Most reports on prostate cryoablation are, however, those pertaining to whole-gland ablation without much emphasis on imaging for cryoprobe placement or treatment monitoring.[41,42] Hemi-gland and focal cryoablations have also been reported under US guidance with high biochemical failure rates of 50% to 75%.[43] Reports describing the use of MR imaging to guide and monitor whole-gland and focal prostate cryoablation started to surface only in the last few years.[44–46] Gangi and colleagues[44] performed MR imaging–guided whole-gland cryoablation on 11 subjects diagnosed with multifocal prostate cancer with Gleason scores ranging between 5 and 8 and no extracapsular disease. They used the transperineal approach with a freehand technique, rather than a perineal template, to insert 4 to 7 cryoprobes into the prostate gland, spaced at 1-cm distances. Biochemical failure was reported in one subject at the 1-month posttreatment time point. MR imaging–guided transperineal cryoprobe insertion is more commonly performed via a perineal template guidance system. Overduin and colleagues[47] performed MR imaging–guided focal cryoablation on 47 subjects with locally recurrent prostate cancer following primary radiation treatment (**Fig. 1**). They used the transperineal template approach to place a median of 3 cryoprobes (range 2–6) into the recurrent prostate tumor. Local tumor recurrence was reported in 23 of 47 subjects (49%) at a median of 12 months' (range 3–42) follow-up duration. MR imaging–guided transperineal cryoablation has also been performed using the perineal grid system to treat 18 subjects with local tumor recurrence in the surgical bed following radical prostatectomy.[46] A range of 2 to 8 cryoprobes was needed depending on the size and number of recurrent tumor nodules. Treatment outcomes at the 15-month follow-up time point were related to cryoprobe spacing and number of applied freeze-thaw cycles during ablation. A sustained biochemical response was reported in 9 of 18 subjects whereby cryoprobes were spaced 0.5 cm apart and 3 freeze-thaw cycles were applied. Placing cryoprobes placed at 1-cm distances and applying 2 freeze-thaw cycles were associated with biochemical failure in the rest of study subjects (9 of 18).[46]

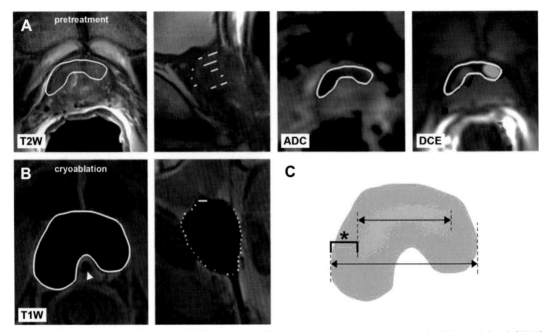

Fig. 1. (*A*) Annotation of a tumor (*outlined in white*) on pretreatment axial and sagittal T2-weighted (T2W), apparent diffusion coefficient (ADC) and dynamic contrast-enhanced (DCE) prostate MR images and (*B*) corresponding ice ball (*outlined in white*) at the end of the second freeze cycle on axial and sagittal intraprocedural T1-weighted (TW1) images, with urethral warming catheter in situ (*arrowhead*). (*C*) The ice ball margin (*asterisk*) was determined by subtracting the radii of the tumor (*yellow*) and ice ball (*blue*) along each direction. (*From* Overduin CG, Jenniskens SF, Sedelaar JP, et al. Percutaneous MR-guided focal cryoablation for recurrent prostate cancer following radiation therapy: retrospective analysis of iceball margins and outcomes. Eur Radiol 2017;27(11):4831; with permission.)

High-Intensity Focused Ultrasound

High-intensity focused US (HIFU) has been used since the 1990s to treat focal prostate cancer with nontargeted whole-gland ablation under US imaging guidance.[48,49] A 5-year disease-free survival rate of 66% was reported, using the Ablatherm-Maxis device, which uses an integrated transrectal probe combining both the diagnostic US imaging and the therapeutic HIFU functionalities.[48] Three recent studies reported MR imaging–guided treatment of localized prostate cancer using high-intensity US. Two of these studies[50,51] used an endorectal focused US ablation system integrated within a 1.5-T MR imaging unit to perform focal ablation of low-volume, low-risk (Gleason score 3 + 3 = 6) prostate cancer with the target areas sonicated during real-time magnetic resonance (MR) thermometry monitoring (**Fig. 2**). Four subjects were treated in the first study[50] with a reported 83% recurrence-free rate at the 6-month follow-up time point. Fourteen subjects were treated in the second study[51] with cancer detected in 7 of 14 men at the 6-month template biopsy and in 8 of 14 men at the 24-month template biopsy.

The third study reporting high-intensity US treatment of focal prostate cancer under MR imaging monitoring[52] used a rigid transurethral high-intensity directional (rather than focused) US system integrated with a 3-T MR imaging system to treat 30 subjects with low- and intermediate-risk prostate cancer. Treatments in this phase I multicenter study involved whole-gland, rather than focal, prostate ablations with cancer detected in 16 of 29 men at the 12-month biopsy (55%), 9 of whom (31%) were positive for clinically significant disease.

Focal Laser Ablation

Laser ablation, as currently practiced, is a newer ablative technique for thermal therapy for localized prostate cancer that started to gain popularity in the recent few years. Lindner and colleagues[53] first reported the use of diode laser fibers, inserted transperineally, to treat 12 subjects with localized low-risk prostate cancer. They, however, used MR imaging only to identify the targets, whereas the actual guidance of fiber placement was achieved via TRUS and the progress of ablation was monitored using thermal

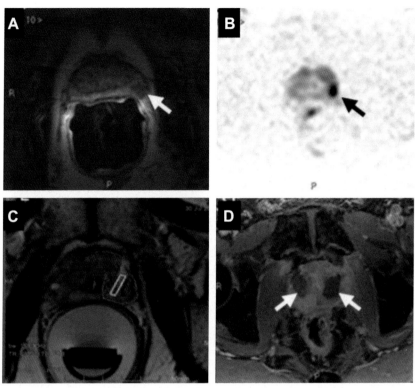

Fig. 2. Images in a 54-year-old man with a PSA level of 7.7 and biopsy-proven Gleason 3 + 3 prostate carcinoma. (A) Pretreatment axial T2-weighted fast spin-echo MR image (repetition time ms/echo time ms, 3300/90) and (B) corresponding axial diffusion-weighted image (105/6000, b = 2000 mm/s²) show a well-demarcated lesion in the left posterior peripheral zone at the midgland level (*white arrow* in [A] and *black arrow* in [B]). A suspicious type 3 curve was seen on dynamic contrast material–enhanced MR images (*not shown*). The other lesion in the right posterior peripheral zone was not seen. (C) Intraoperative MR-guided focused US image shows focused US beam path (*green rectangle*) overlaid on treatment plan for left posterior peripheral zone lesion. (D) T1-weighted contrast-enhanced MR image (400/6) 1 month after treatment shows persistence of nonperfused devascularized ablated volumes in bilateral peripheral zones (*arrows*). (*From* Tay KJ, Cheng CWS, Lau WKO, et al. Focal therapy for prostate cancer with in-bore MR-guided focused ultrasound: two-year follow-up of a phase I trial-complications and functional outcomes. Radiology 2017;285(2):626; with permission.)

sensors. Cancer was detected in 50% of subjects on multicore total prostate biopsy at 6 months. This detection was soon followed by a case study[54] from the same group describing an initial experience of 2 patients with low-risk prostate cancer who were treated with outpatient in-bore transperineal MR imaging–guided focal laser ablation (FLA). No follow-up data are available from this case study. A phase I trial followed by a phase II clinical trial evaluating MR imaging–guided FLA were then conducted at the University of Chicago. Diode laser fibers were inserted transperineally via a brachytherapy template with fiducial markers within the bore of a 1.5-T MR imaging scanner. In the phase I trial, Oto and colleagues[55] reported the treatment of 9 subjects with a Gleason score of 7 or less in 3 or less cores limited to one sextant. At the 6-month follow-up, MR imaging–guided biopsy of

the ablation zone showed no cancer in 7 patients (78%) and a Gleason sore of 6 in 2 patients (22%). In the phase II trial, Eggener and colleagues[56] included 27 men with stage T1c to T2a, PSA less than 15 ng/mL or PSA density less than 0.15 ng/mL³, Gleason score of 7 or less, 25% or less of biopsies, and MR imaging with 1 or 2 lesions concordant with biopsy-detected cancer (Fig. 3). At 3 months, 26 subjects (96%) had no cancer on MR imaging–guided biopsy of the ablation zone. At the 12-month biopsy, cancer was identified in 10 patients (37%), including in the ablation zones in 3 (11%) and outside the ablation zones in 8 (30%) with cancer in and outside the ablation zone in one. In-bore 3.0-T MR imaging–guided transrectal prostate FLA was also recently reported in a brief correspondence by Lepor and colleagues.[57] They included 25 men with stage T1c and T2a

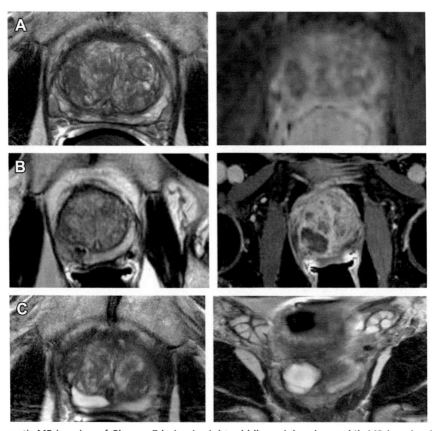

Fig. 3. Diagnostic MR imaging of Gleason 7 lesion in right middle peripheral zone (*A*), MR imaging immediately after FLA (*B*), and MR imaging 1 year after ablation (*C*). (*From* Eggener SE, Yousuf A, Watson S, et al. Phase II evaluation of magnetic resonance imaging guided focal laser ablation of prostate cancer. J Urol 2016;196(6):1672; with permission.)

disease; PSA less than 10 ng/mL; Gleason score less than 8; and 1 to 2 cancer-suspicious regions on mpMRI. At 3 months, targeted biopsy of 28 ablation sites showed no evidence of cancer in 26 (96%). No long-term data are available from this study. The safety and feasibility of performing FLA in a urology clinic (out of bore) using MR imaging–US fusion for guidance has been explored by the University of California, Los Angeles group. In a just-published study, Natarajan and colleagues[58] updated the results of their previous report[59] to include 11 men with intermediate-risk prostate cancer treated with transrectal prostate FLA, with laser fibers inserted into the regions of interest under MR imaging–US fusion imaging and treatment zones monitored via thermal probes. At 6 months, MR imaging–US fusion biopsy of the treatment sites in 10 of 11 successfully completed ablation procedures showed no cancer in 3 subjects, micro-focal Gleason score of 3 + 3 in 3 subjects, and persistent intermediate-risk prostate cancer in 4 subjects.

Photodynamic Therapy

Photodynamic therapy (PDT) is another form of focal treatment that uses laser energy, but the cell death achieved is not the result of direct tissue injury by the laser energy. Rather, PDT uses a low-power laser light to activate an injected photosensitizing drug. The low-power laser is delivered to the prostate gland via optical fibers placed within needles and inserted through a perineal template grid under TRUS guidance. Once the photosensitizer is activated locally by the light, reactive oxygen species form and incite tissue necrosis at the site of interaction between the photosensitizer, light, and oxygen.[60] A recent phase I/II multicenter trial was reported on 30 men with low-volume prostate cancer who underwent hemi-ablation with PDT. Fifteen of 30 patients had a positive biopsy at the 6-month follow up. This rate of positive biopsies decreased to 26.7% when excluding patients who did not receive an optimal dose of photosensitizer.[51]

Irreversible Electroporation

IRE has only been recently used for prostate abla-tion.[61] An initial assessment of safety and clinical feasibility was reported in 2014 whereby the IRE electrodes were inserted via a transperineal approach under TRUS guidance using a brachy-therapy grid. Short-term follow-up was conducted at 6 months following treatment and showed sus-picious residual disease in 6 of 34 subjects on mpMRI. No biopsies were performed.[62] The same group subsequently reported the results of IRE for focal disease limited to the anterior gland using transperineal grid approach under MR imag-ing/US fusion guidance. Seven of 16 subjects had residual disease on the 12-month biopsies, 6 of whom had clinically significant disease.[63] A retro-spective case study of patients with prostate can-cer who underwent prostate gland ablation using IRE as a primary procedure reported 4 of 25 pa-tients with cancer detected in the ablation zone on routine follow-up biopsy at 6 months. The pro-cedures were performed with IRE electrodes placed transperineally under TRUS guidance.[64] The short-term outcomes of 25 men who under-went focal IRE for low-intermediate risk prostate cancer demonstrated the presence of cancer in 5 men on biopsies at 7 months.[65] A series of 16 pa-tients underwent IRE 4 weeks before a scheduled radical prostatectomy; 6 patients were treated with focal, and 10 patients were treated with extended ablation protocol. Procedures were per-formed using transperineally inserted electrodes through a brachytherapy grid under US guidance. The study documented no viable cancer cells within the electrode configuration on whole-mount histopathologic processing the prostatec-tomy specimens.[66]

APPROACHES FOR ABLATIVE DEVICE PLACEMENT UNDER MR IMAGING GUIDANCE

The recent developments in prostate MR imaging has not only led to an improved in vivo mapping of intraprostatic disease burden via identification and targeted biopsy but has also rendered focal treatment of localized cancer a reality. Indeed, much of the momentum behind the currently growing recognition of focal treatment comes from the ability to use MR imaging to guide the ablation procedure and to monitor the effect of treatment.

A prerequisite to successful ablative device guidance is the ability to unequivocally identify the target tumor and to clearly visualize it margins relative to surrounding structures. In that sense, in-bore high-field 3T MRI guidance is preferred in

these procedures due to the improved delineation of target lesions leading to more accurate ablative device placement. Successful in-bore device guidance has also been reported within the 1.5-T MR imaging environment.[55,56] Attempts to simplify the targeting approach by using MR imaging–US fusion data to guide the ablative device have been less successful in both device placement and treatment outcomes.[58] The author's experi-ence from in-bore MR imaging–guided targeted prostate biopsies and focal ablations show that prostate gland displacement and rotation during device guidance can be significant enough to render the acquisition of updated intraprocedural MR imaging scans a necessity. The built-in distor-tion correction algorithms in MR imaging–US fusion systems uses data from historical preproce-dure MR imaging scans and may become less ac-curate with significant displacements, particularly when attempting to target smaller lesions.

Various approaches have been used for ablative device placement under MR imaging guidance, including the transperineal, transrectal, transglu-teal, and transurethral approaches.

Transperineal Approach

In this approach, patients are placed in the supine lithotomy position on the MR imaging table. A sur-face and an endorectal coil are typically used simultaneously. A modified MR imaging–compat-ible brachytherapy grid/template carrying 3 fidu-cial markers is secured against the perineum. An MR imaging scan is performed to localize the grid relative to the prostate targets. The integrated software application facilitates fiducial localization within the stack of axial scans, projects a virtual di-agram of the template on the MR images, and cal-culates the guidance trajectories and appropriate depth of insertion.[67,68] The interventionist then uses the recommended insertion hole of the tem-plate to access the target in a manner analogous to the widely practiced concept of MR imaging–guided breast biopsies. A transperineal freehand technique that does not require the integration of a special software has also been described.[44] In the author's experience, the freehand technique is more suitable for the transgluteal approach, but its application for transperineal prostate inter-ventions is often cumbersome and less accurate.

Transrectal Approach

In this approach, patients are placed in the prone position on the MR imaging table. A phased-array surface body coil is positioned over the gluteal region. A rectal probe is inserted that functions as both a device holder and a fiducial marker. The probe contains a central channel that accommodates a 14-G device, surrounded by a circumferential cavity filled with gadolinium gel that represents the fiducial marker. This rectal probe connects to an MR imaging-–compatible table-mount system that can be manually dialed to direct the probe into any desired trajectory along the x-y-z axes. An MR imaging scan is then acquired to localize the rectal probe location relative to the prostate targets and software application and then recommends the appropriate access trajectories along the 3 axes. The Dyna-TRIM (Invivo Corp, FL, USA) and Sentenelle (Hologic, Toronto, CA) are two presently available systems in the market that are built on this concept. Several robotic systems have also been developed for prostate interventions but are not commonly used in clinical settings.[52–54]

The transrectal approach is most suited for deep and anteriorly located tumors, particularly in larger-size prostate glands.[52] When targeting posterior, capsular-based tumors for focal treatment, the transrectal approach can be quite challenging, as it increases the risk for injury to the anterior rectal wall.

Transgluteal Approach

In this approach, patients are placed in the prone position on a wide-bore MR imaging scanner equipped with interventional accessories. A phased-array surface body coil is positioned over the gluteal region. This technique used in this approach is equivalent to that used during MR imaging–guided interventions in other body organs (eg, liver or kidney), where a freehand technique is used to guide the device into the target tissue while continuously reviewing updates of device placement and tissue displacements on near real-time image updates at the scanner side within the interventional MR imaging suite. After the initial scan identifying the target lesion within the prostate gland, the skin entry point is identified and the coil position is adjusted to bring the entry point to the center of one of the coil openings. The area is then prepped and draped in a sterile fashion and a 14-G MR imaging–compatible introducing needle is advanced through the gluteal musculature and ischiorectal fossa toward the target lesion. This process is monitored under MR-fluoroscopy using a triorthogonal image plane guidance method that has been previously described[52] to interactively monitor the needle on continuously updated sets of true–fast imaging with steady state precession images. Continuous saline infusion may be added through a second introducer needle placed with a similar technique between the prostate and rectum if the tumor abuts the rectal wall. Once the introducing needle position is deemed satisfactory, the author then replaces the introducer stylet with a laser applicator to conduct the thermal ablation procedure (**Fig. 4**). The transgluteal approach is limited by the need for a full interventional MR imaging suite setup and preexisting training on the freehand guidance technique. It does, however, offer a safe technique to treat posterior lesions with a quick targeting approach that enjoys the flexibility to modify the access trajectory on the fly while advancing the introducing needle and reviewing the continuously updated scans.

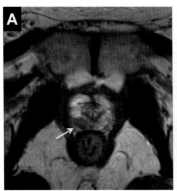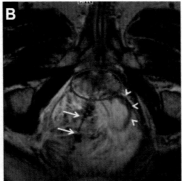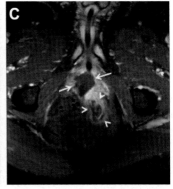

Fig. 4. A 67-year-old man with a PSA level of 4.92 ng/mL. (*A*) Axial turbo spin-echo (TSE)–T2 scan: focal biopsy-proven prostate cancer (Gleason 4 + 3 = 7) in the right peripheral zone apex (*arrow*). (*B*) Axial TSE-T2 scan: Laser fiber (*arrows*) has been introduced via the right transgluteal approach, with its tip within the target lesion (*oval*). Note that saline has been infused to displace the rectum (*arrowheads*) and provide room to generate a thermal ablation zone sufficient to encompass the target tumor without causing rectal injury. (*C*) Axial postgadolinium TSE-T1 scan obtained immediately following the FLA procedure showing the thermal ablation zone (*arrows*) replacing the target tumor. The rectum (*arrowheads*) started to move back to its anatomic location.

Transurethral Approach

In this approach, patients are placed in the supine position on the MR imaging table. Posterior and anterior multichannel phased-array coils are used. The MR imaging–guided transurethral approach for prostate ablation has only been reported with high-intensity US prostate ablation.[42,52] A rigid US applicator carrying an array of 10 independent US transducers is inserted manually into the urethra. An MR imaging scan is then acquired and used to adjust the position of the US applicator within the prostatic urethra to maintain a 3-mm safety margin between the US transducers and sphincter plane at the prostate apex.[42] A suprapubic catheter is inserted to avoid prostate displacement between treatment planning and execution. High-intensity US energy is then delivered to the prostate in one complete rotation of the US applicator under active MR imaging thermometry feedback control.

MR IMAGING MONITORING DURING FOCAL PROSTATE TREATMENT

Once MR imaging has been used to guide the placement of the ablative device and high-resolution scans have confirmed a final satisfactory position with respect to the 3-dimensional geometry of the target tumor, MR imaging plays an essential role during the actual treatment phase. In this phase, the temperature sensitivity of MR imaging sequences is exploited to titrate the ablative dose of the used energy source and to determine the treatment end point based on the actual tissue response of individual tumors. This approach represents a conceptual departure from the earlier versions of prostate ablations where a predetermined ablative dose was applied without imaging feedback. The collective experience and lessons learned from thermal ablations using various energy sources in various body organs clearly indicate that applying a recipe dose of thermal energy is not the best strategy for a successful treatment outcome. Tumor morphology, pathologic type and grade, perfusion, and structure of the adjacent tissues are some examples of the variables that exist and do impact the response of a given tumor to a given ablative dose.

MR imaging is used to monitor the ablative treatment both indirectly, by imaging the phenomena associated with changing tissue temperature, and directly, by imaging the actual tissue destruction resulting from thermal injury.

MR imaging has been reported to provide a reliable interactive visualization of the growing ice ball during cryoablation procedures. Early experiences with this phenomenon have been primarily based on monitoring of MR imaging–guided renal cryoablations,[52–54] with subsequent similar experiences reported during MR imaging monitoring of prostatectomy bed cryoablations of recurrent tumors[36] and of postradiation focal recurrences in native prostate glands.[35] MR imaging monitoring has been useful in this context by providing the real-time feedback necessary to adjust the gas flow to individual cryoprobes in order to modify the size and shape of the forming ice ball, thereby maximizing the treatment effect and minimizing the risk of collateral injury. When using MR imaging to monitor cryoablation procedures, it is important to note that the visualized leading edge of the ice ball during the procedure corresponds to 0°C, which is a sublethal freezing point and results in incomplete treatment if used to indicate the treatment margin. Therefore, the margin of the visualized ice ball should be planned to encompass a margin beyond the desired treatment area to ensure adequate delivery of the lethal isotherms to the tumor border. The threshold for lethal isotherm is thought to be at −40°C.[69,70] Experts recommend at least a 5-mm margin, which may be increased in the vicinity of large vessels, urethral warmers, or other factors that may confound the cooling process.[52,54,55] A recent study evaluating the margin of visualized ice ball during MR imaging–guided salvage cryoablation of postradiation recurrent prostate cancer reported a significantly improved local progression-free survival at 1 year among patients with larger ice ball margins (minimum margin >10 mm = 100%, 5–10 mm = 84%, and <5 mm = 15%).[47]

Monitoring ablative procedures that use tissue heating, rather than cooling, such as high-intensity US and laser ablations, is enabled by applying temperature-sensitive MR imaging sequences[54–56] for direct on-line monitoring of heat deposition. The proton resonance frequency shift method[54–56] is a common technique that continuously acquires phase-sensitive images during treatment, measures the changes in chemical shift resulting from changes in tissue temperature, and displays the resultant data as a color-coded thermal map to visually delineate the temperature distribution over the treatment area. The time-varying temperature maps may be used to calculate a thermal dose map[54] that can be displayed over the magnitude (ie, anatomic) image featuring the target tumor to facilitate an overall estimate of thermal tissue destruction.

In addition to monitoring the changes associated with tissue cooling or heating, MR imaging can be used for direct imaging of tissue injury at the conclusion of the ablation procedure. This ability serves as a second line of assessment of the treatment effect before the target tumor is deemed adequately ablated. This process is based on detecting the changes in the tissue-relaxation parameters that accompany phase transition from a viable to necrotic state.[54,55] Thermally induced tissue injury results in cellular denaturation, shrinkage, aggregation of cytoplasmic proteins, and increased hydrophobic interactions leading to water extrusion.[71,72] Thermal ablation zones demonstrate a T2 hypointense appearance corresponding to tissue necrosis, surrounded by a hyperintense rim of edema and reactive tissue changes. This hypointense appearance of the ablated zone is caused by shortening of T2 relaxation time that likely results from a combination of water extrusion from necrotic tissue along with binding between any residual free water and the denatured proteins. Several studies have previously demonstrated the reliability of MR imaging findings in reflecting the histopathologic changes associated with thermally induced tissue necrosis.[56–60] The rapid loss of T2 signal within the ablated zone is, in the author's experience, less noticeable on immediate postablation prostate scans compared with other parenchymal organ ablations.

Combining the interactive monitoring of ice ball or thermal map with direct imaging of tissue damage at the conclusion of the ablation procedure allows a fairly accurate assessment of the size and configuration of the ablation zone and facilitates the identification of undertreated and thermally resistant foci where additional treatment may need to be directed. This approach for controlled ablation does not only limit potential treatment failures but also guards against unduly aggressive treatment, thereby minimizing the risk of complications.

RECOVERY, COMPLICATIONS, AND MORBIDITY AFTER FOCAL PROSTATE TREATMENT

MRI-guided focal treatment of prostate cancer is typically offered as a same-day surgery procedure that may be performed under moderate sedation or general anesthesia. The procedure is generally viewed as a safe alternative to the more radical forms of prostate interventions, with low morbidity and short recovery time. It is advised, however, to have a detailed discussion with focal treatment candidates to highlight the exact recovery expectations and the possible complications, particularly those related to erectile dysfunction, urine incontinence, and rectal injury.

The incidence of major complications was reported to be less than 2% following focal treatment of localized prostate cancer in 106 patients who underwent HIFU, brachytherapy, cryotherapy, or vascular-targeted PDT.[73] Oto and colleagues[55] reported no significant changes in the average International Prostate Symptom Score (I-PSS) and Sexual Health Inventory for Men (SHIM) scores at 1, 3, or 6 months compared with pretreatment scores during a phase I clinical trial of MR imaging–guided transperineal focal laser ablation of localized prostate cancer. In the phase II trial from the same group, Eggener and colleagues[56] reported no significant changes in the average I-PSS scores over a 12-month follow-up period. They did, however, report the average SHIM score to be lower at 1 month, marginally lower at 3 months, and not significantly changed from baseline at 12 months. Tay and colleagues[51] recently reported a slight insignificant deterioration of Expanded Prostate Index Composite (EPIC) urinary symptom scores at 1 month in 14 patients who underwent MR imaging–guided focused US treatment. The EPIC scores returned to baseline by 3 months and were not significantly changed from baseline at 24 months.

Forty-seven percent of patients who underwent MR imaging–guided transurethral whole gland high-intensity US ablation experienced erectile dysfunction after 1 month. This percentage decreased to 35% after 3 months, 29% after 6 months, and 15% after 12 months.[52] Following MR imaging–guided transrectal HIFU ablations, a trend for insignificant deterioration in sexual function scores was reported that normalized at 3 months.[51]

Three of 9 patients who underwent an aggressive protocol of MR imaging–guided cryoablation to treat prostatectomy bed recurrences experienced progressive urine incontinence.[46] Mild urine incontinence was reported in 3 of 4 patients who underwent MR imaging–guided transrectal focal US ablation.[50] Mild and moderate urine incontinence was reported in 4 of 30 patients who underwent MR imaging–guided transurethral whole-gland US ablation. Of these, only one patient continued to have mild pad-free incontinence at the 12-month follow-up time point.[52]

The most significant complication reported in the literature was a single case of urethrorectal fistula following MR imaging–guided whole-gland cryoablation.[34] This fistula healed on conservative management after 8 weeks. Although this was a complication of ablative therapy, it was associated with a whole-gland, rather than focal, treatment.

Several other minor complications have been reported following MR imaging–guided prostate ablations. These complications include (in a decreasing order of frequency) hematuria, urinary tract infection, urine retention, obstructive micturition, urinary stricture, mild proctalgia, transient dysuria, scrotal pain, focal paresthesia of the glans penis, and epididymitis.[44–46,50,52,55] Two patients in the author's practice also reported mild necroturia a few weeks following MR imaging–guided focal laser ablation of lesions abutting the urethra.

FOLLOW-UP AFTER FOCAL PROSTATE TREATMENT

Long-term monitoring after focal prostate ablation should be offered as an integral part of the initial treatment plan. Before embarking in focal therapy, potential treatment candidates need to understand that this is a relatively new and promising concept that still lacks the long-term evidence available for other established standard-of-care treatment options. The plan for long-term follow-up should typically monitor patients' morbidity and treatment efficacy.

Morbidity

Posttreatment morbidity is preferably evaluated by recognized symptom scores, such as the EPIC urinary symptom score and the American Urological Association's I-PSS and SHIM scores. Using these scores to quantify posttreatment morbidity and to compare symptoms with baseline status facilitates a measurable assessment of outcomes, helps place the recovery expectations in perspective relative to other treatment options, and establishes a common language between treating physicians from various specialties.

Efficacy

Monitoring treatment efficacy entails the acquisition of periodic multi-parametric MR imaging scans, ideally reproducing the same imaging protocol obtained before treatment; analysis of serum PSA trend; and possibly obtaining incremental prostate biopsies.

MULTI-PARAMETRIC MR IMAGING FOLLOW-UP

Acute thermal ablation zones within the prostate gland may demonstrate a hypointense, isointense, or slightly or markedly hyperintense signal on precontrast T1-weighted MR imaging. This reduction of T1 relaxation time results from the inevitable hemorrhage occurring at the treatment site and varies with the degree of target tissue vascularity.[55] These T1-weighted signal changes are usually observed as early as the intraprocedural

or immediate postprocedure scans and typically involute gradually over several months following the ablation procedure. On T2-weighted images, the hypointense appearance of the ablation zone that starts to appear during the ablation procedure continues to evolve and becomes more conspicuous on the early follow-up scans before it starts to gradually decrease in size with the involution of the chronic ablation zone. The ablative device track is typically seen as a linear high T2-weighted signal within the ablation zone, particularly on the early postablation scans.

The margins of the thermal ablation zone demonstrate an acute inflammatory response on the immediate and early posttreatment scans. This reactive tissue change consists of edema, hyperemia, and foci of hemorrhage when examined on histopathology.[57–61] On MR imaging, this inflamed margin is represented by a bright rim surrounding the area of necrosis on T2-weighted scans and demonstrates enhancement on the postgadolinium T1-weighted scans. The inflammatory process encircling the ablation zone has a typically sharp inner and fading outer margin.[57] The author has previously shown that the extent of actual cell death following radiofrequency thermal ablation does eventually extend to the outer margin of the inflammatory rim.[57] To ensure a complete treatment during thermal ablation regardless of the used energy source, the author does, however, advocate the use of the sharp inner margin as an unequivocal indicator of the definite extent of tissue necrosis.

In chronic thermal ablation zones, the treatment margins demonstrate a gradual replacement of the inflammatory response by concentrically laid granulation tissue, which subsequently matures into fibrous tissue in a concentric fashion proceeding from the periphery of the ablation zone toward the center.[57] These tissue changes are represented on MR imaging by the resolution of the T2 hyperintense rim and the development of a thick T2 hypointense (likely fibrotic) rim. It has been the author's experience that this change occurs as early as 3 weeks following prostate focal ablations as opposed to the previously reported gradual resolution of the T2 hyperintense rims surrounding renal ablation zones.[74]

Postgadolinium scans demonstrate rim enhancement around the thermal ablation zone, reflecting hyperemia or enhancing granulation tissue in the acute/subacute phase or enhancing mature fibrotic tissue in the chronic phase. Some residual vessel enhancement may normally be seen within cryoablation beds for several months following treatment[75]; otherwise, rim enhancement should be fairly uniform without any focal hyperperfusion at the ablation site on dynamic contrast-enhanced–MR imaging.

Any pretreatment focal restricted diffusion on diffusion-weighted imaging (DWI) scans should not be identified on follow-up imaging. This evaluation may be limited in the immediate posttreatment period while excessive inflammatory changes persist. DWI scans should also be correlated with the corresponding turbo spin-echo–T2-weighted images in order to distinguish a focal tumor recurrence from a T2 shine-through signal associated with liquefied necrotic tissue at the ablation bed.

On longer-term follow-up scans, the chronic thermal ablation zone involutes into an area of featureless mummified coagulated tissue surrounded by a variable amount of fibrous tissue. Eventually, the entire ablation zone may be replaced by a contracted scar, resulting in an asymmetric loss of prostate tissue and an overall shrinkage of prostate volume.

PROSTATE-SPECIFIC ANTIGEN FOLLOW-UP

The term *biochemical failure* is used to describe a failed response to prostate cancer treatment, manifested by an increase in the serum PSA level. PSA levels used to define failures after radical prostatectomy and radiation therapy are well studied and, despite minor variations, represent a standardized science. Following radical prostatectomy, the optimal definition of biochemical failure for patients with 5-year progression-free probability of less than 50%, 50% to 75%, 76% to 90%, and greater than 90% is a single PSA of 0.05 ng/mL or greater, 2 or more increasing PSAs of 0.05 ng/mL or greater, PSA of 0.2 ng/mL or greater and increasing, and PSA of 0.4 ng/mL or greater and increasing, respectively.[76] Following radiation therapy, with or without hormonal therapy, an increase by 2.0 ng/mL or more greater than the nadir PSA is considered the standard definition for biochemical failure.[77]

These exact definitions of biochemical failure do not currently exist for follow-up after focal prostate ablation treatment. A handful of studies have reported a decrease in the mean or median PSA levels over follow-up durations of up to 24 months,[51,56,58] with one study showing an initial increase in the mean PSA level at 1 month following treatment,[56] which has been the observation at the author's practice as well. No significant PSA differences were, however, reported among patients with documented treatment failures in 2 studies.[51,56] Furthermore, one study found no significant difference in the mean PSA levels before treatment and at the 1, 3, or 6 months after treatment across the study cohort.[55] The interpretation of PSA values following focal treatment remains, therefore, a subject of further study; the PSA trends of individual patients should be assessed in conjunction with mpMRI findings and correlated with the results of incremental prostate biopsies. Given the presence of residual prostate tissue and the variability in treatment extent, the eventual definition of biochemical failure following focal treatment will likely follow that used for radiation therapy, with the exact threshold for the PSA increase greater than the nadir to be determined based on future documented tumor recurrences.

BIOPSY FOLLOW-UP

Targeted prostate biopsies should conceivably be obtained from any suspicious foci identified on follow-up mpMRI scans, either via direct in-bore MR imaging–guided biopsy or MR imaging–US fusion biopsy. Prostate cancer has, however, been documented by several investigators on routinely scheduled biopsies following focal treatment.[47,52,56] In fact, a recent study reported the detection of cancer in 8 out of 14 men treated with MR imaging–guided focal HIFU at 24-month template biopsies, surprisingly without corresponding positive mpMRI findings detected in any subject.[51] The addition of incremental biopsies, not prompted by suspicious findings, during the posttreatment follow-up may, therefore, be necessary, at least for the time being and until the clear parameters of biochemical failure have been established and used to identify patients who may need to be further evaluated with biopsies.

The optimal method, timing, and frequency of these biopsies remain largely uncertain. Published studies report markedly inconsistent approaches to these follow-up biopsies, including targeted MR imaging–guided biopsies of the ablation zones performed at 3 months,[56] 6 months,[55] or 12 months[47]; MR imaging–US fusion biopsies performed at 6 months targeting the original tumor site, the ablation zone, margins of the ablation zone, any new finding, and 6 template sites throughout the ipsilateral prostate[58]; standard 12-core TRUS biopsies performed at 6 months[50] or 12 months[52,56]; and robotic transperineal mapping biopsies performed at 6 and 24 months.[51]

FINAL NOTES AND FUTURE OUTLOOK

Focal treatment of prostate cancer has evolved from a concept to a practice in the recent few years and is projected to fill an existing need, bridging the gap between conservative and radical traditional treatment options. The idea of organ-sparing treatment of localized prostate cancer has been modestly entertained since Onik and colleagues reported[1] a small series of focal nerve-sparing cryosurgery for the treatment of primary prostate cancer as a new approach to preserving potency in 2002. Onik[78] subsequently introduced the term "*male lumpectomy*" in 2004[79] to illustrate the similarity of the concept of targeted prostate cancer treatment to lumpectomy surgery that had revolutionized breast cancer care. The application of this concept remained limited by the inability to accurately visualize and sample focal prostate cancer. The advent of mpMRI and the integration of interventional MR imaging technology in prostate cancer care have been the major catalysts behind the recently revived interest in focal treatment because of a significantly improved ability to visualize, sample, and treat localized disease within the prostate gland.

With its low morbidity and rapid recovery time compared with whole-gland treatment alternatives, focal therapy is poised to gain more acceptance among patients and health care providers. In the meantime, more work is needed to streamline procedural workflow, reduce recurrence rates, improve evidence, and achieve insurance recognition. The importance of proper candidate selection for focal therapy cannot be overstated, as it is critically linked to treatment outcomes and, hence, to future perception and dissemination of this emerging treatment concept.

Diligent preprocedure workup should ensure that the index or clinically significant lesion has been identified and should unequivocally rule out the presence of significant/high-risk disease in the untreated parts of the gland. At the current stage of knowledge, this entails direct tissue sampling, not only from highly suspicious foci on MR imaging but also from low-suspicion foci and from a normal-appearing gland particularly in the contralateral lobe. A focal lesion on MR imaging may represent a high-risk cancer, located just next to a low- or intermediate-risk cancer diagnosed on a systematic TRUS biopsy. Caution should, therefore, be exercised when offering focal treatment based on the result of a systematic TRUS biopsy supplemented by subsequent mpMRI, particularly in patients with large-volume glands. In these cases, additional targeted sampling would be strongly advised before offering focal treatment.

As our experience with focal treatment matures and evidence continues to accrue, the landscape of this practice might look quite different in the future. Focal high-risk disease may or may not remain a contraindication for focal therapy. Furthermore, novel prognostic factors might render what we currently consider a low- or intermediate-risk tumor inappropriate for focal ablation. In fact, the current prostate cancer risk stratification systems using Gleason grading, PSA, and clinical staging alone (see **Table 1**) are likely going to adapt to the vast developments in prognostic tools, leading to the emergence of new risk stratification paradigms that emphasize the value of genomic profiling scores, novel biochemical markers, and mpMRI findings.

REFERENCES

1. Onik G, Narayan P, Vaughan D, et al. Focal "nerve-sparing" cryosurgery for treatment of primary prostate cancer: a new approach to preserving potency. Urology 2002;60(1):109–14.
2. Budaus L, Spethmann J, Isbarn H, et al. Inverse stage migration in patients undergoing radical prostatectomy: results of 8916 European patients treated within the last decade. BJU Int 2011; 108(8):1256–61.
3. Silberstein JL, Vickers AJ, Power NE, et al. Reverse stage shift at a tertiary care center: escalating risk in men undergoing radical prostatectomy. Cancer 2011;117(21):4855–60.
4. Wilt TJ, Brawer MK, Jones KM, et al. Radical prostatectomy versus observation for localized prostate cancer. N Engl J Med 2012;367(3):203–13.
5. Wilt TJ, Jones KM, Barry MJ, et al. Follow-up of prostatectomy versus observation for early prostate cancer. N Engl J Med 2017;377(2):132–42.
6. Miller DC, Gruber SB, Hollenbeck BK, et al. Incidence of initial local therapy among men with lower-risk prostate cancer in the United States. J Natl Cancer Inst 2006;98(16):1134–41.
7. Klotz L. Active surveillance for intermediate risk prostate cancer. Curr Urol Rep 2017;18(10):80.
8. Savdie R, Aning J, So AI, et al. Identifying intermediate-risk candidates for active surveillance of prostate cancer. Urol Oncol 2017;35(10):605.e1–8.
9. Tosoian JJ, Mamawala M, Epstein JI, et al. Intermediate and longer-term outcomes from a prospective active-surveillance program for favorable-risk prostate cancer. J Clin Oncol 2015;33(30):3379–85.
10. Whitson JM, Porten SP, Hilton JF, et al. The relationship between prostate specific antigen change and biopsy progression in patients on active surveillance for prostate cancer. J Urol 2011;185(5):1656–60.
11. Klotz L, Vesprini D, Sethukavalan P, et al. Long-term follow-up of a large active surveillance cohort of patients with prostate cancer. J Clin Oncol 2015;33(3):272–7.

12. Bul M, Zhu X, Valdagni R, et al. Active surveillance for low-risk prostate cancer worldwide: the PRIAS study. Eur Urol 2013;63(4):597–603.

13. Pickles T, Ruether JD, Weir L, et al. Psychosocial barriers to active surveillance for the management of early prostate cancer and a strategy for increased acceptance. BJU Int 2007;100(3):544–51.

14. Gomez-Veiga F, Mariño A, Alvarez L, et al. Brachytherapy for the treatment of recurrent prostate cancer after radiotherapy or radical prostatectomy. BJU Int 2012;109(Suppl 1):17–21.

15. Society, A.C. 2017. Available at: https://www.cancer.org/cancer/prostate-cancer/about/key-statistics.html. Accessed September 20, 2017.

16. Arora R, Koch MO, Eble JN, et al. Heterogeneity of Gleason grade in multifocal adenocarcinoma of the prostate. Cancer 2004;100(11):2362–6.

17. Wise AM, Stamey TA, McNeal JE, et al. Morphologic and clinical significance of multifocal prostate cancers in radical prostatectomy specimens. Urology 2002;60:264–9.

18. Johansson JE, Andrén O, Andersson SO, et al. Natural history of early, localized prostate cancer. JAMA 2004;291(22):2713–9.

19. Albertsen PC, Hanley JA, Gleason DF, et al. Competing risk analysis of men aged 55 to 74 years at diagnosis managed conservatively for clinically localized prostate cancer. JAMA 1998;280(11):975–80.

20. Chodak GW, Thisted RA, Gerber GS, et al. Results of conservative management of clinically localized prostate cancer. N Engl J Med 1994;330(4):242–8.

21. Sakr WA, Haas GP, Cassin BF, et al. The frequency of carcinoma and intraepithelial neoplasia of the prostate in young male patients. J Urol 1993; 150(2 Pt 1):379–85.

22. Yin M, Bastacky S, Chandran U, et al. Prevalence of incidental prostate cancer in the general population: a study of healthy organ donors. J Urol 2008;179(3):892–5 [discussion: 895].

23. Jemal A, Siegel R, Ward E, et al. Cancer statistics, 2006. CA Cancer J Clin 2006;56(2):106–30.

24. Klotz L. Expectant management with selective delayed intervention for favorable risk prostate cancer. Urol Oncol 2002;7(5):175–9.

25. Noguchi M, Stamey TA, McNeal JE, et al. Prognostic factors for multifocal prostate cancer in radical prostatectomy specimens: lack of significance of secondary cancers. J Urol 2003;170(2 Pt 1):459–63.

26. Eggener SE, Scardino PT, Carroll PR, et al. Focal therapy for localized prostate cancer: a critical appraisal of rationale and modalities. J Urol 2007;178(6):2260–7.

27. Simma-Chiang V, Horn JJ, Simko JP, et al. Increased prevalence of unifocal prostate cancer in a contemporary series of radical prostatectomy specimens: implications for focal ablation. J Urol 2006;175:374.

28. Ohori M, Eastham JA, Koh H, et al. Is focal therapy reasonable in patients with early stage prostate cancer (CaP)—an analysis of radical prostatectomy (RP) specimens. J Urol 2006;175(suppl):507.

29. Porten SP, Whitson JM, Cowan JE, et al. Changes in prostate cancer grade on serial biopsy in men undergoing active surveillance. J Clin Oncol 2011; 29(20):2795–800.

30. Motamedinia P, RiChard JL, McKiernan JM, et al. Role of immediate confirmatory prostate biopsy to ensure accurate eligibility for active surveillance. Urology 2012;80(5):1070–4.

31. McClure TD, Margolis DJ, Hu JC. Partial gland ablation in the management of prostate cancer: a review. Curr Opin Urol 2017;27(2):156–60.

32. Barzell WE, Melamed MR. Appropriate patient selection in the focal treatment of prostate cancer: the role of transperineal 3-dimensional pathologic mapping of the prostate–a 4-year experience. Urology 2007;70(6 Suppl):27–35.

33. Onik G, Barzell W. Transperineal 3D mapping biopsy of the prostate: an essential tool in selecting patients for focal prostate cancer therapy. Urol Oncol 2008; 26(5):506–10.

34. Weinreb JC, Barentsz JO, Choyke PL, et al. PI-RADS prostate imaging - reporting and data system: 2015, version 2. Eur Urol 2016;69(1):16–40.

35. Kim SH, Choi MS, Kim MJ, et al. Validation of prostate imaging reporting and data system version 2 using an MRI-ultrasound fusion biopsy in prostate cancer diagnosis. AJR Am J Roentgenol 2017; 209(4):800–5.

36. Seo JW, Shin SJ, Taik Oh Y, et al. PI-RADS version 2: detection of clinically significant cancer in patients with biopsy Gleason score 6 prostate cancer. AJR Am J Roentgenol 2017;209(1):W1–w9.

37. Barentsz JO, Weinreb JC, Verma S, et al. Synopsis of the PI-RADS v2 guidelines for multiparametric prostate magnetic resonance imaging and recommendations for use. Eur Urol 2016;69(1):41–9.

38. Cash H, Maxeiner A, Stephan C, et al. The detection of significant prostate cancer is correlated with the prostate imaging reporting and data system (PI-RADS) in MRI/transrectal ultrasound fusion biopsy. World J Urol 2016;34(4):525–32.

39. Filson CP, Natarajan S, Margolis DJ, et al. Prostate cancer detection with magnetic resonance-ultrasound fusion biopsy: the role of systematic and targeted biopsies. Cancer 2016;122(6):884–92.

40. Vargas HA, Hötker AM, Goldman DA, et al. Updated prostate imaging reporting and data system (PIRADS v2) recommendations for the detection of clinically significant prostate cancer using multiparametric MRI: critical evaluation using whole-mount pathology as standard of reference. Eur Radiol 2016;26(6):1606–12.

41. da Silva RD, Jaworski P, Gustafson D, et al. How I do it: prostate cryoablation (PCry). Can J Urol 2014; 21(2):7251–4.

42. Govorov AV, Vasil'ev AO, Ivanov VIu, et al. Treatment of prostate cancer using cryoablation: a prospective study. Urologiia 2014;(6):69–72, 74. [in Russian].

43. Truesdale MD, Cheetham PJ, Hruby GW, et al. An evaluation of patient selection criteria on predicting progression-free survival after primary focal unilateral nerve-sparing cryoablation for prostate cancer: recommendations for follow up. Cancer J 2010; 16(5):544–9.

44. Gangi A, Tsoumakidou G, Abdelli O, et al. Percutaneous MR-guided cryoablation of prostate cancer: initial experience. Eur Radiol 2012;22(8):1829–35.

45. Bomers JG, Yakar D, Overduin CG, et al. MR imaging-guided focal cryoablation in patients with recurrent prostate cancer. Radiology 2013;268(2): 451–60.

46. Woodrum DA, Kawashima A, Karnes RJ, et al. Magnetic resonance imaging-guided cryoablation of recurrent prostate cancer after radical prostatectomy: initial single institution experience. Urology 2013;82(4):870–5.

47. Overduin CG, Jenniskens SF, Sedelaar JP, et al. Percutaneous MR-guided focal cryoablation for recurrent prostate cancer following radiation therapy: retrospective analysis of iceball margins and outcomes. Eur Radiol 2017;27(11):4828–36.

48. Blana A, Rogenhofer S, Ganzer R, et al. Eight years' experience with high-intensity focused ultrasonography for treatment of localized prostate cancer. Urology 2008;72(6):1329–33 [discussion: 1333–4].

49. Thuroff S, Chaussy C, Vallancien G, et al. High-intensity focused ultrasound and localized prostate cancer: efficacy results from the European multicentric study. J Endourol 2003;17(8):673–7.

50. Ghai S, Louis AS, Van Vliet M, et al. Real-time MRI-guided focused ultrasound for focal therapy of locally confined low-risk prostate cancer: feasibility and preliminary outcomes. AJR Am J Roentgenol 2015;205(2):W177–84.

51. Tay KJ, Cheng CWS, Lau WKO, et al. Focal therapy for prostate cancer with in-bore MR-guided focused ultrasound: two-year follow-up of a phase I trial-complications and functional outcomes. Radiology 2017;285(2):620–8.

52. Chin JL, Billia M, Relle J, et al. Magnetic resonance imaging-guided transurethral ultrasound ablation of prostate tissue in patients with localized prostate cancer: a prospective phase 1 clinical trial. Eur Urol 2016;70(3):447–55.

53. Lindner U, Weersink RA, Haider MA, et al. Image guided photothermal focal therapy for localized prostate cancer: phase I trial. J Urol 2009;182(4): 1371–7.

54. Raz O, Haider MA, Davidson SR, et al. Real-time magnetic resonance imaging-guided focal laser therapy in patients with low-risk prostate cancer. Eur Urol 2010;58(1):173–7.

55. Oto A, Sethi I, Karczmar G, et al. MR imaging-guided focal laser ablation for prostate cancer: phase I trial. Radiology 2013;267(3):932–40.

56. Eggener SE, Yousuf A, Watson S, et al. Phase II evaluation of magnetic resonance imaging guided focal laser ablation of prostate cancer. J Urol 2016;196(6): 1670–5.

57. Lepor H, Llukani E, Sperling D, et al. Complications, recovery, and early functional outcomes and oncologic control following in-bore focal laser ablation of prostate cancer. Eur Urol 2015;68(6):924–6.

58. Natarajan S, Jones TA, Priester AM, et al. Focal laser ablation of prostate cancer: feasibility of MRI/US fusion for guidance. J Urol 2017;198(4):839–47.

59. Natarajan S, Raman S, Priester AM, et al. Focal laser ablation of prostate cancer: phase I clinical trial. J Urol 2016;196(1):68–75.

60. Moore CM, Pendse D, Emberton M. Photodynamic therapy for prostate cancer–a review of current status and future promise. Nat Clin Pract Urol 2009; 6(1):18–30.

61. Onik G, Rubinsky B. Irreversible electroporation: first patient experience focal therapy of prostate cancer. In: Rubinsky B, editor. Irreversible electroporation. Series in biomedical engineering. Berlin: Springer; 2010. p. 235–47.

62. Valerio M, Stricker PD, Ahmed HU, et al. Initial assessment of safety and clinical feasibility of irreversible electroporation in the focal treatment of prostate cancer. Prostate Cancer Prostatic Dis 2014;17(4):343–7.

63. Valerio M, Dickinson L, Ali A, et al. Nanoknife electroporation ablation trial: a prospective development study investigating focal irreversible electroporation for localized prostate cancer. J Urol 2017;197(3 Pt 1):647–54.

64. Murray KS, Ehdaie B, Musser J, et al. Pilot study to assess safety and clinical outcomes of irreversible electroporation for partial gland ablation in men with prostate cancer. J Urol 2016;196(3):883–90.

65. Ting F, Tran M, Böhm M, et al. Focal irreversible electroporation for prostate cancer: functional outcomes and short-term oncological control. Prostate Cancer Prostatic Dis 2016;19(1):46–52.

66. van den Bos W, de Bruin DM, Jurhill RR, et al. The correlation between the electrode configuration and histopathology of irreversible electroporation ablations in prostate cancer patients. World J Urol 2016;34(5):657–64.

67. Woodrum DA, Gorny KR, Mynderse LA, et al. Feasibility of 3.0T magnetic resonance imaging-guided laser ablation of a cadaveric prostate. Urology 2010;75(6):1514.e1–6.

68. Penzkofer T, Tuncali K, Fedorov A, et al. Transperineal in-bore 3-T MR imaging-guided prostate biopsy: a prospective clinical observational study. Radiology 2015;274(1):170–80.

69. Gage AA, Baust J. Mechanisms of tissue injury in cryosurgery. Cryobiology 1998;37(3):171–86.

70. Baust JG, Gage AA, Klossner D, et al. Issues critical to the successful application of cryosurgical ablation of the prostate. Technol Cancer Res Treat 2007;6(2): 97–109.

71. Merkle EM, Nour SG, Lewin JS. MR imaging follow-up after percutaneous radiofrequency ablation of renal cell carcinoma: findings in 18 patients during first 6 months. Radiology 2005;235(3):1065–71.

72. Graham SJ, Stanisz GJ, Kecojevic A, et al. Analysis of changes in MR properties of tissues after heat treatment. Magn Reson Med 1999;42(6): 1061–71.

73. Barret E, Ahallal Y, Sanchez-Salas R, et al. Morbidity of focal therapy in the treatment of localized prostate cancer. Eur Urol 2013;63(4):618–22.

74. Lewin JS, Nour SG, Connell CF, et al. Phase II clinical trial of interactive MR imaging-guided interstitial radiofrequency thermal ablation of primary kidney tumors: initial experience. Radiology 2004;232(3): 835–45.

75. Porter CA 4th, Woodrum DA, Callstrom MR, et al. MRI after technically successful renal cryoablation: early contrast enhancement as a common finding. AJR Am J Roentgenol 2010;194(3):790–3.

76. Mir MC, Li J, Klink JC, et al. Optimal definition of biochemical recurrence after radical prostatectomy depends on pathologic risk factors: identifying candidates for early salvage therapy. Eur Urol 2014; 66(2):204–10.

77. Roach M 3rd, Hanks G, Thames H Jr, et al. Defining biochemical failure following radiotherapy with or without hormonal therapy in men with clinically localized prostate cancer: recommendations of the RTOG-ASTRO Phoenix Consensus Conference. Int J Radiat Oncol Biol Phys 2006;65(4):965–74.

78. Onik G. The male lumpectomy: rationale for a cancer targeted approach for prostate cryoablation. A review. Technol Cancer Res Treat 2004;3(4):365–70.

79. Siegel RL, Miller KD, Jemal A. Cancer statistics, 2016. CA Cancer J Clin 2016;66(1):7–30.

80. D'Amico AV, Whittington R, Malkowicz SB, et al. Biochemical outcome after radical prostatectomy, external beam radiation therapy, or interstitial radiation therapy for clinically localized prostate cancer. JAMA 1998;280(11):969–74.

81. Thompson I, Thrasher JB, Aus G, et al. Guideline for the management of clinically localized prostate cancer: 2007 update. J Urol 2007;177(6):2106–31.

82. Heidenreich A, Aus G, Bolla M, et al. EAU guidelines on prostate cancer. Eur Urol 2008;53(1):68–80.

Role of Prostate MR Imaging in Radiation Oncology

Cynthia Ménard, MD[a,b,*], Eric Paulson, PhD[c,d,e],
Tufve Nyholm, PhD[f], Patrick McLaughlin, MD[g],
Gary Liney, PhD[h], Piet Dirix, MD[i,j],
Uulke A. van der Heide, PhD[k]

KEYWORDS

- Radiotherapy • Brachytherapy • Image-guidance • Prostate cancer • MR imaging

KEY POINTS

- Diagnostic MR imaging can lead to more accurate risk-grouping and appropriate selection of radiotherapeutic approach.
- MR imaging can be directly integrated in the treatment-planning process to design a patient-specific dose plan.
- Key quality indicators (QIs) for the practice of MR imaging simulation in prostate cancer have been derived by expert consensus.
- MR imaging shows promise as a potential surrogate biomarker of response to radiotherapy.
- The central role of MR imaging on radiotherapy workflow will increase as MR–guided radiation delivery systems are implemented.

INTRODUCTION

The role of prostate MR imaging in radiotherapy has long been the subject of interest in the context of the continued evolution of higher-precision radiation delivery techniques. Although uncertainties at the millimeter scale are increasingly scrutinized in high-dose planning for localized prostate cancer, concerns regarding the poor performance of standard planning computed tomography (CT) in guiding an accurate manual segmentation of the prostate boundary have been raised for two decades.[1]

Studies generally demonstrate that prostate volumes segmented on MR imaging are 10% smaller than those segmented on CT,[2–6] with improved performance at the apex and base of the prostate gland.[1,6–10] MR imaging–based segmentations generally lead to reduced dose exposures to adjacent organs at risk,[11–14] but the clinical impact of such dosimetric advantages

Disclosures: No conflicts to disclose.
[a] Centre Hospitalier de l'Université de Montréal (CRCHUM), 900 St-Denis, Room 11.442, Montréal, QC H2X 0A9, Canada; [b] TECHNA Institute, University of Toronto, 124-100 College Street, Toronto, ON M5G 1L5, Canada; [c] Radiation Oncology, Medical College of Wisconsin, 9200 Wisconsin Avenue, Milwaukee, WI 53226, USA; [d] Radiology, Medical College of Wisconsin, 9200 Wisconsin Avenue, Milwaukee, WI 53226, USA; [e] Biophysics, Medical College of Wisconsin, 9200 Wisconsin Avenue, Milwaukee, WI 53226, USA; [f] Department of Radiation Sciences, Umeå University, Umeå SE-90187, Sweden; [g] Department of Radiation Oncology, University of Michigan, 1500 East Medical Center Drive, Ann Arbor, MI 48109, USA; [h] Medical Physics, Ingham Institute for Applied Medical Research and Liverpool Cancer Therapy Centre, 1, Campbell Street, Liverpool NSW 2170, Australia; [i] Department of Radiation Oncology, Iridium Cancer Network, Oosterveldlaan 24, 2610 Wilrijk (Antwerp), Belgium; [j] Department of Molecular Imaging, Pathology, Radiotherapy and Oncology (MIPRO), University of Antwerp, Prinsstraat 13, 2000 Antwerp, Belgium; [k] Department of Radiation Oncology, The Netherlands Cancer Institute, Plesmanlaan 121, 1066 CX Amsterdam, The Netherlands
* Corresponding author. 900 St-Denis, Room 11.442, Montréal H2X 0A9, Canada.
E-mail address: Cynthia.Menard@UMontreal.ca

Radiol Clin N Am 56 (2018) 319–325
https://doi.org/10.1016/j.rcl.2017.10.012

has not been convincing in standard dose fractionation regimens, where reductions in toxicity have been marginal at best.[15,16]

In contrast, the impact of prostate MR imaging in radiotherapy is likely to hinge on its depiction and characterization of cancer burden within the prostate gland. This begins at diagnosis, where the emergence of a tumor-targeted and more representative biopsy sampling will undoubtedly lead to a migration of risk-grouping and subsequent treatments.[17] In addition, evidence now supports the premise that local recurrences after radiotherapy correspond to sites of disease burden at diagnosis, lending credence to a more personalized dose-painted approach to radiation delivery.[18–21]

This review addresses three distinct roles of prostate MR imaging in radiation oncology. First, as a diagnostic tool for more accurate characterization of disease and risk grouping to select the most appropriate therapy. Second, as images directly integrated in the dose-planning process, enabling improved depiction of treatment targets and organs-at-risk. In this context, quality indicators (QIs) for MR simulation (MR-Sim) procedures were derived by expert consensus from the annual MR in RT symposium and are presented here. Finally, the potential role of MR imaging as a better-performing early surrogate biomarker of response to radiotherapy is discussed.

DIAGNOSTIC MR IMAGING FOR RISK GROUPING AND TREATMENT SELECTION

Diagnostic prostate MR imaging examinations have matured and gained widespread acceptance in urologic oncology. The recently updated Prostate Imaging Reporting and Data System version 2 (PIRADSv2) has promoted global standardization and diminished variation in the acquisition, interpretation, and reporting of prostate MR imaging examinations.[22] Since its recent release, publications have confirmed its high diagnostic performance against prostatectomy specimens, and superior performance to PIRADSv1.[23] The value of PIRADSv2 scoring in predicting outcomes has yet to be reported in patients receiving radiotherapy or brachytherapy, and is the subject of ongoing work.

It is known that MR imaging findings, more specifically the amount of extracapsular extension, the presence of seminal vesicle invasion, and the volume of disease, are strong independent predictors of treatment failure after radiotherapy and brachytherapy.[19,21,24,25] Its predictive utility routinely outperforms more conventional predictive factors, such as prostate-specific antigen (PSA) and Gleason grade. Poor outcomes with advanced disease on MR imaging are most likely attributable

to a more aggressive underlying biology, but the contribution of marginal geographic miss during delivery of precision radiotherapy may also contribute.

MR imaging therefore invariably results in migration of stage, and consequently migration of risk-grouping. This is most evident in patients with seemingly intermediate-risk disease, regrouped high-risk because of seminal vesicle invasion (17%) or extracapsular invasion (5%) identified on MR imaging.[26] Targeted biopsies are also increasingly performed, and are associated with an increase in Gleason grade, also resulting in risk-group migration (Fig. 1).

It is important to emphasize the central importance of risk-grouping for the selection of a radiotherapeutic approach. The National Comprehensive Cancer Network identifies high-risk patients as T3a or any Gleason score 8 to 10 or PSA greater than 20, and very-high-risk patients as T3b-4 or primary Gleason pattern 5 or greater than four cores with Gleason 8 to 10. Such patients should be offered hormonal therapy as an adjunct to radiotherapy, and/or a brachytherapy boost to external beam radiotherapy. Very-high-risk patients may also be offered adjuvant docetaxel chemotherapy. For patients whose risk-grouping

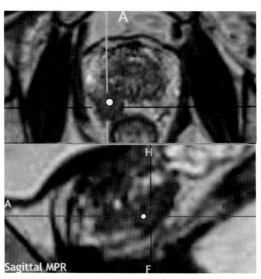

Fig. 1. Patient with intermediate-risk prostate cancer (Gleason 4 + 3 in 3 of 12 samples, PSA 7, T1c) planned for HDR brachytherapy boost to external beam radiotherapy. Planning MR imaging identified a PIRADSv2 = 5 tumor at the right base stage T3a. Targeted biopsy at the time of brachytherapy revealed Gleason 4 + 5 disease. Hormonal therapy was therefore initiated before external beam radiotherapy. A, anterior; F, foot; H, head; lines, planed of MPR reconstruction on three-dimensional axial T2-weighted SPACE image with isotropic 1-mm voxels acquired at 1.5 T. HDR, high-dose-rate; MPR, multi-planar reconstruction; SPACE, sampling perfection with application optimized contrasts using different flip angle evolution.

migrates from low-risk to intermediate-risk, the addition of external beam radiotherapy to brachytherapy should be considered.

DEDICATED MR IMAGING FOR SIMULATION AND TREATMENT PLANNING

MR imaging can be directly integrated in the treatment-planning process to design a patient-specific dose plan. As a first step, images are acquired to create a patient model that is representative of treatment conditions (pelvic position and states of bladder/bowel filling). Targets and organs at risk are segmented, dose-objectives are prescribed, and a plan is then generated and approved.

Conventional dose-planning is performed on CT, on which complementary images (eg, MR imaging) are registered to guide segmentation (**Figs. 2** and **3**). More recently, MR imaging–only planning is gaining acceptance through techniques that model electron density from MR imaging data, enabling dose calculation (**Fig. 4**).[27] When devising an MR imaging acquisition protocol dedicated to treatment planning, it is important to explicitly state imaging goals, because they are often distinct from diagnostics. Goals typically include a clear definition of the prostate gland boundary, depiction of implanted fiducial markers to assist in image-registration (**Fig. 5**) and/or online guidance, and mapping of disease. Multiple sequences may be required to meet all three goals.

As a general principle, acquisition for treatment planning should be performed in a manner that balances reproducing treatment conditions (bowel preparation, bladder preparation, ± immobilization devices), without compromising signal to noise ratio (SNR) (ie, surface coils should be applied as close as possible to the patient surface). A prostate-to-prostate local registration is recommended, because registration of the pelvis is insufficient due to variation in bladder and bowel filling states that are difficult to control and reproduce.

Reproducing exact pelvic position is therefore not required, but should be approximated.

Endorectal coil acquisitions are not recommended, unless a robust deformable registration solution is available or a similar intrarectal immobilization device is applied at the time of treatment delivery. Acquisition time should be optimized to reduce the risk of motion blurring (ideally each acquisition <5 minutes). Bladder filling state should also be comfortable to reduce motion. A rectal enema before imaging can be considered, and buscopan or glucagon to limit peristalsis unless contraindicated. If images show motion artifacts, they should be repeated. Finally, activation of vendor-provided gradient distortion correction and optimization of bandwidth essential to ensure geometrically fidelity.

Diffusion-weighted imaging (DWI) is particularly susceptible to geometric distortions, especially if acquired using a conventional, single-shot spin-echo echo-planar imaging (EPI) sequence. These distortions risk propagation of errors in targeting of tumor subvolumes within the prostate gland. In general, it is recommended that the QIBA profile (qibawiki.rsna.org) be followed. Additional steps specific to prostate imaging can also reduce such distortions in DWI, including (1) left-right phase-encode prescription (in this way, susceptibility effects introduced by rectal air immediately posterior the prostate are not propagated into the prostate gland), (2) careful volume shimming over the gland, and (3) minimization of echo-train length (including use of parallel imaging, partial Fourier, and optimized receiver bandwidths set to minimize effective echo-spacing). Finally, recently introduced segmented EPI[28] methods (or other non-EPI-based techniques) should be strongly considered in the context of radiotherapy planning when available to further improve geometric integrity of DWI.

A more detailed list of QIs for MR imaging simulation was derived by expert consensus using a modified Delphi method and is provided in **Table 1**. An initial list of QIs was drafted and

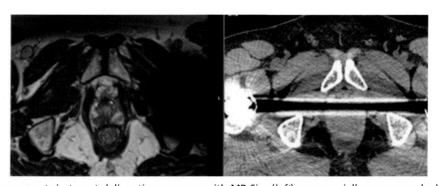

Fig. 2. Improvements in target delineation accuracy with MR-Sim (*left*) are especially pronounced when CT images are degraded by artifacts from metal hip implants (*right*).

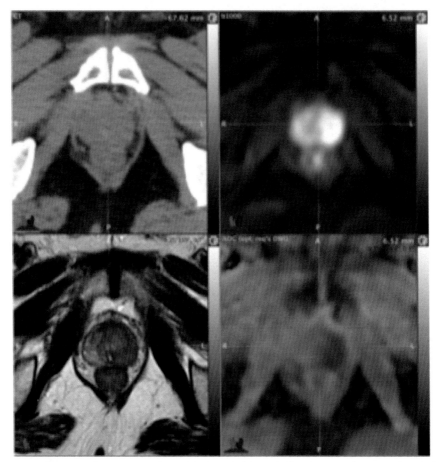

Fig. 3. Improved soft tissue contrast with T2-weighted TSE (*bottom left*) compared with planning CT (*top left*) for target boundary definition. Functional/physiologic information (high b-value DWI *top right*; ADC map *bottom right*) assists in defining disease. A GTV is evident in the left lobe of the prostate gland. Images acquired at 3 T. GTV, gross target volume; TSE, turbo spin echo.

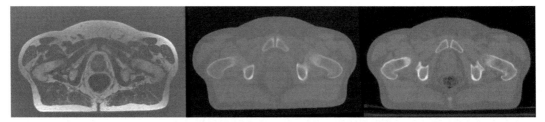

Fig. 4. T2-weighted MR imaging (*left*), synthetic CT (*middle*) generated using MR imaging-Planner (Spectronics Medical, Helsingborg, Sweden), and CT (*right*). (*From* Siversson C, Nordström F, Nilsson T, et al. Technical note: MRI only prostate radiotherapy planning using the statistical decomposition algorithm. Med Phys 2015;42(10):6090–7; with permission.)

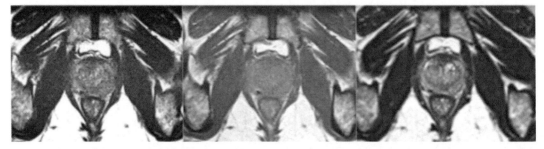

Fig. 5. Implanted fiducial marker clearly depicted as an area of signal void in the right peripheral zone of the prostate gland on a proton-density image acquired using a dual-echo TSE technique (*center*). The corresponding two-dimensional T2-weighted TSE image (*left*), and three-dimensional axial T2-weighted volumetric acquisition using isotropic voxels (1 mm, *right*). Images acquired at 1.5 T for radiotherapy planning. TSE, turbo spin echo.

Table 1
Key quality indicators for MR imaging simulation of prostate cancer

	Quality Indicator	Importance Rating (0–9) 9 = Essential
Indications	When CT image quality is compromised (eg, prosthetic hip implants) or absent from the treatment planning workflow.	7.8
	When PTV margins are small (<5 mm).	7
	In post-planning of LDR prostate brachytherapy to improve dosimetric accuracy.	7.3
	When delineating distinct gross MR imaging–visible tumor volume and clinical target volume targets.	9
Preparation and set-up	Endorectal coil acquisitions should be avoided in the absence of robust deformable image registration tools.	8
	Administration of antiperistaltic agents should be strongly considered to improve image quality, unless contraindicated.	7.3
	Bladder-filling state must be comfortable to reduce motion-related artifacts.	7.1
	Patient set-up should approximate treatment conditions (bowel preparation, bladder preparation, ± immobilization devices), while *maximizing SNR* (ie, surface coils should be applied as close as possible to the patient surface).	8
Acquisition	MR imaging acquisition protocols should generally follow PIRADSv2 guidelines (acr.org) to facilitate diagnostic reporting.	7.7
	Replacing coronal and sagittal T2-weighted images with an isotropic T2-weighted three-dimensional axial acquisition is justified in radiotherapy planning, especially at 1.5 T.	6
	When implanted FMs or brachytherapy seeds must be resolved, strategies to augment the FM signature on above images may suffice (eg, increase voxel resolution, PD via dual-echo acquisition, intermediate TE).	7
	A separate image may be acquired to more clearly highlight FMs (eg, GRE, PD, SSFP, UTE).	7
	DWI is recommended to assist in depiction of tumors if needed.	9
	DCE is considered optional except for salvage of recurrence.	7
	Activation of vendor-provided gradient distortion correction and optimization of bandwidth (fat/water pixel shift <1 mm) is recommended to maintain geometric fidelity.	8
	DWI should follow the QIBA profile (qibawiki.rsna.org). Distortion is minimized using (1) R-L phase-encode direction, (2) volume shimming over the gland, (3) minimizing effective echo-spacing, and (4) considering segmented or other non-EPI techniques.	8.5
	Motion-related artifacts should be mitigated by limiting acquisition time to <5 min when possible. Sequences should be repeated if motion-related artifacts.	7.8
Registration	MR imaging registration to CT consists of a prostate-to-prostate local registration. Bone-to-bone registration of the pelvis is discouraged.	8.7
	The quality of image registration must be evaluated by a physicist and/or physician before treatment planning. Rotations should be carefully scrutinized. Errors in registration translate to systematic errors that propagate through the treatment course, and must be minimized.	7.8
	Intersequence motion of the prostate gland during an MR imaging examination may occur. Such displacements must be evaluated and corrected if present. DWI may require registration to T2-weighted when distortions are observed.	7.2
	In salvage after prostatectomy, users should use great care to consider and mitigate variation in bladder and bowel filling between CT and MR imaging, and to reproduce treatment conditions. The potential for registration error is considered large in this setting. Accurate registration at the level of the external urethral sphincter and gross recurrent tumor (if present) is prioritized.	7.7

Abbreviations: DCE, dynamic contrast enhanced; FM, fiducial markers; GRE, gradient echo; LDR, low dose rate; PD, proton density; PTV, planning target volume; SNR, signal to noise ratio; SSFP, steady state free precession; UTE, ultra-short echo time.

circulated to a panel of experts ahead of the annual MR in RT meeting. Coauthors provided feedback by email, and QIs were discussed and refined for clarity and completeness during a face-to-face meeting. A revised list of QIs was again circulated ahead of the second meeting, where experts scored each QI for importance from 0 to 9 (9 = essential) on a Likert scale, with an opportunity to further refine the language. A third revision of the QIs occurred at the second face-to-face meeting, and assigned a final score of importance.

It is important to recognize that standardization of tumor-target delineation (eg, PIRADS-RT) and optimal dose-painting objectives are the subject of ongoing work. Robust computational tools that map dose requirements, in lieu of poorly reproducible manual tumor segmentations, will undoubtedly become essential. A consensus in this regard is considered premature, and constitutes an urgent unmet need in the field.

MR IMAGING AS A BIOMARKER OF RESPONSE

The gold standard end point for the ultimate measure of success of radiotherapy is failure-free survival. Unfortunately given the long natural history and evolution of disease, this end point lags the cadence of technological advancements in radiotherapy. For this reason, much effort has been invested in validating earlier surrogate end points that are predictive of prostate cancer–specific survival. Prostate biopsy at 2 to 3 years, although informative, is hindered by its invasiveness, risk, and associated sampling error. Biochemical response (and failure) is an imperfect surrogate to measure improvements in local therapy, because a rise in PSA is frequently unrelated to local cancer control.

Prostate MR imaging as an early surrogate measure of success (or failure) in the years ensuing radiotherapy may therefore have a role. The high diagnostic performance of MR imaging in identifying local recurrence has already been demonstrated in patients with biochemical failure.[29–33] It remains to be evaluated in patients without rise in PSA, and compared with prostate cancer–specific survival in large series.

FUTURE DIRECTIONS

The potential impact of MR imaging on radiotherapy workflow and prostate cancer outcomes is important. However, future applications hinge on continued improvements in image quality. Only then can advanced workflows that integrate auto segmentation, quantitative cancer probability mapping, and adaptive dose-painting within a deep-learning engine be realized. This is especially relevant with the emergence of MR imaging–guided radiotherapy systems,[34] where daily MR images have the potential to inform on response and guide adaptation of treatment during a course of radiation delivery.

REFERENCES

1. Milosevic M, Voruganti S, Blend R, et al. Magnetic resonance imaging (MRI) for localization of the prostatic apex: comparison to computed tomography (CT) and urethrography. Radiother Oncol 1998; 47(3):277–84.
2. Roach M 3rd, Faillace-Akazawa P, Malfatti C, et al. Prostate volumes defined by magnetic resonance imaging and computerized tomographic scans for three-dimensional conformal radiotherapy. Int J Radiat Oncol Biol Phys 1996;35(5):1011–8.
3. Kagawa K, Lee WR, Schultheiss TE, et al. Initial clinical assessment of CT-MRI image fusion software in localization of the prostate for 3D conformal radiation therapy. Int J Radiat Oncol Biol Phys 1997;38(2):319–25.
4. Debois M, Oyen R, Maes F, et al. The contribution of magnetic resonance imaging to the three-dimensional treatment planning of localized prostate cancer. Int J Radiat Oncol Biol Phys 1999; 45(4):857–65.
5. Rasch C, Barillot I, Remeijer P, et al. Definition of the prostate in CT and MRI: a multi-observer study. Int J Radiat Oncol Biol Phys 1999;43(1):57–66.
6. Smith WL, Lewis C, Bauman G, et al. Prostate volume contouring: a 3D analysis of segmentation using 3DTRUS, CT, and MR. Int J Radiat Oncol Biol Phys 2007;67(4):1238–47.
7. Wachter S, Wachter-Gerstner N, Bock T, et al. Interobserver comparison of CT and MRI-based prostate apex definition. Clinical relevance for conformal radiotherapy treatment planning. Strahlenther Onkol 2002;178(5):263–8.
8. Parker CC, Damyanovich A, Haycocks T, et al. Magnetic resonance imaging in the radiation treatment planning of localized prostate cancer using intraprostatic fiducial markers for computed tomography co-registration. Radiother Oncol 2003;66(2):217–24.
9. Villeirs GM, De Meerleer GO, Verstraete KL, et al. Magnetic resonance assessment of prostate localization variability in intensity-modulated radiotherapy for prostate cancer. Int J Radiat Oncol Biol Phys 2004;60(5):1611–21.
10. Nyholm T, Jonsson J, Söderström K, et al. Variability in prostate and seminal vesicle delineations defined on magnetic resonance images, a multi-observer, -center and -sequence study. Radiat Oncol 2013;8:126.
11. Sannazzari GL, Ragona R, Ruo Redda MG, et al. CT-MRI image fusion for delineation of volumes in

three-dimensional conformal radiation therapy in the treatment of localized prostate cancer. Br J Radiol 2002;75(895):603–7.

12. Chen L, Price RA Jr, Nguyen TB, et al. Dosimetric evaluation of MRI-based treatment planning for prostate cancer. Phys Med Biol 2004;49(22):5157–70.

13. Buyyounouski MK, Horwitz EM, Price RA, et al. Intensity-modulated radiotherapy with MRI simulation to reduce doses received by erectile tissue during prostate cancer treatment. Int J Radiat Oncol Biol Phys 2004;58(3):743–9.

14. McLaughlin PW, Narayana V, Meirovitz A, et al. Vessel-sparing prostate radiotherapy: dose limitation to critical erectile vascular structures (internal pudendal artery and corpus cavernosum) defined by MRI. Int J Radiat Oncol Biol Phys 2005;61(1):20–31.

15. Ali AN, Rossi PJ, Godette KD, et al. Impact of magnetic resonance imaging on computed tomography-based treatment planning and acute toxicity for prostate cancer patients treated with intensity modulated radiation therapy. Pract Radiat Oncol 2013;3(1):e1–9.

16. Sander L, Langkilde NC, Holmberg M, et al. MRI target delineation may reduce long-term toxicity after prostate radiotherapy. Acta Oncol 2014;53(6):809–14.

17. Ahmed HU, El-Shater Bosaily A, Brown LC, et al. Diagnostic accuracy of multi-parametric MRI and TRUS biopsy in prostate cancer (PROMIS): a paired validating confirmatory study. Lancet 2017;389(10071):815–22.

18. Chopra S, Toi A, Taback N, et al. Pathological predictors for site of local recurrence after radiotherapy for prostate cancer. Int J Radiat Oncol Biol Phys 2012;82(3):e441–8.

19. Fuchsjager MH, Pucar D, Zelefsky MJ, et al. Predicting post-external beam radiation therapy PSA relapse of prostate cancer using pretreatment MRI. Int J Radiat Oncol Biol Phys 2010;78(3):743–50.

20. Arrayeh E, Westphalen AC, Kurhanewicz J, et al. Does local recurrence of prostate cancer after radiation therapy occur at the site of primary tumor? Results of a longitudinal MRI and MRSI study. Int J Radiat Oncol Biol Phys 2012;82(5):e787–93.

21. Joseph T, McKenna DA, Westphalen AC, et al. Pretreatment endorectal magnetic resonance imaging and magnetic resonance spectroscopic imaging features of prostate cancer as predictors of response to external beam radiotherapy. Int J Radiat Oncol Biol Phys 2009;73(3):665–71.

22. Weinreb JC, Barentsz JO, Choyke PL, et al. PI-RADS prostate imaging - reporting and data system: 2015, Version 2. Eur Urol 2016;69(1):16–40.

23. Vargas HA, Hötker AM, Goldman DA, et al. Updated prostate imaging reporting and data system (PIRADS v2) recommendations for the detection of clinically significant prostate cancer using multiparametric MRI: critical evaluation using whole-mount pathology as standard of reference. Eur Radiol 2016;26(6):1606–12.

24. Westphalen AC, Koff WJ, Coakley FV, et al. Prostate cancer: prediction of biochemical failure after external-beam radiation therapy–Kattan nomogram and endorectal MR imaging estimation of tumor volume. Radiology 2011;261(2):477–86.

25. Riaz N, Afaq A, Akin O, et al. Pretreatment endorectal coil magnetic resonance imaging findings predict biochemical tumor control in prostate cancer patients treated with combination brachytherapy and external-beam radiotherapy. Int J Radiat Oncol Biol Phys 2012;84(3):707–11.

26. Chang JH, Lim Joon D, Nguyen BT, et al. MRI scans significantly change target coverage decisions in radical radiotherapy for prostate cancer. J Med Imaging Radiat Oncol 2014;58(2):237–43.

27. Gustafsson C, Nordström F, Persson E, et al. Assessment of dosimetric impact of system specific geometric distortion in an MRI only based radiotherapy workflow for prostate. Phys Med Biol 2017;62(8):2976–89.

28. Foltz WD, Porter DA, Simeonov A, et al. Readout-segmented echo-planar diffusion-weighted imaging improves geometric performance for image-guided radiation therapy of pelvic tumors. Radiother Oncol 2015;117(3):525–31.

29. Zattoni F, Kawashima A, Morlacco A, et al. Detection of recurrent prostate cancer after primary radiation therapy: an evaluation of the role of multiparametric 3T magnetic resonance imaging with endorectal coil. Pract Radiat Oncol 2017;7(1):42–9.

30. Alonzo F, Melodelima C, Bratan F, et al. Detection of locally radio-recurrent prostate cancer at multiparametric MRI: can dynamic contrast-enhanced imaging be omitted? Diagn Interv Imaging 2016;97(4):433–41.

31. Abd-Alazeez M, Ramachandran N, Dikaios N, et al. Multiparametric MRI for detection of radiorecurrent prostate cancer: added value of apparent diffusion coefficient maps and dynamic contrast-enhanced images. Prostate Cancer Prostatic Dis 2015;18(2):128–36.

32. Menard C, Iupati D, Publicover J, et al. MR-guided prostate biopsy for planning of focal salvage after radiation therapy. Radiology 2015;274(1):181–91.

33. Haider MA, Chung P, Sweet J, et al. Dynamic contrast-enhanced magnetic resonance imaging for localization of recurrent prostate cancer after external beam radiotherapy. Int J Radiat Oncol Biol Phys 2008;70(2):425–30.

34. Menard C, van der Heide U. Introduction: systems for magnetic resonance image guided radiation therapy. Semin Radiat Oncol 2014;24(3):192.

Future Perspectives and Challenges of Prostate MR Imaging

Baris Turkbey, MD, Peter L. Choyke, MD*

KEYWORDS

• Prostate • MR imaging • Prostate cancer • Clinically significant cancer • Imaging modalities

KEY POINTS

- MR imaging has become an important part of prostate cancer diagnosis.
- As with any new modality that combines unassailable logic with reasonably good data, it has been rapidly adopted.
- With such rapid growth there are also problems.
- Beyond the carefully controlled environments of academic centers, variations in quality and skill become evident and results in general practice are usually not as impressive.
- However, this very observation provides an impetus to improve the method and make it "bullet proof" and, thus, more widely available and more broadly robust.

INTRODUCTION

Prostate cancer is a major cause of morbidity and mortality worldwide.[1] However, unlike other more aggressive cancers, such as lung and pancreatic cancers, which are almost always aggressive, prostate cancers exhibit a broad range of biology ranging from indolent to highly aggressive. The term "clinically significant" prostate cancer has recently been introduced to distinguish those tumors likely to lead to death from those likely to be indolent and have no impact on survival.[2,3] However, the line of demarcation between these 2 categories of prostate cancer remains unclear and in any given patient can vary.

As a result of this categorization of prostate cancer, management can range from active surveillance to aggressive multimodal radical surgical and radiation therapies. The essential challenge for men diagnosed with prostate cancer is to accurately establish where in this broad spectrum of disease their tumor lies and what its likely trajectory is. This trajectory, which often spans 10 to 20 years, may well overlap and be superseded by the trajectories of other health conditions the patient may have.[4] For instance, in a 75-year-old man with severe cardiovascular disease and hypertension in whom a new intermediate risk prostate cancer is discovered, the former disease is more likely to be a cause of death than the latter; therefore, treatment of the prostate cancer might not be warranted.

It would be comforting if we could foresee exactly what would happen to a patient in the future were their prostate lesions to go undetected or, if detected, untreated. That problem will remain a future challenge for the diagnosis of prostate cancer. However, there is inherent uncertainty over the true aggressiveness of all cancers and new technologies are needed to address this problem. Part of the uncertainty arises simply from sampling issues. For instance, a biopsy may miss a lesion or undersample a lesion.[5] Therefore, more accurate biopsies will ameliorate part of the problem. But the problems go well beyond that. The lesion itself can be interpreted differently

Molecular Imaging Program, National Cancer Institute, National Institutes of Health, 10 Center Drive, Room B3B69, Bethesda, MD 20892, USA
* Corresponding author.
E-mail address: pchoyke@mail.nih.gov

Radiol Clin N Am 56 (2018) 327–337
https://doi.org/10.1016/j.rcl.2017.10.013
0033-8389/18/Published by Elsevier Inc.

by different pathologists using standard Gleason scoring.[6–8] Even establishing the correct interpretation, the prediction of patient outcome is not yet satisfactory. Thus, although the concept of tumor aggressiveness is conceptually clear, the reality of establishing it is more difficult. Nonetheless, given the multifocality of prostate cancer and the heterogeneity of tumor type within any given tumor, accurate tissue sampling is a fundamental limitation in establishing the aggressiveness of a cancer.[9]

Over the past 50 years, there have been several major developments in the assessment of prostate cancer. The most important was the development of the Gleason scoring system by Dr Donald Gleason in the 1960s. Dr Gleason established 5 patterns of prostate cancer. He suggested that prostate cancers be scored by adding the 2 major histologic patterns together. Gradually, Gleason patterns 1 and 2 were recognized as benign features with no clinical impact and, therefore, are almost never used in Gleason scoring today. Thus, the original Gleason scoring scale, which encompassed scores between 2 and 10, has been reduced to a scale of 6 to 10 in current usage. A Gleason score of 6 represents pattern 3 + 3, whereas a Gleason score of 7 can represent either a 3 + 4 or a 4 + 3 tumor.[10] The amount of pattern 4 in a specimen is associated with likelihood of recurrence after treatment, which serves as an imperfect surrogate of aggressiveness. The vast majority of Gleason 6 and some Gleason 3 + 4 tumors are low grade and are rarely associated with disease-specific mortality. Thus, except for large-volume, low-grade prostate cancers, most patients with Gleason 6 tumors are recommended to follow active surveillance.[11–13] Intermediate risk cancers are those containing some degree of Gleason pattern 4, and the higher the 4 component, generally the worse the outcome. This is a large group of patients and encompasses the full range of biologic aggressiveness. Many men with these Gleason 7 disease (3 + 4, 4 + 3) are probably overtreated. However, aside from Gleason scoring there is no generally accepted good prognostic biomarker for these cancers. Multiple revisions of the Gleason scoring system have tended to increase the Gleason 3 + 4 category at the expense of Gleason 6 tumors. However, this has the undesirable effect of causing more cancers to be treated because of the increased risk associated with pattern 4. Cancers with higher Gleason scores (Gleason score of $\geq$8) are considered high risk and have a reasonable expectation of aggressiveness and mortality if untreated. The most recent innovation in pathologic assessment involving the Gleason scoring system is the International Society of Urogenital Pathology's (ISUP) system, which is a 1 to 5 score (whereby Gleason 3 + 3 is the equivalent of a ISUP 1, Gleason 3 + 4 equivalent of ISUP2, and so forth) that has largely been a rebranding of the existing system.[2,14] Thus, Gleason or its equivalent ISUP score, despite multiple limitations, remains the preeminent method of assessing the aggressiveness of prostate cancer. Numerous methods of assessing genomics of tumors ranging from whole genome sequencing to select subsets of genes have been introduced to help characterize the aggressiveness of prostate cancers. However, none of these has proven superior to the others and only a minority of patients undergo this test. Moreover, the interpretation of the scores of these gene tests is entirely subjective. Thus, better methods of characterizing prostate cancer aggressiveness are needed.

The second big innovation in prostate cancer management was the introduction of the prostate-specific antigen (PSA) serum test, which was introduced in the late 1980s.[15,16] The introduction of PSA as a serum test led to an explosion of diagnoses of prostate cancer. Initially, PSA testing was very popular and led to popular screening campaigns. Unfortunately, because PSA is secreted by normal hyperplastic and malignant tissue, it tends to have many false-positive results, especially in men with benign prostatic hyperplasia or inflammation. When a patient has an elevated PSA level they are commonly recommended to have a random biopsy (also known as the systematic biopsy or a 12-core biopsy). The combination of PSA and random biopsy led to a rapid increase in the diagnosis of prostate cancer, but mostly low-risk, indolent cancers. Because Gleason 6 disease was not understood to be as indolent in the 1990s as it is understood today, these patients were often treated with radical surgery or radiation with resultant loss in quality-of-life indices. A series of trials from the United States and Europe in the 2000s explored the value of PSA. They generally showed a mild decrease in mortality in subjects undergoing PSA screening, but this was only achieved at the cost of significant decreases in quality of life. Cumulatively, these studies seemed to indicate that the minimal mortality benefit was canceled out by the decline in quality of life.[17,18] Even before the decision of the US Preventive Services Task Force (USPSTF) in 2012 to recommend against screening with PSA, there was a growing disenchantment with PSA screening. In 2012, when the USPSTF discouraged the use of PSA by assigning a letter grade of "D," there was a further decrease in screening.[19] However, reports began emerging after the USPSTF decision against PSA screening regarding an increase in the rate of metastatic disease at the time of presentation, suggesting that decreases in PSA screening are leading to more advanced disease at presentation.[20–25] Further criticism of the USPSTF decision included the fact that the PLCO (Prostate Lung Colon Ovary) study, the largest study of PSA screening in the United States, and one that weighed heavily in the decision to recommend against PSA screening, was flawed because the majority of those in the control arm (no PSA screening) had actually had PSA testing during the study, even though they were reportedly unscreened.[26] This factor serves to invalidate the results of the PLCO trial for prostate screening. In the spring of 2017, the USPSTF upgraded PSA testing to a grade of "C," meaning that it should be offered for selected patients depending on individual circumstances and after discussion with the physician.[27] However, the use of PSA screening remains controversial with the majority of urologists considering it worthwhile and the majority of primary care physicians remain dubious of its benefits. There is a major need for a serum or urine test that more accurately identifies patients harboring clinically significant prostate cancers.

Another major development in prostate cancer diagnosis was the introduction of MR imaging for diagnosis. Throughout the 1990s, MR imaging was principally recommended for staging of prostate cancer, a task for which it proved not particularly well-suited. Specifically, the ability to detect extraprostatic extension and local nodal disease are limited with MR imaging. It was only when MR imaging began to be used to localize prostate cancer for the purposes of diagnosis that its popularity increased.[28,29] There was a gradual recognition that MR imaging was capable of detecting lesions that random needle biopsies were missing. This finding made sense; random biopsies tend to sample mainly the posterior part of the prostate gland, and many of the MR imaging-positive lesions were located anteriorly. At first T2-weighted imaging and dynamic contrast-enhanced MR imaging were the sequences used to diagnose prostate cancers. Eventually, by the mid 2000s, it became clear that diffusion-weighted MR imaging was the most sensitive pulse sequence for detecting prostate cancer. In the late 2000s, the value of high b value MR imaging was shown (**Fig. 1**). Thus arose the multiparametric MR imaging or mpMRI that is in wide use today.[30]

Of course, it was clear that simply diagnosing a cancer on MR imaging was not enough; the lesion still had to be biopsied. Because the lesion was discovered on MR imaging, it was logical that the lesion be biopsied under MR imaging. A variety of devices were developed to direct needle biopsies in-gantry using MR imaging guidance. The patient had to lie prone and the procedure was inherently time consuming, because it is difficult to manipulate the needle while the patient is in the center of the magnet. Thus, a series of steps were required, whereby the patient had to be moved in and out of the gantry multiple times while the needle was properly positioned and imaged. This was time consuming for both the radiologist and the scanner, both of which added cost. Nonmagnetic needles and other MR imaging–compatible equipment were needed to safely perform in-gantry biopsies.[31,32] Importantly, urologists, who were referring patients to radiology practices for such MR imaging–guided biopsies, were not eager to give up the prostate biopsy, which was a key element of their practice. Thus, alternatives were sought.

The first alternative was to perform what came to be known at "cognitive fusion" whereby the location of the lesion on MR imaging was estimated on the transrectal ultrasound (TRUS) image using spatial cues on the image. Because the plane of imaging of the MR imaging and TRUS are rarely aligned, this maneuver can be quite challenging and requires operators who are adept at estimating and triangulating locations on scans using internal fiducial markers, such as cysts or calcifications.[33,34] Naturally, there are some operators who are quite good at doing this, but the majority of users find it difficult. It is certainly difficult to teach. Thus, although cognitive fusion has its strong advocates and is very cost effective, it has given way to software- and hardware-driven solutions, namely the MR imaging-TRUS fusion biopsy.

The MR imaging-TRUS fusion biopsy was first described in 2007 by Xu and colleagues.[35] The basic concept was that biopsies could be performed under ultrasound while using MR imaging for guidance after registration and tracking. The first step was to segment the prostate on MR imaging. This was initially done manually, but is now done in a semiautomated manner on commercial software. When the patient arrives for the biopsy, having previously undergone an MR imaging study, a TRUS is performed in a 3-dimensional mode. The prostate is segmented on the ultrasound image and then it is superimposed on the segmented MR image.[36] This "fusion" was initially done using "rigid" registration, but eventually "elastic" registration was implemented, in which to the shapes of the prostate on MR imaging and TRUS examinations were warped to each other

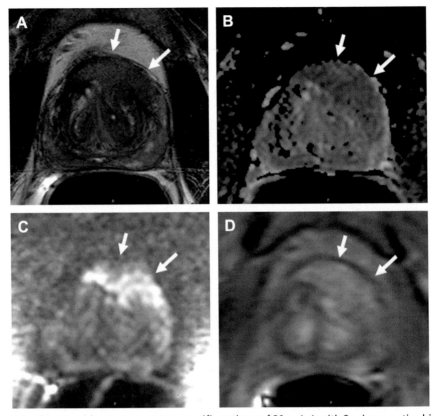

Fig. 1. A 55-year-old man with a serum prostate-specific antigen of 30 ng/mL with 2 prior negative biopsies. Axial T2-weighted MR imaging shows a lesion in the anterior transition zone (*arrows*) (*A*), which shows restricted diffusion on apparent diffusion coefficient mapping (*B*) and b2000 diffusion-weighted MR imaging (*C, arrows*) and early contrast enhancement on dynamic contrast-enhanced MR imaging (*D, arrows*). The lesion underwent transrectal ultrasound examination/MR imaging fusion-guided biopsy, which revealed Gleason 4 + 4 prostate adenocarcinoma.

so that there was good overlap. Once the MR imaging and the TRUS segmentations are fused, the TRUS probe must then be tracked so as to maintain the spatial integrity of the MR imaging superimposed on the ultrasound image, regardless of the position of the TRUS probe. As the TRUS probe is moved by the user, sensors on the probe or attached to the probe update the fusion image so that the operator constantly sees the updated MR imaging superimposed on the ultrasound image in the same plane. This can be accomplished in a number of ways: radiofrequency tagging of the probe, holding the probe using an articulated arm, or by image registration.[31] Regardless of how the TRUS probe is tracked, needles can then be introduced under real-time ultrasound imaging and samples can be obtained from the MR imaging-defined prostate lesions. This entire process adds 5 to 10 minutes to a routine TRUS biopsy and with experience can be done very quickly, and outside of the MR imaging suite.[31] The biopsy

is generally performed by urologists and as a result it has become widely accepted.

There have been a number of other developments in prostate cancer diagnosis that are too early in development to be considered paradigm shifting and, therefore, are not discussed in detail here. They are discussed in more detail in the final section regarding the future of prostate MR imaging. Briefly, they include serum or urine tests that help to define the risk that the patient harbors a clinically significant prostate cancer. These tests generally use some combination of kallikrein derivatives or specific RNA markers and are used to define which patient population with an increased PSA should undergo biopsy.[37] They are being introduced slowly into general practice. Another group of new tests are genomic tests of biopsy tissue. These tests purport to give an added indication of the aggressiveness of the cancer independent or in addition to that of the Gleason score.[38] The full impact of these tests remains unclear because they can add considerable cost to the workup for prostate cancer and it is unclear how the data they produce should be used. For this reason, they are not yet playing a major role in diagnosis.

THE CURRENT STATUS OF MR IMAGING

mpMRI imaging is in relatively wide use today. An enormous boost was received when the second version of the Prostate Imaging-Reporting and Diagnosis System (PI-RADS v2) was introduced in 2015. The PI-RADS v2 enabled standardized reporting and provided an important framework for educating radiologists and enhancing communication with urologists. It has been widely adopted by clinicians and imagers alike.[30]

The use of prostate mpMRI has been guided by several major studies. Siddiqui and colleagues[39] documented more than 1000 cases who had undergone both MR imaging and MR imaging-TRUS fusion biopsy and compared these data with the results from 12-core biopsies. They found a 30% increase in the rate of detection of clinically significant cancers and a 17% decrease in the rate of detection of indolent cancers. Thus, combined with the unassailable logic that one should see what one is biopsying, this study lent credence to the idea that MR imaging–guided biopsies were superior to random 12-core biopsies.

The PROMIS trial (Diagnostic accuracy of mpMRI and TRUS biopsy in prostate cancer) was a large multicenter trial in which mpMRI followed by targeted biopsy versus 12-core versus saturation biopsy (which was the ultimate validation in this study). This study showed that multiple centers could achieve excellent sensitivities for clinically significant cancers but at the same time pointed out that a negative MR imaging was a strongly positive predictor of the absence of clinically significant cancer. Thus, the authors of this study concluded that MR imaging could be used as a gatekeeper for biopsy.[40] So far, these recommendations have not been adopted by most practitioners, but it shows that PIRADS scoring has evolved from a lesion scoring system for purposes of selecting lesions for biopsy, to the early stages of a prostate cancer biomarker.

MR imaging has been recommended for patients who have had a prior negative biopsy but continue to exhibit evidence of rising PSA. A joint American Urologic Association–Society of Abdominal Radiology white paper endorsed the use of MR imaging in this setting on the premise that the original biopsy may have missed a clinically significant cancer. This is the preeminent indication for prostate MR imaging.[41] Additionally, the role of MR imaging before placing patients on active surveillance is well accepted, because 20% to 30% of AS candidates on purely clinical grounds are found to have tumors that make them ineligible for active surveillance. Numerous studies have documented this advantage in properly selecting patients for active surveillance.[42,43]

Thus, MR imaging is now considered an important adjunct in the diagnosis of prostate cancer. An increasing number of patients are undergoing MR imaging before their first biopsy, but the most common scenarios are that the patient undergoes MR imaging for the first time after either a negative systematic biopsy with persistently rising PSA or after receiving a positive biopsy indicating low-grade (Gleason 3 + 3, 3 + 4 with small amount of pattern 4, ISUP 1 or 2) cancer. In this setting, MR imaging is used to determine if the patient is truly a candidate for active surveillance.

Despite considerable enthusiasm for the use of MR imaging and MR imaging-TRUS fusion biopsy, and its wide adoption, a number of concerns have been raised as it has become more disseminated. The problems can be divided into those pertaining to the MR imaging technique and those pertaining to the biopsy. Among those pertaining to the MR imaging technique include the quality of the MR imaging, the quality of the interpretation, and certain inherent limitations of MR imaging and the current PIRADS v2 scoring system. Among the problems relating to the biopsy include quality of the registration between the MR imaging and the TRUS, and problems relating to the actual performance of the biopsy and its interpretation. We detail these issues before concluding with a future look at prostate MR imaging and image guided biopsy that seeks to address these current issues.

It is clear that the quality of MR imaging is not uniform across centers. The genesis of nonuniform image quality is complex. It includes the use of outdated equipment, but also the improper use of up-to-date equipment. Technical issues such as excessive gas in the rectum can degrade the diffusion-weighted sequences, rendering the scan difficult to interpret. Inappropriate imaging parameters, particularly suboptimal gradient strength, can lead to artifacts that render the images difficult to interpret. Movement and metallic artifacts are additional issues with image quality. Some MR imaging units perform markedly better with the use of an endorectal coil; however, these coils are both expensive and uncomfortable, so they are often not used.[44–46]

A second factor influencing success is radiologist expertise in interpreting the MR imaging.

Because MR iamging of the prostate is still relatively new for most radiologists, there is heterogeneous experience across centers. This factor can lead to disappointing local results. Fortunately, there are a plethora of training courses and educational materials that are available for radiologists to improve their skills. The advent of the PIRADS v2 system of scoring creates an easily taught scale for lesion suspicion that guides clinician with regard to the recommendation for biopsy (Fig. 2). The PIRADS v2 system also provides advice on the performance of prostate MR imaging, thereby improving the general outcome. However, there are criticisms of PIRADS v2, particularly its high interreader variability and its low predictive value for PIRADS 3 and 4. These factors pose challenges to the future of MR imaging of the prostate.

Regardless of image quality and interpretive skills, there are known limitations of MR imaging. Approximately 5% to 20% of MR imaging lesions that harbor clinically significant cancers are either invisible or greatly underestimated by MR imaging.[47–50] Some centers report false-negative rates on MR imaging (on a per-lesion basis) as high as 30%, but more typically this rate is 5% to 15%. These false-negative results arise when clusters of tumors are separated by swatches of normal tissue and, thus, the tumor is volume averaged to the point that it is indistinguishable from normal. This means that if MR imaging alone is used to guide biopsies, a significant minority of clinically significant tumors will be missed. Thus, despite the improvement in guidance afforded by imaging, there remains a general recommendation that random biopsies also be included along with targeted biopsies. This recommendation commonly results in more biopsy needle passes than before, from an average of 12 to an average of 18 with image guidance (2 biopsies for each MR imaging lesion, with a mean number of 3). Naturally, this causes more trauma, bleeding, and infection opportunities. One hopeful indicator is that completely negative MR imaging studies have a very low risk (<5%) of harboring clinically significant cancers. However, completely negative MR imaging studies are relatively uncommon.

In addition to these false-negative results, MR imaging has a lot of false-positive results relating to coexisting conditions such as infection, inflammation, prior trauma, and hyperplasia. This is especially true in the transition zone. As a result, even highly suspicious lesions (PIRADS 4 and 5)

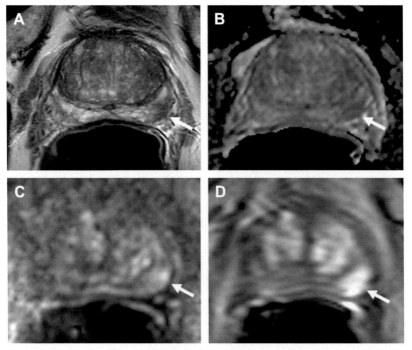

Fig. 2. A 59-year-old man with a serum prostate-specific antigen of 6 ng/mL and no prior biopsy history. Axial T2-weighted MR imaging shows a lesion in the left mid peripheral zone (arrow, A), which shows mild diffusion restriction on apparent diffusion coefficient mapping (B) and b2000 diffusion-weighted MR imaging (C, arrow) with marked early enhancement on dynamic contrast-enhanced MR imaging (D, arrow). The lesion underwent transrectal ultrasound examination/MR imaging fusion-guided targeted biopsy, which revealed Gleason 3 + 4 prostate adenocarcinoma.

have a considerable false-positive rate. For instance, in a compilation of studies the false-positive rate for PIRADS 4 lesions (which are considered high risk) was 60% to 80%.[51] Thus, many biopsies prove to be negative for cancer and, therefore, the patient was put at risk for no benefit. Finally, although MR imaging-directed biopsies reduce the number of low-grade (Gleason 6) cancers, MR imaging does not eliminate them and a moderate number of PIRADS 4 and 5 lesions return as low-grade cancers.[51]

Concerns have also been raised regarding the biopsy component of the MR imaging-TRUS biopsy. Segmentations must be accurately performed, and their quality must be checked. Importantly, the quality of the fusion between the MR imaging and TRUS images is especially important at the level of the lesion. This is even more important for smaller lesions, where even subtle fusion mismatches can lead to missing the lesion during the biopsy.

Finally, the accuracy of the tracking and patient movement between the image fusion and the actual time of biopsy can cause problems leading to less than ideal results. The accuracy with which the operator directs the needle to the lesion can be another source of error. This is especially true for the platforms that allow freehand motion of the TRUS probe, where the user can be significantly off track from the planned biopsy route.

THE FUTURE OF MR IMAGING OF THE PROSTATE

Although MR imaging has introduced a much-needed rationality into the diagnosis of prostate cancer there is still room for improvement. It is clear that standards need to be established for what constitutes an MR imaging study of sufficient quality to be used in diagnosis. It is likely that a combination of phantom imaging and analytics of patient prostate imaging will provide quantitative and objective assessments of image quality. Automated systems of image quality assessment would provide a more objective test of sufficient image quality. It is likely that certifications from centralized authorities will need to be established, specifying quality controls needed to perform MR imaging. The same certification process may also apply to radiologists who wish to interpret prostate MR imaging. This process would follow the history of mammography and MR imaging of the breast that was initially performed by generalists but evolved into a specialty of its own with its own regulatory and quality control processes.

The problems of false-positive results, false-negative results, and interreader variability may be addressed with computer-aided diagnosis (CAD) algorithms. Using machine learning methods, algorithms can be trained to recognize intermediate and high-risk cancers.[52–54] When used as an adjunct to a radiologist's interpretation, they enable more clinically significant cancers to be detected and fewer low grade tumors. They can be trained against Gleason or ISUP grading, immunohistochemistry, and even genomics. As an output, they can better predict where clinically significant lesions are likely to be. Early experience with CAD suggests that it leads to more uniform interpretations across readers with lower experience levels and can better predict where the most worrisome part of the tumor is. Currently, biopsies are aimed at the geometric center of a lesion; in the future, CAD methods may help to direct biopsies to the most biologically significant part of the tumor (**Fig. 3**). Moreover, because CAD systems can recognize subtle changes in the image not directly visible, it tends to reflect more accurately the true extent of the tumor. This is of particular importance for focal therapy where, if the visible lesion alone is treated, there is a 10% to 30% of local recurrence owing to incomplete ablation. Treatment based on CAD findings may result in more complete treatments with lower rates of recurrence. The rate of false-negative MR imaging studies should also decrease, because CAD algorithms can detect subtle textural abnormalities that are below the detection threshold of the human eye.

The PIRADS system requires revision. Although it has been widely accepted, it is variably interpreted owing to the subjective criteria it uses.[55–57] One approach might be to rely on more quantitative aspects of MR imaging including apparent diffusion coefficient, T2 values, and kinetic information from dynamic contrast-enhanced MR imaging. The development of CAD tools has also taught that some features such as lesion heterogeneity, prostate shape, and lesion shape and dimensions, currently not standardized as "imaging parameters" may also provide useful quantitative information that could be more reproducible among readers. Further, reducing the high false-positive rate of MR imaging studies for PIRADS 4 lesions is a desirable goal. More focus on additional criteria suggested here may improve this situation.

A very important development in prostate cancer detection will be an improvement in the definition of clinically significant prostate cancer. Current definitions include many cancers that prove to be indolent especially when patient comorbidities are considered. Thus, a redefinition of clinically significant cancers may have a

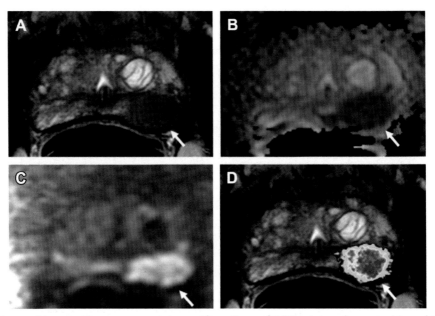

Fig. 3. A 57-year-old man with a serum prostate-specific antigen of 5.87 ng/mL and no prior biopsy history. Axial T2-weighted MR imaging shows a lesion in the left mid peripheral zone (*arrow, A*), which shows diffusion restriction on apparent diffusion coefficient mapping (*B*) and b2000 diffusion-weighted MR imaging (*C, arrows*). A computer-aided diagnosis map derived from mpMRI (overlaid on axial T2-weighted MR imaging) localizes the suspicious lesion (*D, arrow*). The lesion underwent transrectal ultrasound examination/MR imaging fusion-guided targeted biopsy, which revealed Gleason 4 + 4 prostate adenocarcinoma.

profound influence on the ability of MR imaging studies to detect them. This change will inevitably entail less reliance on the Gleason scoring formulation to assess aggressiveness and more reliance on laboratory markers, such as immuno-histochemistry or genomics. For instance, more aggressive tumors tend to be larger, lower in apparent diffusion coefficient and T2 value, and enhance more readily than less aggressive tumors. In contrast, although the majority of patients with low-risk disease are offered active surveillance, many patients who might benefit from active surveillance are treated radically. MR imaging is very useful in confirming that they are indeed active surveillance candidates. However, a large number of patients are considered intermediate risk, including those with Gleason 3 + 4 and Gleason 4 + 3 lesions (ISUP 2 and 3). The majority of these cancers are not lethal, but the presence of grade 4 disease in the specimen causes sufficient concern that active treatment is often recommen-ded. This outcome is unfortunate, because many of those tumors will never progress to metastatic disease. However, the Gleason scoring system, although predictive for low- and high-risk cancers, is not highly predictive for intermediate-risk disease. New genomic tests of biopsy tissue may serve to divide intermediate patients into intermediate- to high-risk and intermediate- to

low-risk disease, thus encouraging intervention in the former and surveillance in the latter. The ability to obtain an accurate sample of the tissue is vital for accurate genomics. Thus, multiple samples from different parts of an index lesion may be important in predicting the outcome in a given patient.

The fusion biopsy process itself is also ripe for improvement. The current system relies heavily on the operator to properly register the images and move the biopsy prove. One can easily envision future devices in which the CAD not only segments the prostate MR imaging and ultra-sound examination, recognizes the most suspi-cious lesions but also performs the registration and monitors it continuously. Robotic arms could be used to direct the course of the biopsy needle more accurately into predetermined targets. Accu-rate mapping of lesions could be performed and could be archived for future use. Alternatively, virtual reality headsets could be used to improve the "cognitive" biopsy be creating virtual overlays of the MR imaging on the ultrasound image in real time, and allowing the user to direct the needle into the lesion.

The advent of new PET agents targeted to pros-tate cancer may usher in a new era wherein both PET and MR imaging are used to detect and stage cancers. For instance, prostate-specific membrane antigen (PSMA)–targeted PET probes show remarkable sensitivity for aggressive cancers both within and outside the prostate gland.[58–61] Currently, and for the foreseeable future, PSMA PET imaging will likely be too costly to be used routinely in the diagnosis of prostate cancer, except for high-risk patients (high PSA and Gleason/ISUP Score). PSMA scans may be used for staging. In this regard, the opportunity to either fuse the PSMA scan to the MR image or to obtain both scans in a PET/MR imaging scanner will provide improved anatomic information (MR imaging) as well as improved specificity (PET).[62]

SUMMARY

MR imaging has become an important part of prostate cancer diagnosis. As with any new modality that combines unassailable logic with reasonably good data, it has been rapidly adopted. With such rapid growth, there are also problems. Once the method is out of the carefully controlled environments of academic centers, great variations in quality and skill become evident and results in general practice are usually not as impressive as they were in academic centers. However, this very observation provides an impetus to improve the method and make it "bullet proof" and, thus, more widely available and more broadly robust. Improved quality assurance for MR imaging scans, including a certification process, will likely result in better outcomes. The wider use of computer assisted diagnosis and other machine learning techniques promise to bring the inexperienced reader up to the level of an experienced reader while decreasing inter-reader variability. Improved characterization of clinically significant prostate cancer may assist in making MR imaging more useful in patient management. Improved methods of registering MR imaging to TRUS and robotic arms controlling the biopsy should reduce the impact of inexperienced operators and make the entire system of MR-guided biopsies more robust. Indeed, the same tools that go into guiding accurate biopsies can also be used, outside the MR gantry, to direct focal therapies. The possibility of combining PET using prostate-targeting probes such as PSMA-directed tracers with MR imaging portends a future where the need for biopsy will be reduced and the true extent of the cancer can be assessed more accurately. The future of MR imaging in the prostate will build on the current challenges and imperfections to make a more robust and useful tool in the coming decade.

REFERENCES

1. Siegel RL, Miller KD, Jemal A. Cancer statistics, 2017. CA Cancer J Clin 2017;67(1):7–30.
2. Epstein JI, Amin MB, Reuter VE, et al. Contemporary Gleason grading of prostatic carcinoma: an update with discussion on practical issues to implement the 2014 International Society of Urological Pathology (ISUP) Consensus Conference on Gleason Grading of Prostatic Carcinoma. Am J Surg Pathol 2017;41:e1–7.
3. Schulman AA, Howard LE, Tay KJ, et al. Validation of the 2015 prostate cancer grade groups for predicting long-term oncologic outcomes in a shared equal-access health system. Cancer 2017;123(21):4122–9.
4. Litwin MS, Tan HJ. The diagnosis and treatment of prostate cancer: a review. Jama 2017;317(24):2532–42.
5. Marberger M, Barentsz J, Emberton M, et al. Novel approaches to improve prostate cancer diagnosis and management in early-stage disease. BJU Int 2012;109(Suppl 2):1–7.
6. Ozkan TA, Eruyar AT, Cebeci OO, et al. Interobserver variability in Gleason histological grading of prostate cancer. Scand J Urol 2016;50(6):420–4.
7. Kweldam CF, Nieboer D, Algaba F, et al. Gleason grade 4 prostate adenocarcinoma patterns: an interobserver agreement study among genitourinary pathologists. Histopathology 2016;69(3):441–9.
8. Sadimin ET, Khani F, Diolombi M, et al. Interobserver reproducibility of percent Gleason pattern 4 in prostatic adenocarcinoma on prostate biopsies. Am J Surg Pathol 2016;40(12):1686–92.
9. Lin D, Ettinger SL, Qu S, et al. Metabolic heterogeneity signature of primary treatment-naive prostate cancer. Oncotarget 2017;8(16):25928–41.
10. Gleason DF. Classification of prostatic carcinomas. Cancer Chemother Rep 1966;50(3):125–8.
11. Wenger H, Weiner AB, Razmaria A, et al. Risk of lymph node metastases in pathological Gleason score</=6 prostate adenocarcinoma: analysis of institutional and population-based databases. Urol Oncol 2017;35(1):31.e1-6.
12. Anderson BB, Oberlin DT, Razmaria AA, et al. Extraprostatic extension is extremely rare for contemporary Gleason score 6 prostate cancer. Eur Urol 2016;72(3):455–60.
13. Moschini M, Carroll PR, Eggener SE, et al. Low-risk prostate cancer: identification, management, and outcomes. Eur Urol 2017;72(2):238–49.
14. Epstein JI, Egevad L, Amin MB, et al. The 2014 International Society of Urological Pathology (ISUP) Consensus Conference on Gleason Grading of Prostatic Carcinoma: definition of grading patterns and proposal for a new grading system. Am J Surg Pathol 2016;40(2):244–52.

15. Papsidero LD, Kuriyama M, Wang MC, et al. Prostate antigen: a marker for human prostate epithelial cells. J Natl Cancer Inst 1981;66(1):37–42.

16. Wang MC, Papsidero LD, Kuriyama M, et al. Prostate antigen: a new potential marker for prostatic cancer. Prostate 1981;2(1):89–96.

17. Schroder FH, Hugosson J, Roobol MJ, et al. Prostate-cancer mortality at 11 years of follow-up. N Engl J Med 2012;366(11):981–90.

18. Andriole GL, Crawford ED, Grubb RL 3rd, et al. Prostate cancer screening in the randomized prostate, lung, colorectal, and ovarian cancer screening trial: mortality results after 13 years of follow-up. J Natl Cancer Inst 2012;104(2):125–32.

19. Carlsson S, Vickers AJ, Roobol M, et al. Prostate cancer screening: facts, statistics, and interpretation in response to the US Preventive Services Task Force review. J Clin Oncol 2012;30(21):2581–4.

20. Halpern JA, Shoag JE, Artis AS, et al. National trends in prostate biopsy and radical prostatectomy volumes following the US Preventive Services Task Force guidelines against prostate-specific antigen screening. JAMA Surg 2017;152(2):192–8.

21. Fleshner K, Carlsson SV, Roobol MJ. The effect of the USPSTF PSA screening recommendation on prostate cancer incidence patterns in the USA. Nat Rev Urol 2017;14(1):26–37.

22. Alam R, Tosoian JJ, Okani O, et al. Metastatic prostate cancer diagnosed by bone marrow aspiration in an elderly man not undergoing PSA screening. Urol Case Rep 2017;11:7–8.

23. Eapen RS, Herlemann A, Washington SL 3rd, et al. Impact of the United States Preventive Services Task Force 'D' recommendation on prostate cancer screening and staging. Curr Opin Urol 2017;27(3):205–9.

24. Lee DJ, Mallin K, Graves AJ, et al. Recent changes in prostate cancer screening practices and prostate cancer epidemiology. J Urol 2017;198(6):1230–40.

25. Haider MR, Qureshi ZP, Horner R, et al. What have patients been hearing from providers since the 2012 USPSTF recommendation against routine prostate cancer screening? Clin Genitourin Cancer 2017;15(6):e977–85.

26. Shoag JE, Mittal S, Hu JC. Reevaluating PSA testing rates in the PLCO trial. N Engl J Med 2016;374(18):1795–6.

27. Van der Kwast TH, Roobol MJ. Prostate cancer: draft USPSTF 2017 recommendation on PSA testing - a sea-change? Nat Rev Urol 2017;14(8):457–8.

28. Turkbey B, Pinto PA, Mani H, et al. Prostate cancer: value of multiparametric MR imaging at 3 T for detection–histopathologic correlation. Radiology 2010;255(1):89–99.

29. Futterer JJ, Heijmink SW, Scheenen TW, et al. Prostate cancer: local staging at 3-T endorectal MR imaging–early experience. Radiology 2006;238(1):184–91.

30. Barentsz JO, Weinreb JC, Verma S, et al. Synopsis of the PI-RADS v2 guidelines for multiparametric prostate magnetic resonance imaging and recommendations for use. Eur Urol 2016;69(1):41–9.

31. Brown AM, Elbuluk O, Mertan F, et al. Recent advances in image-guided targeted prostate biopsy. Abdom Imaging 2015;40(6):1788–99.

32. Pondman KM, Fütterer JJ, ten Haken B, et al. MR-guided biopsy of the prostate: an overview of techniques and a systematic review. Eur Urol 2008;54(3):517–27.

33. Puech P, Rouvière O, Renard-Penna R, et al. Prostate cancer diagnosis: multiparametric MR-targeted biopsy with cognitive and transrectal US-MR fusion guidance versus systematic biopsy–prospective multicenter study. Radiology 2013;268(2):461–9.

34. Puech P, Ouzzane A, Gaillard V, et al. Multiparametric MRI-targeted TRUS prostate biopsies using visual registration. Biomed Res Int 2014;2014:819360.

35. Xu S, Kruecker J, Guion P, et al. Closed-loop control in fused MR-TRUS image-guided prostate biopsy. Med Image Comput Comput Assist Interv 2007;10(Pt 1):128–35.

36. Xu S, Kruecker J, Guion P, et al. Real-time MRI-TRUS fusion for guidance of targeted prostate biopsies. Comput Aided Surg 2008;13(5):255–64.

37. Dani H, Loeb S. The role of prostate cancer biomarkers in undiagnosed men. Curr Opin Urol 2017;27(3):210–6.

38. Loeb S, Ross AE. Genomic testing for localized prostate cancer: where do we go from here? Curr Opin Urol 2017;27(5):495–9.

39. Siddiqui MM, Rais-Bahrami S, Turkbey B, et al. Comparison of MR/ultrasound fusion-guided biopsy with ultrasound-guided biopsy for the diagnosis of prostate cancer. JAMA 2015;313(4):390–7.

40. Ahmed HU, El-Shater Bosaily A, Brown LC, et al. Diagnostic accuracy of multi-parametric MRI and TRUS biopsy in prostate cancer (PROMIS): a paired validating confirmatory study. Lancet 2017;389(10071):815–22.

41. Rosenkrantz AB, Verma S, Choyke P, et al. Prostate magnetic resonance imaging and magnetic resonance imaging targeted biopsy in patients with a prior negative biopsy: a consensus statement by AUA and SAR. J Urol 2016;196(6):1613–8.

42. Alberts AR, Roobol MJ, Drost FH, et al. Risk-stratification based on magnetic resonance imaging and prostate-specific antigen density may reduce unnecessary follow-up biopsy procedures in men on active surveillance for low-risk prostate cancer. BJU Int 2017;120(4):511–9.

43. Turkbey B, Mani H, Aras O, et al. Prostate cancer: can multiparametric MR imaging help identify

patients who are candidates for active surveillance? Radiology 2013;268(1):144–52.

44. Turkbey B, Merino MJ, Gallardo EC, et al. Comparison of endorectal coil and nonendorectal coil T2W and diffusion-weighted MRI at 3 Tesla for localizing prostate cancer: correlation with whole-mount histopathology. J Magn Reson Imaging 2014;39(6): 1443–8.
45. Caglic I, Hansen NL, Slough RA, et al. Evaluating the effect of rectal distension on prostate multiparametric MRI image quality. Eur J Radiol 2017;90:174–80.
46. Borofsky S, Haji-Momenian S, Shah S, et al. Multiparametric MRI of the prostate gland: technical aspects. Future Oncol 2016;12(21):2445–62.
47. Marks LS. Some prostate cancers are invisible to magnetic resonance imaging! BJU Int 2016;118(4): 492–3.
48. Le JD, Tan N, Shkolyar E, et al. Multifocality and prostate cancer detection by multiparametric magnetic resonance imaging: correlation with whole-mount histopathology. Eur Urol 2015;67(3):569–76.
49. Priester A, Natarajan S, Khoshnoodi P, et al. Magnetic resonance imaging underestimation of prostate cancer geometry: use of patient specific molds to correlate images with whole mount pathology. J Urol 2017;197(2):320–6.
50. Muthigi A, George AK, Sidana A, et al. Missing the mark: prostate cancer upgrading by systematic biopsy over magnetic resonance imaging/transrectal ultrasound fusion biopsy. J Urol 2017;197(2):327–34.
51. Mehralivand S, Bednarova S, Shih JH, et al. Prospective Evaluation of Prostate Imaging Reporting and Data System, version 2 using the International Society of Urological Pathology Prostate Cancer Grade Group System. J Urol 2017;198(3):583–90.
52. Wang S, Burtt K, Turkbey B, et al. Computer aided-diagnosis of prostate cancer on multiparametric MRI: a technical review of current research. Biomed Res Int 2014;2014:789561.
53. Lay N, Tsehay Y, Greer MD, et al. Detection of prostate cancer in multiparametric MRI using random forest with instance weighting. J Med Imaging (Bellingham) 2017;4(2):024506.
54. Peng Y, Jiang Y, Yang C, et al. Quantitative analysis of multiparametric prostate MR images: differentiation between prostate cancer and normal tissue and correlation with Gleason score–a computer-aided diagnosis development study. Radiology 2013;267(3):787–96.
55. Rosenkrantz AB, Oto A, Turkbey B, et al. Prostate Imaging Reporting and Data System (PI-RADS), version 2: a critical look. AJR Am J Roentgenol 2016;206(6):1179–83.
56. Rosenkrantz AB, Ayoola A, Hoffman D, et al. The learning curve in prostate MRI interpretation: self-directed learning versus continual reader feedback. AJR Am J Roentgenol 2017;208(3):W92–100.
57. Rosenkrantz AB, Babb JS, Taneja SS, et al. Proposed adjustments to PI-RADS version 2 decision rules: impact on prostate cancer detection. Radiology 2017;283(1):119–29.
58. Vinsensia M, Choyke PL, Hadaschik B, et al. 68Ga-PSMA PET/CT and volumetric morphology of PET-positive lymph nodes stratified by tumor differentiation of prostate cancer. J Nucl Med 2017; 58(12):1949–55.
59. Rowe SP, Gage KL, Faraj SF, et al. (1)(8)F-DCFBC PET/CT for PSMA-based detection and characterization of primary prostate cancer. J Nucl Med 2015;56(7):1003–10.
60. Zamboglou C, Schiller F, Fechter T, et al. (68)Ga-HBED-CC-PSMA PET/CT versus histopathology in primary localized prostate cancer: a voxel-wise comparison. Theranostics 2016;6(10):1619–28.
61. Budaus L, Leyh-Bannurah SR, Salomon G, et al. Initial experience of (68)Ga-PSMA PET/CT imaging in high-risk prostate cancer patients prior to radical prostatectomy. Eur Urol 2016;69(3):393–6.
62. Eiber M, Weirich G, Holzapfel K, et al. Simultaneous 68Ga-PSMA HBED-CC PET/MRI improves the localization of primary prostate cancer. Eur Urol 2016; 70(5):829–36.

Moving?

Make sure your subscription moves with you!

To notify us of your new address, find your **Clinics Account Number** (located on your mailing label above your name), and contact customer service at:

Email: journalscustomerservice-usa@elsevier.com

800-654-2452 (subscribers in the U.S. & Canada)
314-447-8871 (subscribers outside of the U.S. & Canada)

Fax number: 314-447-8029

Elsevier Health Sciences Division
Subscription Customer Service
3251 Riverport Lane
Maryland Heights, MO 63043

*To ensure uninterrupted delivery of your subscription, please notify us at least 4 weeks in advance of move.

ELSEVIER